A comparative approach to policy analysis

A
comparative approach to policy analysis

Health care policy in four nations

Howard M. Leichter

Assistant Professor of Political Science
University of Houston

Cambridge University Press

Cambridge
London   New York   Melbourne

Published by the Syndics of the Cambridge University Press
The Pitt Building, Trumpington Street, Cambridge CB2 1RP
Bentley House, 200 Euston Road, London NW1 2DB
32 East 57th Street, New York, NY 10022, USA
296 Beaconsfield Parade, Middle Park, Melbourne 3206, Australia

First published 1979

Printed in the United States of America

Library of Congress Cataloging in Publication Data
Leichter, Howard M
A comparative approach to policy analysis.
Bibliography: p.
1. Policy sciences.
2. Medical policy – Case studies.   I. Title.
H61.L42 300'.1'8   79-50625
ISBN 0 521 22648 1 hard covers
ISBN 0 521 29601 3 paperback

For
Elisabeth,
Laurel, and
Alexandra

Contents

Preface

In the decade of the 1970s the comparative, or cross-national, study of public policy came into its own as a field of academic inquiry. Like their colleagues in the field of American politics, students of comparative politics had come to recognize that the analysis of political systems will remain incomplete as long as the questions of what government does, why, and with what consequences remain unanswered. In addition, the comparative approach to the study of public policy recommended itself because it reflects the reality in the policy-making process of most nations. Policy makers throughout the world constantly engage in comparative inquiry when seeking solutions to common public problems. One need only consider the frequent references by American policy makers to the health care experiences of other nations, during the course of the debate on an American national health care program, to appreciate the importance of cross-national policy influences. This book reflects the desire both to achieve academic completeness in the study of national political systems and to document and underscore the importance of cross-national diffusion in the policy-making process.

Although the utility of comparative policy studies is generally acknowledged, no such agreement has developed concerning the best way to approach the matter. No effort is made in this book to establish the primacy of one approach over another. My position is that no single approach is inherently or demonstrably superior to any other and that the study of public policy is best served by the use of a variety of analytical tools. The first part of this book, which introduces the reader to the comparative study of public policy, includes a discussion of various approaches and the application of one of these: the multinational, aggregate data approach. The second part of the book, however, uses a case study approach in examining a single area of public policy: national health care.

In the course of writing this book I received assistance, advice, and encouragement from a variety of sources. Professors Roger Durand, Donald Lutz, and Joseph Nogee of the University of Houston read various portions of the manuscript and made many useful suggestions. Professors John Ambler and Gaston Rimlinger of Rice University read an early version of the manuscript. Both were far more generous and gracious with their time and advice than I had any right to expect. Professor Alan Stone of the University of Houston is a friend and colleague. At various stages in the development of the manuscript he performed both roles in superb fashion.

I am also heavily indebted to several persons for clerical, technical, and research assistance. While doing research in West Berlin on the German medical system, I was fortunate in having the talented assistance of Lawrence Lehmann. Judy Myers of the University of Houston Library System proved an extraordinarily knowledgeable and resourceful research librarian. Sally Becker and her associates at the University of Houston Typing Service somehow managed to produce a virtually flawless product, meet the publisher's deadline, and remain thoroughly pleasant. Any shortcomings that remain are solely the responsibility of the author and do not reflect upon the talents of those mentioned above.

I should also like to note the generous financial assistance provided by the University of Houston through its Research Initiation Grant program. This aid allowed me the time and resources to conduct much of the research that went into the book.

I would like to thank Sage Publications for permission to include here material that was presented in my article "Comparative Public Policy: Problems and Prospects," in Stuart S. Nagel (ed.), *Policy Studies Review Annual* (Beverly Hills: Sage Publications, 1977), pp. 138–50.

Ultimately, however, it was not professional or institutional assistance, but rather the support, encouragement, and patience of my family that contributed most to this enterprise. My daughters Laurel and Alexandra, and my wife Elisabeth, were constant reminders of what is truly important in the world. I dedicate this book to them.

H.M.L.

June, 1979

Part I

Comparative policy analysis

1

Introduction

There has always been debate over the appropriate nature and extent of the state's role in the lives of people throughout the world. Consider, for example, the following descriptions of medical organization in three major nations.

The majority of the population in England consider it not only not a disgrace, but the most natural thing in the world, when they fall ill, to demand and receive free treatment without question or delay.

Americans hold rightly that no person is entitled to occupy a free bed unless or until he can prove beyond dispute that he is unable to pay something for the treatment he receives in the hospital ward.

There is relatively little free medical relief anywhere in America.

The entire hospital system in Russia is now under the control of the State and municipal corporations.[1]

Presumably the reader does not find these descriptions particularly surprising – until he notes that they are from a book published in 1893.

Compare these descriptions of medical care with the diversity of opinions expressed, in America and England, on the issue of free public education. The first statement, written in 1871, is by Henry Fawcett – prominent Cambridge University professor, member of Parliament, and later postmaster general of England – and reflects a view of free public education not uncommonly held by the British elite at the time.

Additions are constantly being made to the list of those things which people ought to do for themselves, but which they desire others to do for them. One of the latest examples is the demand, which so many of the working classes are now making, that parents should not be required to pay for their children's education, but that all schools should be free. It will be found that these demands simply show how many there are who will always try to escape from the responsibility of their own acts. The extent to which they are permitted to do this will in no small degree determine the amount of poverty and misery which will exist in a country.[2]

The second statement, written in 1876 by the American poet Ralph Waldo Emerson, reflects the historical commitment on the part of most Americans to the principle of public education.

The poor man, whom the law does not allow to take an ear of corn when starving, nor a pair of shoes for his freezing feet, is allowed to put his hand into the pockets of the rich, and say, you shall educate me, not as you will, but as I will . . . The child shall be taken up by the State and taught, at the public cost, the rudiments of knowledge, and at last the ripest results of art and science.[3]

These comments reveal, not only the diversity of opinion and fact on such policy matters as medical care and education, but also the dangers and difficulties of generalizing about the provision of public goods and services, across time, for particular political systems and ideologies. As the first set of comments indicates, the provision of free medical care for the needy predates both communism in Russia and socialism in Great Britain – yet both countries lagged behind the United States in providing free public education. The United States, on the other hand, although one of the earliest nations to adopt programs of free, compulsory public education, stood alone among modern nations in the mid-1970s in not providing comprehensive medical care for the majority of its people. In most respects, Emerson's comment and the earlier description of medical care are as accurate today as they were for nineteenth-century America.

How does one explain the enormous diversity in the ability and/or willingness of governments throughout the world to provide the goods and services necessary to satisfy basic human needs and wants? The fact that great policy differences exist among nations, and within nations over time, raises a number of questions that can best be answered by the cross-national, or comparative, analysis of public policy. For example, which type of government or political regime is most effective in providing for the education, safety, or health of its people – communist or noncommunist, military or civilian, presidential or parliamentary systems? Why do some nations commit a greater proportion of their resources to education than to medical care? How and why does the capacity or willingness of a government to provide certain public goods and services change over time? The task of comparative policy analysis, and the purpose of this book, is to address these and related questions.

The policy orientation in comparative politics

A prominent scholar in the field of comparative politics wrote in 1975 that comparative policy analysis "is a field of study that does not yet exist."[4] This comment is already outdated.[5] It is true, to be sure, that until quite recently there were few studies in comparative politics that dealt specifically and systematically with the comparison of public policies or the comparison of political systems in terms of their public policies. Moreover, most introductory or survey texts in the field of comparative politics have paid only scant attention to similarities and differences in public policy as a basis for comparing political systems.[6]

In recent years this neglect has been partially remedied as students of comparative politics increasingly have turned their attention to the cross-national study of public policy. The impetus for this new policy orientation comes from the field of state and local politics in the United States, where recent academic research has produced a deluge of studies dealing with comparisons of local politcal units and their public policies.[7] The debt students of comparative politics owe their colleagues in American state and local politics is evident in the similarity of research questions and techniques used in the earliest efforts at comparative policy analysis.[8]

The antecedents of the recent policy orientation among political scientists, of whom students of comparative politics are merely the most recent converts, are for the most part esoteric and need not detain us.[9] One factor, however, stands out and does require our attention. The most significant factor contributing to the emphasis on public policy is the vastly expanded role government now plays in the lives of people in this country and throughout the world. Governments in virtually every nation in the world today are regulating more activities, providing a greater variety and proportion of the goods and services produced, and employing a larger percentage of the work force than they did 100, 50, or even 10 years ago. Consider, for instance, one measure of this growth of government: public expenditures as a percentage of the gross national product (GNP) in six selected countries since 1900 (Table 1-1). In all six nations government expenditures as a percentage of GNP have increased tremendously since the turn of the century. Clearly, Richard Hofferbert's explanation for the increased interest in public policy by students of American politics is equally appropriate and valid for those studying comparative politics. "Political scientists are also social scientists, and as such they quite naturally focus their attention on the circumstances that matter most in society. Increasingly, policies made by public – primarily governmental – decision makers have come to constitute a key directional force in our collective and individual lives."[10]

Whatever the explanations for its development, the subfield of comparative policy analysis is on its way to becoming an integral part of the field of comparative politics. However, because it is a relatively new enterprise, the comparative study of public policy has suffered from several problems that have thus far inhibited its development. One such problem has been the absence of agreement on a definition of public policy. A second takes the form of often conflicting and contradictory conclusions in the literature concerning the alleged primacy of political, social, or economic factors in influencing public policy. If one accepts, as this author

Table 1-1. *Growth in government expenditure as a percentage of gross national product: selected countries; 1900-74*

Year	United States	Japan	United Kingdom	India	Germany	Mexico
1900	7.7[a]	21.5	14.4	10.4	14.9	6.3[b]
1960	28.1	33.2	42.0	17.6	38.6[c]	13.7
1974	41.7	35.1	55.0	27.2	47.4	26.9

[a]1902; [b]1925; [c]1958.

Sources: K. N. Reddy, "Growth of Government Expenditure and National Income in India: 1872–1966," *Public Finance*, 25 (1970), 81–95; Shibskankar P. Gupta, "Public Expenditure and Economic Growth: A Time Series Analysis," *Public Finance*, 22 (1967), 423–61; Frederick C. Mosher and Orville F. Poland, *The Cost of American Governments* (New York: Dodd, Mead, 1964), p. 157; James W. Wilkie, *The Mexican Revolution* (Berkeley: University of California Press, 1970), p. 7; *Annual Statistical Yearbook* (New York: United Nations, 1975).

does, that the ultimate aim of the comparative study of public policy is the development of theory – that is, statements about the relationship between public policy on the one hand, and political, social, and economic systems variables on the other – then it is necessary to deal with these problems at the outset.

What is public policy?

"No term in social science has suffered more ambiguity and abuse in the 1960s and 1970s than 'policy.' "[11] Having alerted us to the problem, Feldman, in a review of three recent books on comparative public policy, stops short of remedying the situation. Considering the penchant of political scientists for getting enmeshed in definitional imbroglios, such "ambiguity and abuse" are not at all surprising. Given the general lack of cooperative research and the absence of a common analytical framework in political science, it is unlikely that we shall ever have a universally accepted or acceptable definition of public policy. Nevertheless, it is necessary for authors to specify what they are studying so as to provide direction for other scholars as well as understanding for the general reader. Wherever adequate and useful definitions exist, they should be used. The definitions of public policy (and of such derivative concepts as policy decision, output, and impact) adopted here build upon the existing literature.

Public policy is defined here as a series of goal-oriented actions taken by authoritative (usually governmental) actors. Like Heclo's and Alford's, this definition emphasizes state activity.[12] As such, public policies are usually contained in legislative enactments, including budgets, executive and administrative orders and decisions, judicial decisions, and the like. However, like Heclo, we recognize also that "a policy, like a decision, can consist of what is *not* being done."[13] For example, the absence of a national health care system in the United States is as much a statement and a measure of public policy as is the series of decisions that led to the establishment of the British National Health Service. Finally, by contrast, a *policy decision* is a single binding act by an authoritative entity "that authorize(s) or give(s) direction and content to public policy actions."[14] For example, the government of a less developed country might adopt a policy of eradicating illiteracy. The adoption of this policy presumably would be followed by a series of legislative or executive actions or decisions providing for the creation of adult education courses, increased teacher training, and the expansion of educational facilities.

Public policies and policy decisions are for the most part, however, merely statements of governmental intent. The fact that authoritative actors have proclaimed their desire to eradicate illiteracy does not guarantee that any steps actually will be taken in that direction. Thus, the study of public policy must also be concerned with *policy output:* what governments in fact do to enforce their intentions (i.e., policies). To continue the example of the policy to eradicate illiteracy, the policy outputs one would expect might include actual increases in expenditures for education, enrollments in adult education courses, numbers of new teachers, and classroom construction.

But the study of public policy is still not complete, for one must also be concerned with the consequences of governmental activity: *policy impact,* or performance. After all has been said and done, has the rate of illiteracy actually declined? Unfortunately, the measurement of policy impact is often complicated by the fact that the consequences of a policy may be both immediate and long-range, intended and unintended. The immediate and presumably intended consequence of the illiteracy eradication policy was to achieve a totally – or nearly so – literate population. An implicit and long-range consequence might be the development of a population with the skills necessary for the modernization of the society. However, increases in literacy in modernizing societies may have the unplanned and unintended consequence of creating political instability. As Huntington has noted, an increase in literacy is among those factors that "give rise to enhanced aspirations and expectations which, if unsatisfied, galvanize individuals and groups into politics. In the absence of strong and adaptable political institutions, such increases in participation mean instability and violence."[15] Of course, unintended policy consequences may be of a positive nature. There is, for example, some evidence to suggest that the rising literacy rate in Sri Lanka has helped slow the rapid population growth in that country. The high literacy rate (about 86 percent) has apparently facilitated the dissemination of birth control information and led to a change in attitudes concerning large families.[16] It is, of course, sometimes as difficult for the researcher to identify and measure the unintended consequences of public policies as it is for the decision makers to anticipate them. Nevertheless, policy analysts must be alerted to such consequences.

In sum, public policy is a set of related state activities (or inactivity where the state could or might be expected to act). Such activity may occur over a short period of time or may span many years. When we study the German, British, Russian, and Japanese health care systems, we will examine a series of state decisions spanning several decades. Because public policy has several dimensions, the study of public policy must include an analysis of the intended purpose of state activity, steps taken to enforce these intentions, and measures of their consequences. Furthermore, as viewed here, the purpose of the study of public policy is to explain or account for why states have taken the actions they have. Obviously, this is not the only reason for studying public policy. One may do so for the purpose of recommending courses of action to decision makers. In this study we will limit ourselves to an explanation of state activity. Lastly, the comparative study of public policy has the additional obligation of explaining similarities and differences in policies among political systems.

This last point, accounting for policy and policy differences, introduces a second problem that has characterized early studies of comparative public policy: the apparently chaotic state of the art.

Approaches to comparative policy analysis

The study of public policy reminds one of the popular Indian folktale about the four blind men who are led to an elephant. Each is positioned at a different part of the animal: One feels the elephant's leg, another the tail, the third an ear, and the last one the body. As a result of their tactile experiences, each in turn describes what he has felt as a log, a rope, a fan, and a wall.

Students of public policy are much like the four blind men: Each tends to examine a small part of a very large animal. The diversity of conclusions concerning the alleged primacy of social, economic, or political factors in the policy process has in large measure been a product of the particular part of the elephant each one has examined. But the problems for the student of *comparative* public policy are potentially more severe than those facing the four blind men. Presumably the four – given a reasonable amount of time, the ability to move around the beast, some degree of intelligence, and the opportunity to compare their findings – would ulti- mately arrive at an accurate conclusion about what it was they had actually felt. Consider the complexity of the problem if the four men had been presented, not with one elephant but with an elephant, a giraffe, a hippo- potamus, a gazelle, and so on.

Students of comparative public policy are like blind men in a corral of exotic animals. They are asked to explain the behavior of a large number of nation-states and an almost infinite variety of policy activities. Further- more, they approach the task from different analytical perspectives.

Given the enormous range of policy areas, the number and variety of political systems, and the different analytical approaches, it is hardly surprising that research results have been so confusing and conflicting. For example, Anthony King concludes that political culture is the key to explaining why the state has played a more active role in Western Europe than in the United States.[17] Caiden and Wildavsky, however, dismiss political culture as a residual category with little value in explaining planning and budgeting in poor countries.[18] Frederic Pryor, in a compari- son of public spending in communist and capitalist nations, concludes that there are few policy differences that can be attributed to the differ- ences in economic systems.[19] Guy Peters, however, finds in a comparative study of social policy in France, Sweden, and the United Kingdom, that whereas political factors are important in influencing economic security policy, socioeconomic factors are dominant in the area of education.[20] And so it goes. For some, political factors account for policy; for others, socio- economic factors; and for still others, the responsible factor depends upon the area of policy and the historical period.

This author is neither surprised nor concerned about the state of the art. It would be extraordinary indeed if a single factor, say political culture, was found responsible for all policies, at all times, in all nations. Clearly, some of the diverse and conflicting evidence is a function of the type and level of analysis. Robert Jackman, studying social policy in 60 nations, could not possibly go into the detail that Hugh Heclo did in his study of social policy in two nations. Each has studied different dimensions of the social policy-making process and each has contributed to our understand- ing of that process.

What is disturbing, however, is the seemingly haphazard and disjointed fashion in which comparative policy analysis has proceeded. Obviously, both aggregate data analysis and case studies have much to offer. Yet until both types of studies are integrated into a common analytical frame- work, their utility will be limited and theory building unlikely. The purpose of this book is to provide a modest first step toward both the integration of various approaches to the study of comparative public policy and the process of theory building in the field. This can be accomplished best by first establishing a common analytical framework. Let us be more specific by outlining the plan of this book.

The plan of this book

At first glance a book on comparative policy analysis may appear an overly ambitious and immodest undertaking. How can one possibly compare the full range of national public policies, in any meaningful detail, for over 140 nations. The answer, quite simply, is that one cannot – at least not in a single volume. How, then, can one approach the task? As suggested above, cross-national studies of public policy usually have taken one of two general approaches. The first has been to study a limited number of comparable political systems (e.g., Western or industrialized) and a limited range of policy areas (e.g., pollution or social welfare).[21] This approach is typically rich in details dealing with the development of policy problems and solutions, the dynamics of the policy process, and the content and consequences of particular policies. However, the limited geographical and substantive focus of these studies has imposed severe restrictions on the authors' self-avowed intentions to produce ''generalizations'' or hypotheses that are applicable to or testable on a larger and more diverse group of nations and policy areas.

The second major approach, referred to here as the aggregate data approach, seeks greater cross-national generalizability in terms of the causes and consequences of public policy by examining a much larger number and variety of nations. Employing aggregate data and various statistical techniques, these studies have dealt with the relationships among various political, social, and economic factors and policy outputs and impacts for many nations. However, whatever this approach accomplishes in breadth of coverage it often sacrifices in substance and insight into the content of the policies and the dynamics of the policy process. It is not at all unusual for these studies virtually to ignore the individual nations. For example, in a book dealing with social equality in 60 nations, Robert Jackman makes only the briefest reference to 14 nations.[22] In addition, these studies tend to produce generalizations of a rather high level of abstraction and of questionable utility. For example, a major conclusion of one of the earliest and most frequently cited studies dealing with the relationship between systems variables and public policy in 76 nations was: ''The effect of different levels of political representativeness on the development of national social security programs varied with the level of economic development enjoyed by the nation.''[23] What is needed, particularly in an introductory analysis, is an approach to comparative public policy that draws upon and integrates the virtues of both the multination studies, and the broad-range generalizations they produce, and the more narrowly focused, but richly detailed, analyses of specific case studies.

The first requirement is to bring some semblance of order to the seemingly infinite variety of policy activities in which governments engage. In another study, we offered a typology of public policy intended to do just this. The scheme categorizes policies into five major types: (1) distributive – policies that involve the allocation of goods and services and the necessary appropriation of funds to provide those goods and services, (2) extractive – policies that provide for the collection of revenues, (3) symbolic – policies that allocate status and acknowledge achievement, (4) regulatory – policies that seek to control some aspect of human behavior, and (5) administrative – policies that concern the organization or administration of government.[24] This book concentrates on the first of these policy areas: distributive policies. We do not think it is possible to say that one type of policy is more important than another. It seems clear, however, that the distribution of goods and services occupies a good deal of the time and energies of policy makers, the resources of society, and the interest of citizens. It is by any standard an important area of state activity. We feel that at this stage in the development of comparative policy studies it is better to explain one important policy activity well than several poorly. Thus, Chapter 4 examines public spending in three major areas – defense, education, and health. However, because of the previously mentioned limitation of the aggregate data approach (namely, a high level of generality and superficiality), Part II delves more deeply into one specific area of distributive policy: health care.

Having limited the analysis to distributive policy, we are still left with the problem of bringing some order to the infinite variety of policy-relevant variables in order to make the comparative study of public policy more manageable. To accomplish this, Chapter 3 provides an accounting or organizing scheme. The scheme is intended to supply a common classificatory system, without which comparison and ultimately theory building in policy analysis are impossible. Although the scheme is applied ultimately only to the area of distributive policy, it is applicable to other types of policy, and some examples in Chapter 3 are from these other areas.

It is necessary to digress here in order to demonstrate the role played by classificatory schemes in theory building. The process of theory building may be viewed as involving four stages: (1) problem selection, (2) systematic observation (entailing the classification of variables), (3) generalization, and (4) explanation.[25] The problem-selection stage requires a decision about what is worth studying and what is not. Such decisions usually involve value judgments based, in large measure, on informed opinion. For example, a decision to study electoral behavior in the nations of Asia and Africa would be academically questionable given the relatively unimportant, meaningless, or nonexistent nature of electoral behavior in most nations in these areas. We have made the informed judgment that distributive policies, and in particular health care, are important. We know of few things in life that are as important to people throughout the world as good health and its maintenance.

Having decided what to study, one proceeds systematically to collect and analyze data. And it is at this point that classification of independent and dependent variables becomes critical. The importance of this stage of theory building is underscored by Arthur Kalleberg, who reminds us that "classification is the basic type of concept-formation in science. Neither comparison (non-metrical ordering) nor measurement proper can take place without it."[26]

Only after systematic observation, governed by the formal classification of phenomena, has occurred can one discover relationships among variables. The next step in the process is to formulate generalizations about, and explanations for, the relationship among variables.

The systematic observation/classification stage of theory building is, to be sure, a relatively primitive one. However, it is also indispensable – without it theory is impossible. It is our feeling that most studies in comparative policy analysis have ignored these first two stages. They have not told us why they have chosen particular policies for analysis and, more seriously, have not placed either the dependent variable (i.e., public policy) or the independent variables (i.e., political, economic, or social system factors) in an analytical framework.

We believe that the fivefold classification of policy types and the accounting scheme presented in Chapter 3 are appropriate ways to begin the process of theory building in comparative policy analysis.

The book, then, is divided into two parts. Part I deals with various generalizations about the factors that help account for public policy and applies some of these to an analysis of distributive or expenditure policy in over 130 nations. Part II analyzes a specific policy (and one that is of particular current concern to Americans) – national health care – in four nations. In each case we try to explain or account for the nature and development of health care policy in terms of the accounting scheme discussed in Part I.

Specifically, Chapter 2 traces the origins of the state as a major supplier of goods and services throughout the world. We see, for example, that war and internal insecurity, along with the concern for economic development, have provided a major stimulus to the growth of state functions. By placing the phenomenon of the positive state in historical perspective, we try to shed some light on its current manifestations, particularly in developed countries, and on its potential implications for newly emerging nations. Chapter 3 offers an accounting scheme that the student of public policy may use to examine systematically and comparatively some of the political, social, and economic factors that have been found to explain why governments do what they do. Although no attempt is made definitively to resolve the debate over the primacy of political versus socioeconomic factors in the determination of public policy, emphasis is placed on political explanations for policy selection. This emphasis reflects both the author's bias and the fact that this is a book on political science and comparative politics. Chapter 4 examines public expenditures for defense, education, and health care in more than 130 nations. Unlike most multination studies, which tend to ignore individual nations and national differences, the data are presented in unaggregated form to allow the reader to see where each nation ranks. Wherever possible we try to explain the differences in policy priorities among nations.

Chapters 5 through 8 (Part II) examine the development of health care policy in four nations of quite different geographical, political, and social backgrounds. The introduction to Part II explains the selection of each country. Suffice it here to note that the countries and periods of time studied are (1) Germany since 1883 – the year the world's first national health insurance system was started; (2) Great Britain since 1905 – the year generally considered to mark the beginning of the modern welfare state; (3) the Soviet Union since the Bolshevik Revolution of 1917; and (4) Japan since the Meiji restoration of 1868. Although emphasis is placed on these specific time periods, we examine the question of whether these political watersheds resulted in significant departures in health policy from the previous regime or era in each country. Finally, in each case we integrate the general propositions and hypotheses discussed in Part I with the causes, content, and consequences of health care policy in these four countries. Unlike the analysis of expenditure policy in Chapter 4, which deals with one year only (1973), these case studies trace the evolution of health care over the course of several decades. By taking a historical perspective in these case studies, we wish to demonstrate that the courses of action open to policy makers are to a great extent limited by the decisions and conditions inherited from their predecessors. Policy decisions in most political systems, democratic or otherwise, are rarely totally new and independent courses of action. Even under revolutionary circumstances, the past cannot be totally abandoned. At issue here is not that policy innovation and change do not occur – they obviously do – but rather that one of the crucial reference points for any policy maker is the accumulation of past decisions and the historical milieus in which these decisions were taken.

The book concludes (Chapter 9) with an attempt to apply the findings concerning the development of health care policy in the four nations studied to the future direction of American national health care policy.

2

The origins and evolution
of the positive state

If one were to compile a list of activities performed by governments in the world today, it would include the most extraordinary range and variety of items. There are governments, for example, that prohibit men from wearing their hair long (Singapore) and women from wearing their skirts short (Malawi); that try to regulate the maximum number of children a family may have (India) and the minimum number of weeks of vacation workers must have (Sweden and Australia); that control prices and wages (Finland, the Netherlands) and monopolize the sale of tobacco (France) and telephone services (Italy). In terms of public policy, the similarities and differences among nations, and therefore one basis for comparing them, lie not in whether the state intervenes in the daily lives of the people, but rather in the nature and extent of that intervention. In Chapter 1 it is noted that, in addition to the range of current state activity, the magnitude of that activity is greater today than in the recent past. This is documented by measuring the increase of state expenditures as a percentage of the gross national product (GNP) in selected nations since the turn of the century. In fact, in most noncommunist, industrial nations, state spending currently accounts for between 35 and 40 percent of the GNP.

The increased scope and magnitude of state activity are viewed differently by different people. For some, state activity represents an unwanted and unwarranted encroachment in their lives and a resulting loss of individual freedom. For others, it suggests the hope of a better life, with greater equality and opportunity for themselves and their children. Our purpose in this chapter is neither to applaud nor to condemn, but rather to explain the worldwide expansion of state activity. What are the origins of the positive state? How, why, when, and where did the state become so important in providing goods and services and regulating behavior? By tracing the origin and evolution of the positive state, we hope to lay the basis for an understanding of its current form: the "general-welfare state."[1] In addition, we wish to disabuse the reader of the notion that the current nature of state activity is unique to our own time or that, indeed, it is necessarily irreversible.

In this chapter we distinguish among three historical periods. The first begins with the emergence of the modern nation-state during the sixteenth century and runs to the latter part of the eighteenth century. During this period, the centralized, positive state first appeared. The political/economic system it fostered was known as mercantilism or, in Germany, cameralism. The policies of governments in this period were directed toward achieving international power and internal peace in order that centralized national economies could develop and thrive. The second period, beginning in some nations early in the nineteenth century, was the time of the Industrial Revolution in much of Western Europe. This period was characterized, in some nations, by a more limited concept of the role the state should perform than existed in the sixteenth through the eighteenth centuries. The third period, beginning roughly in the latter part of the nineteenth century, displayed reaction to problems created by the Industrial Revolution. During this last period the state intervened more frequently and directly in the lives of people and on a much broader scale and in a more effective manner than were necessary or possible in the seventeenth and eighteenth centuries.

By the beginning of the twentieth century, in much of Europe and parts of Asia and the Americas, the notion that the state is the appropriate instrument for ensuring the security and personal well-being of the individual had become firmly fixed. Over the past several decades the concept of the welfare-oriented state has gained nearly universal acceptance and, therefore, provides a common basis for comparing the policies and performances of nations today.

Before proceeding further, two cautionary points must be raised. The first is that these historical stages, like most efforts to categorize history neatly, are rather broadly defined. Some nation-states emerged later than others and industrialized later than others. Thus, these categories are meant to convey general trends or stages in the evolution of state activity and do not always coincide with the experiences of each nation. Second, it is impossible definitively and exhaustively to detail the genesis and evolution of state activity from the sixteenth through the nineteenth centuries. All we hope and need to accomplish here is an outline of the more characteristic and typical features of state activity in each period.

The emergence of the modern state: sixteenth through eighteenth centuries

Beginning in the sixteenth century, the modern nation-state emerged in Europe and parts of Asia. It was during this time that the nation-state acquired the characteristic form of a centralized authority, able to exercise reasonably consistent control over a relatively well-defined territory. If the preceding sentence seems to contain an abundance of qualifiers, it is because in these early years, control often was qualified. In addition to the exercise of control over a territory and a population, it was during this period that many activities we now associate with the modern nation-state began to make their first, albeit tentative, appearance. In some instances these activities appear to bear a remarkable resemblance to current state functions. Consider, for example, one historian's commentary on Prussia prior to 1740.

Perhaps the most intriguing experience for me in describing the areas of state inter-vention in the era before 1740 was the realization of the almost complete identity of these areas with practically every area of regulation by the state in contemporary society. Anti-poverty, consumer protection, minority rights, concern for the moral implications of clothing styles, extension and availability of education to all citizens at all levels, certification of teachers and health practitioners, urban development, anti-pollution measures to protect water and air, draft evasion by university matriculation, concern for the old, the sick, the unemployed, the discharged veteran, sanitation and fire security measures, and, of course, the primary issue of public security, law and order, all equally concern dynastic prince and modern democratic republics.[2]

Although this description is undoubtedly accurate, at least for Prussia, it is also somewhat misleading. There are, to be sure, many similarities between the modern state and its ancestors in the sixteenth through the eighteenth centuries, but there are also profound differences. What were the major characteristics of state activity prior to the Industrial Revolution? How did these differ from current practices?

The range and effectiveness of state activity

As the above description of Prussia suggests, state activity in the sixteenth through eighteenth centuries was sometimes quite extensive. Clearly, given the number of political units and length of time involved, great variation in state involvement occurred, so that a defininitive or detailed characterization is not possible. Nevertheless, certain general features are discernible.

Providing for defense and maintaining internal order

The primary function of the traditional or early modern state was to afford the individual and the society protection and security from external enemies and disruptive forces within the society. This, in turn, would ensure the appropriate environment for developing a prosperous economy. It was in the fulfillment of the primary state function that many of the activities engaged in by governments were undertaken and justi-fied during the formative years of the modern nation-state. It is only a slight overstatement to suggest that most of the other activities performed by the traditional state – taxation and finance, economic regulation, sumptuary legislation, public works – in large part were derivatives of the overriding defense- and order-maintaining function of the state.

The frequency of international war during the sixteenth through eighteenth centuries – over 150 wars were fought between 1500 and 1800[3] – suggests that state leaders had ample opportunity and need to engage and enlarge the state apparatus. "Up to our own time dramatic increases in national budgets, national debts, numbers of governmental employees or any other indicator of governmental scale in European countries have occurred almost exclusively as a consequence of preparations for war."[4] In the sixteenth century, and indeed in our own century, wars have been the major stimulus to the development and expansion of the state. Given the frequency of internal disorders, we must assume that maintaining law and order must also have played a major role in the expansion of state activity. Sorokin, in a study of only eight European nations between the sixteenth and nineteenth centuries, calculated that 395 internal disturbances occurred during that period.[5]

Public finance

Perhaps the most obvious and important of the state's activities relating to the protection of society as well as its economic well-being was the development of public taxation and financing systems. According to Daniel Bell, the modern state

arose in the 16th century and after, primarily out of the needs of the princes and monarchs of the European states to pay the expenses of war . . . Taxes thus came to be levied, and a bureaucratic administrative system arose to collect, and then to spend, these monies. As the newly emergent state acquired a solid framework, taxes came to be used for other than the original purposes.[6]

Bell's comment is equally applicable to the traditional eighteenth-century kingdoms of Burma, Siam, and Vietnam, where tax collection and regional warfare were the main state activities. Raising adequate revenues stretched the ingenuity of the ruler, the activities of the state, and the frequency with which public authority and private individuals came in contact. Illustrative of these revenue-raising devices that began in the seventeenth century are indirect or excise taxes levied in France, England, and Holland on beverages, preservatives, wearing apparel, and textiles.[7] In addition, direct taxes such as the tithe (percentage of a harvest), poll tax (a set tax per person), hearth tax (a fee levied on every home with a chimney), real estate and various forms of income tax were introduced in Europe and parts of Asia in the seventeenth and eighteenth centuries. In fact, the first modern income tax was introduced in Britain in order to finance the war against the American rebels.[8] The frequency of wars and civil disturbances required a steady flow of revenue. This, in turn, required the establishment of a permanent state bureaucracy and more or less regular contact between the individual and the state. Barrington Moore's description of traditional India provides us with a useful summary of the relationship between the state and the masses in many traditional systems: "The fundamental features of the traditional Indian polity were a sovereign who ruled, an army that supported the throne, and a peasantry that paid for both."[9]

Social and economic regulatory policy

Although defense of the nation, maintenance of internal order, and the collection of monies necessary to finance these efforts were of overriding importance in the traditional state, none constituted the most pervasive or intensive source of intervention and activity on the part of the emerging modern state. Rather, it was in the area of regulating socio-economic behavior that the traditional state became most intimately involved with the largest number of people. To a certain extent these regulations, such as those dealing with the production and distribution of food, were themselves intended to support the war-making capacity of the state. For example, "much of the Hohenzollern [i.e., Prussian] grain policy went into building up stores and supply systems for a big standing army, and assuring the free movement of grain into those provinces where the army was concentrated. The riveting of agrarian policy to the war machine held into the nineteenth century." Although Prussia may have been the extreme case, similar demands for food and resulting food policies existed in France, England, Spain, Russia, and the Scandinavian countries.[10] Food policy was related also to the maintenance of internal order. In this regard, state distribution of food was used as a police measure. For example, the Manchu rulers of China (1644–1911) established a system of "imperial storage depots for grain that could be distributed to the population in times of shortage. The rulers recognized very clearly the connection between hunger and peasant rebellion."[11] Similar precautionary strategies to deal with food riots were adopted in Europe. There, as in China, the state became involved in the production and distribution of food in order to prevent internal disorders as well as to supply standing armies.

It would be misleading and historically inaccurate to suggest that the traditional state intervened in the economic life of society solely for the purposes of supplying its armed forces and nonmilitary bureaucracy and forestalling internal disorder. The paternalistic concept of monarchical rule, noblesse oblige, dictated that the ruler provide for the general well-being of his or her subjects. This concern, common in many societies, led to the most incredibly detailed and wide-ranging regulations of economic activity. In sixteenth- and seventeenth-century England, for example, "the crown issued minute rules concerning the quality of hops and malt in brewing, the size of buckets, the type of materials to be used in the manufacture of thread, leather, soap, glass, tobacco and a host of other products." Similarly, in seventeenth- and eighteenth-century France, there were laws "establishing minimal levels of salt consumption and prescribing the number of threads in the warp of a piece of fabric."[12]

Regulations that ostensibly had the purpose of protecting the economic welfare of the community frequently contained social and moral implications as well. The relationship between the economic and moral welfare of the community, and the lengths to which the state was willing to intercede to ensure both, are most clearly illustrated by various actions taken by the Prussian rulers during the sixteenth to eighteenth centuries. Many of the regulations dealt with various life cycle celebrations and ceremonies such as births, christenings, betrothals, weddings, and funerals. In each case, detailed laws were issued for the purpose of restraining "immoral, extravagant, wasteful consumption of food and drink" as well as other personal excesses. It is impossible to do justice to the range and detail of these regulatory efforts, but a few illustrations help capture the essence and purpose of these governmental actions. For example, limitations were placed on the number of persons allowed to attend christenings, betrothals, and weddings and on the amount of food and drink that could be consumed on each occasion. Laws passed in 1551 and 1580 established the following restrictions on wedding celebrations: "Not more than ten tables of twelve guests each were permitted, although an extra table of out-of-town guests and one extra table for small children might be added. The maximum number of courses at each meal was not to exceed four; white and red wine and one foreign beer were allowed." The celebration could not exceed two days, and limits were placed on the fees paid to entertainers, food suppliers, and kitchen help.

In an effort to reduce the amount spent on funerals and related mourning activities, laws in 1604, 1655, and 1716 specified those members of the deceased's family who could wear mourning clothes, the materials to be used, and the duration for which they could be worn. In addition, music was prohibited at the funeral and postburial meals. Finally, a law of 1604 detailed acceptable clothing and personal decorations for members of each social class. "Specifically, the members of the first social rank . . . were forbidden to use velvet, satin, sable, marten or more expensive furs for whole coats . . . jackets or trousers . . . Velvet was allowed for bodices, jackets, collars and hats. Jeweled and gilded decorations were forbidden." Unmarried maidens of first-class families could not wear velvet and satin dresses until their marriage.[13] The content of the legislative activity illustrated above may have been unique to Prussia, but the tendency to integrate economic and moral regulatory policy was not.

State economic regulatory activity during this period was above all committed to the promotion and protection of newly developing national economies.[14] The tendency of the traditional state to intervene in the economic life of a society entailed grandiose efforts aimed at regulating the very nature of a nation's economic character. Such regulations included tariff policies intended to protect a nation's industries, its supply of precious metals and raw materials, and its international trade balance. In large measure, the laws described above specifying the quality and quantity of ingredients for various products (e.g., leather, thread, soap) were an attempt by the state to ensure the quality, hence salability and competitiveness, of exported goods. Collectively, these protectionist and expansionist policies were part of an economic doctrine, later called *mercantilism* (or cameralism in Germany), which dominated much of Europe in the sixteenth through eighteenth centuries. Mercantilism again illustrates the lengths to which the early modern state intervened in the individual and collective economic life of the nation.

The whole host of economic regulations associated with mercantilism, ranging from prohibiting certain imports and exports to specifying the number of threads in a piece of cloth, required state supervision and inspection. Thus, mercantilism contributed to the increased contact between the individual and the state as well as to the size of the state bureaucracy.

Maintaining class distinctions

Another characteristic of state activity prior to the nineteenth century was that public policy often was used as a means of perpetuating social class differences. In the case of the Prussian laws cited above, different provisions were applied to the four clearly defined social ranks in Prussian society: Members of the third and fourth ranks generally were limited to a smaller amount of food and drink on festive occasions, a shorter celebration or mourning period, and less fancy apparel and decorations than those of the first two ranks. Such publicly enforced social distinctions were not unique to Prussia. Similar state-enforced privileges and distinctions existed in other countries. For example, with regard to the Chinese nobility, "their homes, carriages, and clothing were prescribed by government decree so that their style of life would conform with their rank-order in society."[15]

The enforcement problem

Thus far we have tried to demonstrate that the range of state activity during the sixteenth to eighteenth centuries was quite extensive. Indeed, as the description of Prussia quoted at the beginning of this chapter indicates, the range was in some cases apparently as comprehensive as that of the twentieth-century modern nation-state. But if the Prussian case suggests the lengths to which the state was willing to intervene in the lives of people, it also illustrates the difficulty, and frequently the inability, of the traditional state to enforce its intentions. Persistent evasion of all forms of public regulations plagued the Prussian (and English, Japanese, Indian, Burmese, etc.) rulers throughout the sixteenth, seventeenth, and eighteenth centuries. In 1713 Frederick William I of Prussia complained that "a number of ordinances issued by previous rulers concerning police matters have not been observed, to the harm of the common good," and in 1723 he issued the Edict of Failure to Observe Adequately All Previous Fire-Prevention Ordinances in Town and Country.[16]

The frustration of Frederick William was shared by his counterparts in England, Japan, and elsewhere. Holt and Turner note that in England during the sixteenth and seventeenth centuries, "regardless of which aspect of government regulation of the economy is examined, the record in nearly every case forces one to a conclusion which may be summed up in a single sentence: The policy was unsuccessful because it could not be enforced."[17]

The reader should not conclude that the traditional state was completely impotent; obviously, European and Asian rulers were able to collect sufficient taxes, raise large enough armies, and regulate enough behavior to support themselves and protect their nations. Neither would it be accurate to conclude that all states were equally unsuccessful in enforcing their rules. The Chinese and French rulers were apparently more successful than the English or Japanese in enforcing their laws. Finally, we are not suggesting that the distinction between the traditional state and the modern state is that the former could not enforce its rules whereas the latter can; an examination of rates of income tax evasion in many modern nations belies such a contention. However, the indication is that *one* characteristic feature of traditional states, and one that distinguishes them from the modern state, is the relatively greater inability of the traditional leaders to enforce their will. It would take us too far afield to account for the enforcement problem, but among the facts that should be noted are the lack of an effective bureaucracy and primitive communications technology.

Social welfare

If preparation for war, maintaining internal order, and protecting and promoting the nation's economy were the reasons behind much of the regulatory, extractive, and distributive policies of the traditional state, paternalism provided the motivation for much of its redistributive or welfare policy efforts. The paternalistic concept of government, buttressed in Europe by the tenets of Christian morality, was well suited to the development of state-supported welfare or poor-relief programs during the sixteenth to eighteenth centuries. By the seventeenth century, virtually every European state had some sort of centrally established public welfare program. One of the first was the *Grand Bureau des Pauvres* ("Central Relief Office") established in France in 1550. Other early efforts were the Elizabethan Poor Law, passed in 1601; a Russian system of state-operated welfare established during the reign of Peter the Great (1682–1725); and a Prussian system of state poor relief that evolved in various edicts between 1596 and 1703. As in other policy areas, there was considerable variation in control and operation among the programs. Nevertheless, certain distinguishing and common philosophical assumptions and substantive elements could be found in most European welfare systems. The most noteworthy of these features deserve attention because in them we find some direct links to our own modern concept and operation of welfare systems.

The first point to be emphasized is that the motivation behind early welfare systems was not exclusively paternalistic or religious. In many instances, poor relief was an exercise of the state's police power. It was simply another instrument for dealing with the problems of maintaining law and order. Throughout the sixteenth to eighteenth centuries, in Europe and elsewhere, landless peasants, persons uprooted by war, returning and unemployed soldiers resorted to vagrancy, begging, stealing, and extortion to support themselves. In an effort to get these people off the streets, reduce the crime rate, and keep them physically apart from the more respectable members of society, welfare or poor-relief systems were established. Derek Fraser, describing the origins of the famous Elizabethan Poor Laws, captures what was true in other European states: "Laws against vagrancy were . . . the origins of poor relief, and whenever economic conditions prevailed which encouraged men to wander the country in search of employment, the late medieval and early modern English state sought to restrict this mobility for fear of its social consequences."[18]

Early welfare, and particularly health, measures were related also in theory and practice to the doctrine of mercantilism. The reasoning here was that the power and wealth of the state depended on a healthy, vigorous, and large population. Therefore, the national interest required state intervention in the area of public health. In the German states this intervention took the form of "medical police" ordinances that dealt with medical education, disposition of medicines, hospital regulations, and epidemic prevention.[19]

A second common feature of early poor relief systems is the legal distinction between categories or types of needy persons. The primary distinction was between those who were legitimately poor (e.g., the aged, insane, blind, or otherwise physically handicapped) and the ablebodied scoundrels, rogues, and professional beggars who refused honest work. Typically, each category of persons was treated differently. For example, both the Elizabethan Poor Law and the welfare policies of Tsar Feodor II (1676–82) and Catherine the Great (1762–96) provided for institutional relief (almshouses) for the "deserving" poor; workhouses for the ablebodied poor who were willing to work; and punishment for the ablebodied who refused to work (e.g., a house of correction in England; beatings in Russia or Siberia).[20] From the very beginning poor relief was deemed justified only in cases of severe disability.

A third feature of pre-nineteenth-century welfare systems was the assumption that each locality should be held responsible for its own poor and needy. Although early poor-relief laws were centrally promulgated, they were typically financed and/or administered by local agencies. Such responsibility was rarely welcomed by local authorities, who were becoming increasingly burdened by the financial responsibility and who therefore were encouraging recipients to leave their jurisdiction. In an edict of 1696, Frederick III of Prussia prohibited local authorities from evading their responsibility by granting travel permits to beggars.[21] The dispute over local versus central responsibility for maintaining public welfare programs, an issue of considerable current concern in United States localities, has a long tradition.

The final noteworthy feature of these welfare programs is that acceptance of public relief carried with it considerable social stigma, marking the recipient as socially inferior. In some cases, most notably England, a person who received public assistance, became "pauperized" and, therefore, ineligible to perform various civil functions. In addition, paupers often were sent to workhouses. Not only social but legal sanctions were imposed on those who had to turn to public welfare assistance.

Summary

In this section a portrait is sketched of the emerging nation-state prior to the late eighteenth century. In summary:

1. Although public policy in the traditional state was partially based on paternalism (noblesse oblige) and Christian morality, the principal reasons were the overriding functions of defending the nation, maintaining internal peace and order, and protecting and promoting national economic wealth.

2. In pursuance of these functions traditional state leaders undertook such derivative activities as taxation, maintaining social class distinctions, and instituting public welfare programs.

3. The state's activities were sometimes quite extensive and comprehensive, covering in great detail significant areas of social and economic behavior.
4. However, the ability of the state to enforce its policies was severely limited by inadequate bureaucratic and technological development. This is one of the major differences that separates the state before and after the nineteenth century.

Laissez faire: the nineteenth-century attack on the active state

In the nineteenth century the concepts of mercantilism and state activism that had characterized state behavior in the sixteenth through eighteenth centuries came under attack and in many cases were superseded by a new philosophy: the limited state. The set of ideas that supported this view was summarized by the phrase *laissez faire* or *laissez nous faire* ("let it be" or "let us alone") and was first advocated by English and French philosophers and economists during the late eighteenth and early nineteenth centuries. It should be noted that paternalism and aspects of mercantilism generally survived the onslaught of laissez faire in Prussia and Russia. Furthermore, even in Great Britain, where it was most consistently applied in the late eighteenth to mid-nineteenth centuries, acceptance of the doctrine did not result in complete state withdrawal from regulatory activity. In practice, laissez faire resulted in a retreat or lessening, but not total abandonment, of state social and economic intervention. Furthermore and paradoxically, the very doctrine that counseled limited state involvement required a rather vigorous assertion of state activity to achieve its aims, if only because state action was required to rescind the numerous protectionist policies enacted during the heyday of mercantilism. For this reason, one can view laissez faire as another, albeit much diminished, form of state activity.

The doctrine of laissez faire demands our attention for several reasons. First, although not universally adopted, it did exert considerable influence throughout the Old World and ultimately in what is now called the Third World. This influence can be explained by the fact that major European colonizing powers, such as France and England, embraced the doctrine at home and exported it to their colonies. Second, as we soon shall see, laissez faire, in theory and practice, posed the major obstacle the advocates of the modern, activist state had to overcome. And finally, the doctrine, now embodied in modern American conservative political thought, continues to exert influence in the shaping of public policy.

The theory and its implications

The concept of laissez faire as articulated in the nineteenth century denoted a doctrine that opposed intervention by the state in the economic activities of a nation. It was predicated on the assumption that society and the economy were governed by "laws of nature" that imposed a "natural order and harmony" on life. Any tampering or interference by the state would upset this natural order. The state was to play a minimal role: to provide for the national defense, preserve internal order, and generally create an atmosphere conducive to the operation of a free and competitive marketplace. Beyond this, the state was to withdraw and allow the laws of nature to operate unfettered.

The implications and prescription of laissez faire were clear: The mercantilist, interventionist policies of the sixteenth through eighteenth centuries interfered with the natural economic order. The writings of Adam Smith, and particularly his famous *Inquiry into the Nature and Causes of the Wealth of Nations* (1776), provided much of the basis for, and exerted enormous influence over, subsequent laissez-faire doctrine – although Smith himself was far less doctrinaire than his followers. According to Adam Smith, mercantilism had to be replaced with the "obvious and simple system of natural liberty" in which "every man, as long as he does not violate the laws of justice, is left perfectly free to pursue his own interest his own way, and to bring both his industry and capital into competition with those of any other man or order of men."[22] Led by "an invisible hand," each man by pursuing his own economic interests would frequently and unwittingly promote the interests of society in general. Apparently, however, invisible hands were not enough. Karl Polanyi argues quite persuasively that the laissez-faire goal of a self-regulating, free market economy required, at least in England, considerable state intervention. "The road to the free market was opened and kept open by an enormous increase in continuous, centrally organized and controlled interventionism."[23] The apparent incongruity between the theoretical assumptions of laissez faire and its practical requirements were reconciled in and justified by the belief that whatever was done by the state was undertaken in an effort to achieve long-term economic freedom.

The implications of laissez faire extended beyond the realm of economic policy and activity. Just as the advocates of laissez faire condemned state interference in the economy (except when it served their purpose), so too did they attack the social aspects associated with traditional state paternalism. Here again they argued that the laws of nature must operate, unfettered by state intervention. For example, advocates condemned the poor laws in England and elsewhere as an unnecessary and unwise interference with the social order. Thomas Malthus rejected the poor laws on the basis that poor people were "themselves the cause of their own poverty; that the means of redress are in their own hands, and in the hands of no other persons whatever; that the society in which they live and the government which presides over it, are without any *direct* power in this respect."[24] The notion that poverty is the result of personal defects rather than economic conditions or policies and, therefore, not a legitimate concern of the state, was widely held in the nineteenth century.

Another belief widely held by laissez-faire advocates was that not only does the state have no responsibility toward the needy but any public support actually causes greater harm to society in general. Malthus saw the poor laws producing the twin evils of encouraging the poor to multiply and taking resources away from "the more industrious and worthy members" of society.[25] Another and somewhat more extreme expression of the position was made by Herbert Spencer, an Englishman who had an enormous impact on American thinking on this subject. In attacking those who would endorse public support of the needy, Spencer argued that, though well intentioned, these good samaritans were unthinking.

Blind to the fact that under the natural order of things society is constantly excreting its unhealthy, imbecile, slow, vacillating faithless members, those unthinking, though well-meaning, men advocate an interference which not only stops the purifying process, but even increases the vitiation – absolutely encourages the multiplication of the reckless and incompetent by offering them an unfailing provision.[26]

Summary

The doctrine of laissez faire was consistent with the needs of the Industrial Revolution. The old mercantilist system that advocated controlling market forces – labor, trade, competition, capital, etc. – appeared to obstruct industrial growth and its requirements for a mobile labor force, free flow of capital, economic competition, and easy access to world markets and materials. Laissez faire emphasized natural laws and individual rights, rejected government paternalism and intervention, and, therefore, appeared better suited to the needs of the new economic order.

Although never fully adopted as the sole guide for formulating public policy, even in England, laissez faire did have a profound impact on the framework within which policy was made in England, on the Continent, and in the United States during the nineteenth century. The limited state, self-help, and individual liberty were exalted. It was in this atmosphere that industrial growth and the colonization of much of Asia and Africa took place.

But as industrialization proceeded in the more advanced nations, it left in its wake a changing social, economic, and political environment. And just as mercantilism and traditional paternalism appeared incompatible or detrimental to the development of industrialization, so too did laissez faire begin to appear inadequate in the face of the political and social consequences of industrialization. Thus, by the latter part of the nineteenth century a revised concept of state began to appear. This concept, embraced in theory and enshrined in constitutions, although not always put in practice, was the idea of the general-welfare state. In a sense, the general-welfare state concept marked a revitalization of the active state. We now turn to an examination of its origins and manifestations.

The emergence of the positive state

The shift from a primarily agrarian to a primarily industrial economic base produced, and continues to produce, extraordinary societal dislocations and profound social and economic changes. Although the impact of industrialization and responses to it have been as numerous and varied as they have been profound, many similarities exist among the experiences of both the early and late industrializing nations. It is thus possible to draw a composite sketch of the consequences of, and reactions to, industrialization. Because our concern in this section is with the emergence of the general-welfare state as a reaction to the trauma of industrialization, attention is focused on those nations that were the first to industrialize: England, France, the United States, and Germany. Much of what is discussed, however, has clear parallels in, and implications for, recently modernizing nations.

Industrialization and its consequences

Industrialization is a process that both requires and produces fundamental societal change. Among its primary requirements is a relatively large and mobile labor force. Typically, the manpower needs of industrial societies have been recruited from rural populations within the nation itself (e.g., England, France, Germany, and Japan) or from abroad (e.g., the United States, Singapore, and Australia). The process of supplying the manpower needs of industrialization in this manner caused several societal changes. Most obviously, it resulted in high population concentration in industrial (including mining) towns and cities. The magnitude of the demographic changes involved was enormous. Between 1850 and 1900 cities such as Amsterdam, Berlin, Brussels, Chicago, London, Paris, Saint Petersburg, and Vienna, to name just a few, had population increases of between 100 and 300 percent or more. Among the more outstanding examples are Berlin, whose population increased from 419,000 in 1850 to 1.9 million in 1900; London, which grew from 2.7 million in 1850 to 6.6 million in

1900; and Chicago, which in 30 years (1860–90) increased in size from 100,000 to 1 million people.[27]

The nature and magnitude of the social changes that accompanied urbanization were even more dramatic. To begin with, housing conditions in the new industrial towns were deplorable. Overcrowded, rat-infested tenements could not accommodate the rapidly growing urban population. As a result, flimsy and unsafe structures were crowded even closer together, and all available "living" space, including hallways and cellars, was used. According to one source, approximately one-sixth of the entire population of Liverpool lived in cellars during the nineteenth century.[28]

Such overcrowded conditions produced serious public health and sanitation problems. There were inadequate supplies of pure water and food; infant and maternal mortality rates soared; cholera, typhus, and other epidemics were common in the nineteenth century throughout Europe and Asia. All these problems were exacerbated by the inadequacy or nonexistence of sewage and waste removal facilities. Human wastes were frequently disposed of in the streets. Urban crime rates, in the absence of modern police forces, soared. One need only consult the works of Charles Dickens or Karl Marx for ample testimony to the horror of urban life in nineteenth-century England and much of Europe. Perhaps the only saving grace in all this was that one did not have to endure it long: Death came early for industrial urban dwellers. The average age at death for a worker in Manchester, England, in the early nineteenth century was 17 years – about one-half the age of an upper-class citizen.[29]

The movement from rural to urban areas caused another fundamental social change, one that further contributed to the hardships of urban life. Here we are referring to the decline of the extended family structure. In an extended family – parents, grandparents, married children, and their families – the welfare of the individual is the direct concern and responsibility of the family as a unit. During difficult periods, such as those involving physical injury, ill health, economic hardship, marital disputes, it is the family in traditional agrarian society that provides social and economic security. The family also is expected to provide for the welfare of those in positions of "natural dependency": children, pregnant women, and old persons. The movement to cities often separated families and caused the breakdown of the extended family. Thus, urbanization helped undermine one of the very structures that could have absorbed some of the shocks accompanying major social and economic dislocations. This entire process is currently being repeated in virtually identical form throughout Asia and Africa.

Whereas many of the hardships of the nineteenth century derived from the urbanizing process, others could be directly attributed to the employment environment in industrial enterprises. There is no better description of the conditions of employment and the abuses suffered, particularly by women and children, than that contained in the testimony of Samuel Coulson before a parliamentary Select Committee of Factory Children's Labour (1831–32). Mr. Coulson's two daughters, who would have been between 5 and 12 years old, worked in a cloth mill. The committee asked Mr. Coulson to describe the employment conditions of his daughters.

Q At what time in the morning, in the brisk [busy] time, did those girls go to the mills?

A In the brisk time, for about six weeks, they have gone at 3 o'clock in the morning, and ended at 10, or nearly half past at night.

Q What intervals were allowed for rest or refreshment during those nineteen hours of labour?

A Breakfast a quarter of an hour, and dinner half an hour, and drinking a quarter of an hour.

Q Was any of that time taken up in cleaning the machinery?

A They generally had to do what they call dry down; sometimes this took the whole of the time at breakfast or drinking, and they were to get their dinner or breakfast as they could; if not, it was brought home.

Q Had you not great difficulty in awakening your children to this excessive labour?

A Yes, in the early time we had to take them up asleep and shake them, when we got them on the floor to dress them, before we could get them off to their work; but not so in the common hours.

Q Supposing they had been a little too late, what would have been the consequence during the long hours?

A They were quartered in the longest hours, the same as the shortest time.

Q What do you mean by quartering?

A A quarter was taken off.

Q What was the length of time they could be in bed during those long hours?

A It was near 11 o'clock before we could get them into bed after getting a little victuals, and then at morning my mistress used to stop up all night, for fear that we could not get them ready for the time; sometimes we have gone to bed, and one of us generally awoke.

Q What time did you get them up in the morning?

A In general me or my mistress got up at 2 o'clock to dress them.

Q For how long together was it?

A About six weeks it held; it was only when the throng was very much on; it was not often that.

Q The common hours of labour were from 6 in the morning till half-past eight at night?

A Yes.

Q With the same intervals for food?

A Yes, just the same.

Q Were the children excessively fatigued by this labour?

A Many times; we have cried often when we have given them the little victualling we had to give them; we had to shake them, and they have fallen to sleep with the victuals in their mouths many a time.[30]

Later in the testimony Mr. Coulson told the committee how his eldest
daughter lost a finger in one of the weaving machines. The daughter
missed work and wages for 5 weeks.

Similar accounts were given in other countries. A report to the Prussian
government concerning 7- to 9-year-old factory workers described their
"pale faces, dull, inflamed eyes, swollen bodies, puffed cheeks, swollen
lips and nostrils, swollen glands, skin diseases, and asthmatic fits."[31]

It is not possible to do justice to the full range of problems and societal
changes that accompanied the Industrial Revolution. By now, however,
the reader should have some notion of the enormous human costs
involved.

Policy reactions to industrialization

During the course of the nineteenth century, it became clear to many that
the social and economic dislocations and human misery spawned by industrialization required remedial action beyond that which was provided by
private charities, existing poor laws, or "invisible hands." A positive
exertion of state power was needed. Wherever it held sway, laissez faire
provided an ideological and practical obstacle to state intervention on
behalf of the victims of industrialization. A more receptive environment
to state involvement existed in countries like Germany, Austria, and
Russia, where paternalism had persisted over laissez-faire sentiment.
However, even in England, France, and the United States, where laissez
faire had it strongest advocates, the doctrine was losing support in favor of
a more activist and positive concept of state. Increasingly there was the call
for the state to provide protection, not only against external enemies and
internal lawlessness, but also against the evils and insecurities of industrialization. Initially, governments, when they responded at all, did so in a
gradual, piecemeal fashion. There was not as yet, in the late nineteenth
century, a coherent theory of a positive state that was committed to the
general welfare. Only in the twentieth century would such a commitment
emerge.

Many factors influenced the timing, rate, and content of social and
economic activity that eventually became public policy. The remainder of
this chapter examines some of these factors and activities. Subsequent
chapters, and particularly the case studies in Part II, devote greater time
and detail to the evolution of the general-welfare state in the twentieth
century. For now, however, we must be content with taking the narrative
only as far as the first tentative steps in this direction.

Public health and medical services

Perhaps predictably, public health was one of the first areas in which the state began playing an active and decisive role. Although inadequate housing and deplorable working conditions might offend the religious and moral sensibilities of the politically and socially powerful, these offenses need not directly affect them. Epidemic diseases such as cholera, typhus, and smallpox, however, tended to be indiscriminate, affecting rich and poor alike, although those crowded in the urban slums undoubtedly suffered more than those who could escape to country estates. Thus, some of the first positive exertions of state authority came in the area of public health. As early as 1832, France adopted a public health law, and in 1848 a public health act was passed in England that established a general board of health and delegated various public health activities to local boards of health. Five years later, in 1853, Parliament passed a truly extraordinary law that required compulsory smallpox vaccinations for all infants. Derek Fraser underscores the importance of the law, quoting R. J. Lambert's statement that it constituted "the first continuous health activity prompted by the state . . . an extraordinarily early development of state interference: a free, compulsory and nationwide health service in miniature."[32]

The nineteenth century also saw an emerging concern over the differences in the incidence of noncommunicable disease and in mortality rates among socioeconomic groups. Systematically gathered social and medical statistics revealed that the urban poor and working classes were ill more frequently and lived shorter lives than the middle and upper classes and even the rural poor. The evidence demonstrated that these differences were attributable directly to industrial and urban living and working conditions. The various government reports and sociological studies that documented this situation led a number of nineteenth-century reformers, physicians, and public health and other government officials to the conclusion that what society had created, society must remedy. Thus Solomon Neumann, a leading Prussian advocate of state involvement in health care, wrote:

It is the duty of society, i.e., of the state . . . to protect, and when endangered to save, the lives and health of the citizens. If it is the duty of social man to combat and to help endure the dangers which develop precisely because of social life, then it is equally clear that the state is obliged to combat and where possible to destroy not only natural dangers, but as well those dangers to human life.[33]

In addition to Neumann, prominent advocates of this position were Virchow in Germany, Meynne in Belgium, Griscom in America, and Chadwich in England. In 1842, Chadwich, in a report to the Poor Law Commission, advocated locally appointed district medical officers. The above-mentioned 1848 Public Health Act adopted Chadwich's suggestion.[34]

The provision of free, state-supported, and state-administered medical assistance to the needy was another reaction to nineteenth-century industrial- and urban-related health problems. In England such assistance was supplied under the poor laws, but at a social price. Until 1885, to request free medical assistance resulted in *pauperization,* (i.e., losing one's political rights and being subject to placement in a workhouse.) France was one of the first nations in the nineteenth century to provide free medical treatment and hospitalization for the needy. It did so in the National Law for Free Medical Assistance passed in 1893.[35] By the latter part of the nineteenth century, the state in Sweden, Norway, Switzerland, Poland, and Russia was employing doctors to provide free or inexpensive medical services to the needy and to supervise public health programs. In addition, the European colonizing nations introduced the notions of state-run hospitals, salaried doctors, and free medical services for the needy to their African and Asian colonies. It is noteworthy that the practice of a state health care system continued into the independence period in most of these Asian and African countries.[36]

Industrial legislation

Another important area of early state social policy dealt with abhorrent industrial labor practices. Most of these laws concerned the health and safety of women and children. As early as 1813, the French government issued a decree "prohibiting the employment of children under ten years of age in the underground galleries of mines." This was followed by an act in 1841 regulating the working time of children in certain types of factories: 8 hours for children between 8 and 12 years old and 12 hours for those between 12 and 16 years old.[37] In practice, however, this law had little real significance because no provision was made for inspectors. In fact, although subsequent labor laws were passed in 1848 and 1874, France did not adopt meaningful and enforceable factory legislation until 1892 and 1893.

In England, early factory and labor legislation was primarily concerned with the length of working hours, factory safety and sanitation conditions, and education for women and children. Although Parliament had passed a factory act as early as 1802, this law applied only to apprenticed pauper children in certain limited industries and was not intended as a general regulation of industrial working conditions for children. The landmark Factory Act of 1833 was such a law. It set limits on working hours for children under 13 years of age (e.g., children under 13 years old could work only a maximum of 9 hours a day and 48 hours a week), required

health certificates from children as a basis of employment, required working children under 13 years old to attend school, and gave the government
authority to appoint four factory inspectors to ensure compliance with the
law. This act was "clearly a great turning-point in the history of social
policy. It acknowledged the right of the state to intervene where there was
an overwhelming need to protect exploited sections of the community.
The ultimate responsibility for ensuring the welfare of children at work was
centered not on parent or employer but on the community at large."[38]

During the remainder of the century, subsequent English legislation
dealt with conditions of employment for women and adult males, as well
as children. A parliamentary act in 1842 prohibited the employment of
young girls and women in coal mines. In 1844, adult female labor was
restricted to 12 hours per day. And in 1847, a 10-hour bill for both men
and women was enacted, although subsequent legislation was required to
enforce its provisions. Factory acts in 1864, 1867, 1871, and 1874 were
consolidated in the Factory and Workshop Act of 1878, which further
extended protection to women and children by making provisions for their
education, limiting the types of jobs in which they could engage, reducing
the number of working hours, and regulating sanitary conditions at
working places.

Factory legislation in other industrializing nations tended to follow
chronologically and substantively the lead taken by England. The Swiss
Federal Factory Labor Law of 1877 established an 11-hour working day for
adults in factories and workshops. Australia established an 8-hour day for
women and young boys in 1885. In 1889, Belgium limited the number of
hours and type of economic activity in which children under 16 could
engage. This law was not as comprehensive or effective as similar legislation in England, and as late as 1896 children were working up to 11 hours
a day in factories and mines.[39]

By the turn of the century virtually every industrializing nation in the
world had adopted some form of labor and industrial legislation regulating working hours and conditions.

Education
Publicly supported, universal primary education was another by-
product of the nineteenth century. Although public school systems had
appeared earlier in both the American colonies and Prussia, it was only in
the nineteenth century that the practice became widespread.

In the case of the United States, this development was the result of
initiative by colonies rather than a "national" effort. Publicly supported
and operated elementary education was first established in the 1640s in
the Massachusetts Bay Colony. By the time of the Revolution, similar

systems were common throughout the colonies. In Prussia, a state-run educational system began developing in the early eighteenth century, and by 1794 a system of state-run, compulsory education was fully established. In both countries, then, compulsory education preceded industrialization.

On the other hand, in England and on the Continent, state involvement in primary education appears to have been a response to the needs of the Industrial Revolution. At the beginning of the nineteenth century the notion that everyone should be educated was both alien and, for some members of the elite, obnoxious. One such objection was expressed in 1807 during a parliamentary speech against a bill that would have provided free education for pauper children in England.

The scheme would be bound to be prejudicial to the morals and happiness of the labouring classes; it would teach them to despise their lot in life, instead of making them good servants in agriculture and other laborious employments to which their rank in society had destined them; instead of teaching them subordination it would render them factious and refractory as was evident in the manufacturing counties; it would enable them to read seditious pamphlets, vicious books and publications against Christianity; it would render them insolent to their superiors.[40]

Despite such opposition, it became apparent that "there was an urgent need for a literate and better educated population to man the new industries and their supporting services. Universal education became an economic necessity."[41] Gradually the nations of Europe adopted public school systems. Free, compulsory education was established in Sweden in 1842. Between 1870 and 1891 compulsory systems were established in Great Britain, France, Italy, and Japan. By the latter part of the nineteenth century the principle that education is a state responsibility had become part of the political culture of the modern world.

Social insurance

Of all the changes that occurred in the course of the nineteenth century, none was more significant than the shift from the concept of poor law relief to the idea of social insurance. This shift represented a revolutionary change in attitude and practice with regard to who should assume responsibility for certain types of individual misfortune.

We have already seen that poor laws were in part police measures and in part acts of aristocratic benevolence, extended to marginal elements in society not because they had a right to relief but because the community had a right to protection from these elements and the state had a paternal obligation to the needy. Relief tended to be punitive in nature, stigmatizing in effect, and reforming in intent. But the standards of both laissez faire and state paternalism were becoming inappropriate and inadequate as industrialization and socioeconomic insecurity advanced. The increasingly large, vocal, and educated urban working class began organizing, demanding, and receiving greater political power. With the end of the extended family system, the needs of the urban worker for protection from the insecurities associated with urban industrial employment – loss of wages owing to job-related injury, illness, unemployment, and of course, old age – increased. "When social investigations showed that age, illness and involuntary unemployment were the greatest cause of poverty among a wage working population, social means of protection that were free from the punitive stigma of the poor law became inevitable."[42]

Though the urban industrial milieu created the conditions in which the need and demand for social security grew, the motivation, timing, and content varied from one country to another. It is not possible to do justice here to the development of these systems. Part of that story will be told when we examine the development of the health insurance programs of Germany, Great Britain, the Soviet Union, and Japan. Brief attention must, however, be paid to Germany because it was the first nation to adopt a comprehensive social insurance program and thus became the model for many other nations. A full account of the health insurance aspect of the program appears in Chapter 5.

The first modern, comprehensive social security program was developed in Germany during the 1880s. Under the guiding and powerful hand of Chancellor Otto von Bismarck, laws in 1882, 1884, and 1889 established compulsory sickness, accident, old-age, and disability insurance programs. Several factors explain Bismarck's radical social program. The first was the long-standing tradition of the Prussian paternalistic state and its concern for the needy. In addition, certain immediate political factors influenced Bismarck's decision. At the time "Bismarck enjoyed sufficient authority in the Prussian-German State to push through social legislation when he finally decided that there was need for it."[43] Such a need presented itself in the form of a rapidly growing, radical, socialist-oriented party (Social Democrats) that threatened the government, the monarchy, and conservative rule in Germany. In introducing the social insurance measures, "Bismarck's dominant concerns were to woo the workers away from socialism and to preserve the country's authoritarian monarchy."[44] Thus was born, in an authoritarian, conservative, monarchical political system, the concept of modern social insurance.

Shortly after its introduction, several nations followed the German example. Austria and Czechoslovakia established programs for injury insurance in 1887, sickness insurance in 1888, and old-age disability insurance in 1906; Denmark developed a similar set of programs between 1891 and 1896; Italy between 1898 and 1919; and Great Britain between 1897 and 1911. By the second decade of the twentieth century, most advanced nations in the world had relatively comprehensive social insurance programs. The major exception was the United States. It did not

have a job-related injury or illness insurance program until 1908 – several
years after most other modern nations had adopted such programs. An
old-age, disability, and survivor's insurance program was set up in 1935,
almost one-half century after the German law and several years after laws
in such nations as Spain (1919), Uruguay (1919), Brazil (1924), and Chile
(1924). The United States did not adopt a (partial) medical insurance
program until 1965. Today, almost all (128) nations have some type of
work injury insurance program; most (108 nations) have old-age, disability, and survivor's insurance; and about one-half (71 nations) have
medical / maternity insurance programs.

Conclusion

This chapter traces the transformation of the nation-state from its traditional origins in the sixteenth century to its modern form in the late nineteenth century. This period is divided into three stages, and the major
state-related features of each are characterized. Among the major points
emphasized are:

1. The philosophy of the traditional state, a combination of
   paternalism and praetorianism, posited a broad range of activities for the state. Most of these were regulatory in nature and
   related to the primary state responsibility of national defense,
   maintaining internal order, and promoting national economic wealth. Whereas the policy assumptions of the traditional state were almost as ambitious as those of the modern
   state, its enforcement capacity was not.
2. The advent of the Industrial Revolution, beginning in the
   late eighteenth century, changed the social, economic, and
   political order of the nation-states affected. In some countries,
   most notably England, France, and the United States, a new
   theory of state – laissez faire – sought to limit the role of
   government to providing an environment in which the free
   market could best operate. In all countries touched by industrialization, society and economy underwent dramatic changes:
   urbanization, social dislocation, human suffering, and hardship. The relatively secure agrarian life gave way, for many,
   to a much harsher, highly uncertain urban life.
3. Neither state paternalism nor laissez faire was adequate to deal
   with the urgent problems of urban industrial society and the
   political demands of the new urban proletariat. By the late
   nineteenth century a new concept of state began to evolve:
   the general-welfare state. This view is based upon the assumption that individuals have certain "social rights," among

which is the right to be protected from the various uncertainties associated with an urban industrial environment.[45]

By the second decade of the twentieth century, the notion that the state
exists to promote positively the interests and welfare of all citizens had
become established in theory, if not in fact, in most of the world. It is this
concept of government that has been embraced by the newly emerging
states during the twentieth century. And it is by this standard that we
must compare and evaluate the public policies of nations today.

3

Accounting for public policy

Most of us at one time or another have been bewildered by or incredulous over the policies pursued by various governments. Consider for a moment the seemingly incomprehensible policies of the American and French governments with regard to cigarette smoking. Why does the United States government use public taxes to provide tobacco farmers with price supports, commodity loans, and agricultural extension services and at the same time publicly finance research on the dangers of tobacco smoking, support antismoking advertising campaigns, and compel manufacturers to inform the public of the hazards of cigarette smoking? Similarly, one may ask why the French government, through the state-owned tobacco monopoly (SEITA, or Service for the Industrial Exploitation of Tobacco and Matches), actively encourages people to smoke more, while the French Ministry of Health is waging a costly ($500,000 in 1975) antismoking campaign involving advertising, a law against smoking in public places, and mandated health warnings on cigarette packages. Why *do* governments do what they do?

The range and number of factors that influence or determine what governments do or, for that matter, what they choose not to do, are virtually infinite. Public policy may be influenced by prior policy commitments, international tension, a nation's climate, economic wealth, degree of ethnic conflict, historical traditions, the personality of its leadership, the level of literacy of its people, the nature of its party system, and whether it is governed by civilian or military leaders. The list could be extended almost indefinitely. Virtually anything can influence or determine what governments do.

In order to bring some semblance of order to the enormous number of policy-relevant variables and, therefore, make the comparative study of public policy more manageable, we offer an accounting or organizing scheme. As noted in Chapter 1, the purpose of the scheme is to allow the student to proceed systematically, at the observation stage of theory building, in the investigation of why national governments choose or reject various policies. The scheme is an inventory of those factors that influence the making of public policy. It is our belief that at this stage in the development of comparative policy studies it is necessary to categorize, rather than theorize about, the factors that explain public policy. The framework is described and illustrated in this chapter and applied in subsequent chapters.

The accounting scheme

The accounting scheme used here is based on a similar framework introduced by Robert Alford. According to Alford: "Decisions, policies and government roles can be explained by a combination of situational, structural, cultural and environmental factors."[1] Following Alford's lead, we suggest that the first step in trying to explain the decisions and policies of governments is to order the available evidence. The instrument chosen is the four broad categories suggested by Alford, although the definition of each varies somewhat from his. We begin with a definition of each category and an illustrative tabular presentation of the content of the categories.

A *situational* factor is a more or less transient, impermanent, or idiosyncratic condition or event that has an impact on policy making. The qualifier "more or less" is included to alert the reader to the fact that even a seemingly transient event can be relatively long in duration. For example, as discussed below, wars and other violent events are among the most important factors influencing public policy; yet, like World War II, they can be rather lengthy affairs. On the other hand, a race riot in Soweto, South Africa (June 1976), lasting only a few days is illustrative of a situational factor of much shorter duration that nevertheless resulted in significant change in that country's language and educational policy: dropping the mandatory use of Afrikaans as a teaching language in black schools. In addition, it is recognized that at some point an enduring situational factor, such as a change in political regime, becomes a structural factor. Our concern here is with the "relatively" immediate impact of an event or condition on public policy. It is impossible to put a time limit on when a transient event becomes institutionalized and, therefore, part of a nation's social, political, or economic structure.

Structural factors are the "relatively unchanging elements of the society and polity." Structural factors include the more permanent and persistent features of a system, such as its economic base, political institutions, or demographic structure. These features have a more sustaining and, therefore, generally more predictable impact on policy than situational factors.

Cultural factors are the "value commitments of groups within the community or the community as a whole." It appears that Alford, who

appends to his definition the clause "expressed through laws and policies," is primarily concerned with political values or culture (e.g., "norms
attached to political participation"). Our definition of cultural factors
includes both political and general culture values (e.g., religious values).

Environmental factors are events, structures, and values that exist
outside the boundaries of a political system but that influence decisions
within the system. The Arab oil boycott of 1973–4, which resulted in a
decision by the Dutch government to ban all nonemergency gasoline-
burning vehicular traffic on Sundays, is an example of an environmental
event influencing a national political decision.

It is impossible, of course, to deal with all the situational, structural,
cultural, and environmental factors shaping public policy throughout the
world. Instead, we present, in outline form, a list that suggests the range
and variety of the variables (Table 3–1). We then describe and illustrate
the dynamics of a sample of the policy-influencing variables. The sample
includes factors that have been demonstrated to be important in the
comparative policy process. It is important to emphasize here that this
presentation is illustrative, not exhaustive. Our intention is to provide the
reader, in his/her capacity as either a lay observer of events or a researcher
of the comparative policy process, with an instrument or perspective with
which to explain why national governments pursue the policies they do.

Before we examine in detail some of the factors listed in Table 3–1, two
important points must be emphasized. The first is that rarely does any one
factor operate in isolation. The policy context usually involves a simul-
taneous interplay of more than one situational, structural, cultural, or
environmental influence. For example, the Canadian government's decision in July 1976, to prohibit Taiwanese athletes from competing under
the banner of the Republic of China in the 1976 Summer Olympics was
made in a complex policy context. First of all, it was a personal decision by
a prime minister (Pierre Trudeau) in a parliamentary system. Second, it
was the result of pressures by the Peking government, which provides
Canada with an approximately $300 million trade surplus from the sale of
Canadian wheat to the People's Republic of China. Finally, Trudeau was
under pressure from the International Olympic Committee, the United
States government, and the Chinese-Canadian community on the west
coast of Canada. Situational, structural, and environmental factors were all
involved in the decision.

Thus, although this chapter discusses and illustrates the impact of these
factors as if they operate in singular or discrete fashion, the reader must
bear in mind that the policy context actually involves the interplay of
many factors.

Second, these policy-related factors vary (i.e., have greater or lesser influence), according to the policy area. For example, it is probably the

Table 3-1. *A scheme for analyzing public policy*

I. Situational factors
   A. Violent events: international and civil wars, communal conflict, terrorism, assassination
   B. Economic cycles: depression, recession, inflation
   C. Natural disasters: epidemics, droughts, floods, oil spills, earthquakes
   D. Political events and conditions
      1. Political status change: achieving independence, joining or leaving an international association, integration with another political unit
      2. Political regime change: revolution, coup d'etat, election of a radical political party
      3. Change of government: electoral shift in power from conservative to liberal party
      4. Political reform: extending suffrage
      5. Political corruption or scandal: Lockheed scandals, Watergate
      6. Change in political leadership: election of a de Gaulle or an F. D. Roosevelt; death of a Stalin or a Franco
   E. Technological change: inventions such as the automobile, airplane, nuclear weapons
   F. The policy agenda: competition among policy issues and their proponents for the time, attention, and resources available to decision makers
II. Structural factors
   A. Political structure
      1. Type of political regime: military or civilian, socialist or nonsocialist, competitive or noncompetitive party system
      2. Type of political organization: federal or unitary system
      3. Form of government: parliamentary, presidential, nondemocratic
      4. Group activity: number, strength, and legitimacy of interest groups
      5. Political process: legislative–executive relations, budgetary process, nature of bureaucracy
      6. Policy constraints: incrementalism, prior policy commitments
   B. Economic structure
      1. Type of economic system: free market, planned, or mixed economy
      2. Economic base: primarily agrarian or industrial, diversified or one-product dependency
      3. National wealth and income: size and growth rate of GNP, distribution of wealth
      4. Complexity of economic organization: modern or traditional economy
   C. Social, demographic, and ecological structure
      1. Population: age structure, birth rate, geographical distribution, communal divisions, rate of in- and out-migration, level of education
      2. Degree of urbanization: proportion of population living in urban and rural areas
      3. Natural resources: land, water, minerals
      4. Geographic location: island or landlocked, tropical or temperate climate, proximity to militarily strong or weak neighbors
III. Cultural factors
   A. Political culture
      1. National heritage
      2. Political norms and values: concerning the role of the individual and the state

Table 3-1 *(cont.)*

         3. Formal political ideology: Marxist, fascist, democratic
     B.   General culture
         1. Traditional social values: relating to social institutions and arrangements such as marriage, the family, sex roles
         2. Religion: religious values and role of religious institutions in society
IV.   Environmental factors
     A.   International political environment: cold war, détente
     B.   Policy diffusion: emulation and borrowing of policy ideas and solutions from other nations
     C.   International agreements, obligations, and pressures
         1. World public opinion
         2. International affiliations: United Nations, UNESCO, International Olympic Committee, Organization for African Unity
         3. Participation in international conferences and agreements: Stockholm Conference on Man and the Environment
         4. International financial obligations: World Bank loans, Agency for International Development (U.S. AID) assistance
     D.   International private corporations: International Telephone & Telegraph, Chase Manhattan Bank

case that a nation's population structure (i.e., its age distribution, birth rate, etc.) has greater impact on distributive policies like education and social security than on administrative or symbolic policies. And even within the area of distributive policy, demographic structure is more likely to affect social policy than defense policy. Similarly, the determinants of public policy also vary from one time to another. Guy Peters, in a study of social policy in France, Sweden, and the United Kingdom, found that *socioeconomic* factors had a greater impact on policy during the early stages of political development, whereas *political* factors were more important during the transitional stage in these countries.[2]

One of the interesting questions facing public policy analysts is whether the variation in influence, from one policy area to another and from one historical time to another, holds constant cross-nationally. In subsequent chapters some tentative explanations are offered about the relative importance of situational, environmental, cultural, and structural factors on distributive policies. Bearing these points in mind, we can now turn to a discussion of some of the factors outlined in Table 3-1.

The impact of situational factors on public policy

Wars and other national crises

Severe national crises predictably have major impact on national public policy. Among such crises perhaps none has produced more profound and lasting policy consequences than participation in a major war. We have already noted that during the sixteenth through the eighteenth centuries war was a primary contributor to the extension of state activity. Generally such activity was directly related to the war-making capability of the state: raising revenues, conscription, and ensuring adequate military supplies.

In the twentieth century too, war has been responsible for expanding the role of the state. The impact of war on public policy in this century, however, has been more profound than in the past. Recent wars, like those in the past, have required governments to make extraordinary demands on the community. For most people, however, modern warfare has been total warfare in the sense that it has directly affected virtually the entire community. Civilian, as well as military, populations have been directly involved in the conflict through air raids, population evacuations, rationing, civil defense work, employment in defense industries, and of course, higher tax levies. The totality of modern warfare required and produced unprecedented expansion of state activity. Governments were required to generate and collect new sources of revenue, provide various social and protective services, regulate, and in many instances participate in, heretofore private social and economic activities. The relationship between the conduct of modern warfare and the initiation of new state activities is specifically illustrated in the case studies in Part II. Suffice it here to note that the accelerated development of Britain's welfare state, and most clearly its National Health Service, can be traced directly to the impact of World War II on the British homeland.

The significance of the wartime expansion of state activity lies less in those actions taken during the war – after all, people expect and demand extraordinary measures under such circumstances – than in the fact that these activities tend to continue, although at a somewhat diminished level, after the war. Policy studies of Great Britain, the United States, Australia, Canada, Germany, and South Africa all have found the same phenomenon: Public taxing, spending, and the range and scope of state activities never return to their prewar levels. Why should this be the case?

One reason is that periods of crisis tend to condition people to accept or tolerate higher levels of public taxing, spending, and state involvement in various activities. Temporary expedients initiated in times of national crisis, in the name of the national interest, tend to become permanent features of state activity.

A second reason is what Peacock and Wiseman in their study of Great Britain have termed the *inspection process.*

The conduct of war . . . has increasingly instituted a general inspection process for the whole population and economy which has revealed much about social conditions. It has taken the catastrophe of war to bring home to those in power that economic progress does not automatically disseminate the benefits of education and health.[3]

The experience of total war and community sacrifice produced an awareness of the inequalities, at least in British society, and a demand for a
more just distribution of resources. In most instances, it was the state,
which after all had demanded the wartime sacrifice, that was expected to
undertake the redistribution of societal resources.

Lastly, the demands made upon society as a result of twentieth-century
world wars have tended to be socially leveling in nature: for example,
rationing, universal conscription, excess profits taxes. These, in turn,
generated postwar egalitarian impulses and policies. Much of the British
welfare-state legislation of the late 1940s, as well as President Truman's
1948 executive order integrating the U.S. Armed Forces, stemmed, in
large part, from such impulses.

Other social upheavals, such as an economic depression and natural
disasters, have had similar impact on public policy. For example, it was as
a result of the Great Depression of the 1930s that countries such as the
United States, Canada, Chile, Ecuador, Greece, New Zealand, and Peru
introduced major social insurance programs, expanding the role of the state
and establishing new norms concerning the acceptable range and scope of
state activity. It should also be noted that national disasters can have an
entirely different – inhibiting – impact on public policy. We shall see in
Chapter 8, for example, that a severe earthquake in Japan in 1923 forced
postponement of that nation's first health insurance program. In the case
of Japan and other nations, national disasters sometimes strain a nation's
resources and make it difficult to initiate new policies.

Political change

It is likely, although by no means certain, that various types of political
change affect public policy. Is it not obvious that changes in the political
status of nations – say from colony to independent nation – or the acquisi-
tion of power by a new, perhaps revolutionary regime influence public
policy? Actually, a good deal of the policy literature has underscored the
resiliency of established policies and the incremental way, for example,
that public expenditures change even after revolutionary changes in political regimes. Indeed, one student of Latin American public policy, James
Wilkie, reports that:

Students of revolution may suppose that one of the first steps which a revolutionary government might take would involve a dramatic shift in the pattern of public
expenditures. In two of the three Latin American major social and economic revo-
lutions in this century, however, such was not the case. Mexico failed to achieve a
significant shift in state budgetary policy until the 1930s (more than twenty years
after the revolution of 1910). In the late 1960s the pattern of Bolivian central
government finances remained as it had been prior to the 1952 revolution.[4]

Of the third revolution, the Cuban, Wilkie says: "The authoritative
time-series data since 1959 remain unavailable and uninvestigated." However, Rolland Paulston finds in an analysis of state expenditures on public
education that between 1958 (the year before the Cuban Revolution), and
1962, per capita expenditures increased dramatically from 11.5 to 31.3
pesos. Over the same period, the number of schools increased from 7,567
to 13,780 and the number of teachers from 17,355 to 36,613.[5] Clearly,
the revolution made a difference in Cuban education policy.

Other examples can be found to support the thesis that political change
does influence the course and content of public policy. A case study by
Peter Sederberg of changes in public expenditures in Ghana, formerly the
Gold Coast, nicely illustrates the relationship between political change and
policy change. Sederberg describes three important political changes in
Ghana from 1946 to 1969 and the effect these had on national policy
priorities as reflected in public spending. The first change occurred in
1951, when the Gold Coast was given control over its own internal policy.
With this grant of authority there was a relative and absolute increase in
the amount spent on education. As Sederberg explains: "Africans would
naturally attach greater importance to the provision of general education
for their people than would the colonial rulers."[6]

The second important political change occurred in 1956, when Ghana
was granted independence. With sovereignty came control over national
defense and foreign relations and an immediate rise in the proportion of
the budget allocated to these functions. This increase leveled off after
1962.

The third significant change took place in 1966, when the regime of
Kwame Nkrumah was overthrown by a military coup d'etat. Ghanaian
public policy reflected a change in priorities, as military expenditures, as a
percentage of the total budget, again increased.

Two of these changes – achieving independence and experiencing a
coup – represent two of the most common types of political changes
occurring in the last three decades: Since 1945, over 65 nations have won
or been granted their independence, and there have been in excess of 60
successful violent coups since the end of World War II. One suspects,
although this should be empirically confirmed, that policy changes similar
to those that occurred in Ghana can be found in many other cases.

Another common type of political change frequently associated with
policy change is the replacement of one party in power by another. Here
the likelihood, magnitude, and types of policy changes are apt to be functions of the ideological distance between the parties involved. For
example, rather significant policy changes were introduced in Chile
between 1971 and 1973 by the Marxist-oriented Unidad Popular under

Salvador Allende, following its victory over the centrist Christian Democrats in the 1970 elections. Included in Allende's Popular Unity program
were (1) the nationalization of certain foreign-owned enterprises (e.g.,
copper industry); (2) social and economic reforms aimed at achieving an
egalitarian society, including public housing, agrarian reform, and a
nationwide uniform minimum wage law; and (3) a reorientation in Chile's
foreign policy.

Similarly, significant policy changes occurred in Great Britain following
the Labour Party's victory over the Conservatives in 1945. The policy initiatives taken by Labour, and opposed by the Conservatives, included a
commitment to relinquishing Britain's colonial empire: the nationalization of the coal, railway, iron, steel, and domestic airlines industries;
and an elaborate social welfare program. The case of nationalization of
the British iron and steel industries provides an excellent example of
the impact of party change on public policy. In 1946 the Labour Party
nationalized the iron and steel industries; in 1953, when the Conservatives
returned to power, the industries were denationalized; in 1967 Labour
again returned to power, and renationalized the steel industry.

In those cases where little ideological distance separates the parties vying
for power, radical departures in public policy are less likely. The United
States is an obvious example: Change in party at the national level, except
under extraordinary circumstances (e.g., Franklin Roosevelt and the
Depression), rarely leads to fundamental policy departures.

Summary

The point emphasized in this section is that in trying to account for and
compare the content of and changes in public policy, one must be sensitive to various situations and events affecting nations. Among the more
obvious, dramatic, and important events have been major social
upheavals. In these cases, the nature, although not necessarily the specific
content, of the policy change appears to be similar cross-nationally: an
increase in the scope of state activity and responsibility.

In addition, political events of varying magnitude, ranging from revolution to a change in political party, influence the course of public policy.
In these cases, it is much more difficult to generalize about even the
direction, much less the content, of policy change. Clearly, one of the
tasks facing comparative policy analysis in the future is the systematic
study of the impact of various types of political events on the content of
public policy.

The impact of structural factors on public policy

Chapter 1 mentions the debate among political scientists over the relative impact of political versus socioeconomic variables on public policy. Initially, studies in this area tended to conclude that various socioeconomic factors are more important than political variables in accounting for policy outcomes. More recently, however, a "revisionist" school has emerged claiming that, contrary to previous evidence, political process variables are in fact an important influence in the determination of policy outcomes.

As the evidence mounts, it becomes clearer that the issue is not likely ever to be definitively resolved in favor of one set of factors over another. The impact of political or socioeconomic factors is, as suggested earlier, probably a function of the level of political and economic development, as well as of the particular policy area involved. Our purpose here is not to prove the greater importance of one factor over another, but rather to illustrate how different political, social, and economic structural variables influence public policy. The reader is reminded that structural variables are persistent features of a nation-state and provide an enduring part of the context within which public policy is made.

Demographic and ecological structure

Public policy can be viewed as the response on the part of authoritative actors to the demands and needs of people. In some areas of public policy, and at certain times in a nation's development, the demographic and ecological structure of a society determines or dictates the nature of these wants and needs and, therefore, the kinds of policies and decisions that, in some sense, *have to be made.* In addition, demographic and ecological factors influence policy makers in that they represent the resources available for carrying out public policy.

Among the demographic features of a society that influence public policy, the nature of its population is one of the most obvious and important. Consider, for example, the age structure of the population. Many less developed countries have high birth rates and decreasing infant mortality rates. This combination produces a population structure with a disproportionate percentage of minors. For example, the proportion of the nation's population under 15 years old accounts for nearly one-half the total population in such less developed countries as Jordan, Kenya, Mexico, Nicaragua, Niger, Somalia Republic, Sudan, and Swaziland. This compares with an average of about 26 percent under 15 years old in European countries. The more youthful demographic structure of the less

developed countries requires a greater commitment of resources to such
youth-oriented programs as school construction and inoculation programs.
In these countries the "need" for youth-oriented public goods and
services is greater than in countries with a generally older population.
Conversely, in countries with a heavy concentration of persons over 60 or
65 years old, there is a greater need for social security programs, old-age
homes, and geriatric hospitals.

Other population-related factors also influence public policy. For
example, the uneven geographic distribution of a population within a
nation may cause certain problems or conditions that require a policy
response. One such problem, common to many less developed nations, is
the heavy concentration of people in certain regions of the country.
Central Luzon in the Philippines, the Island of Java in Indonesia, and the
Rio de Janeiro–São Paulo megalopolis of Center–South Brazil are examples
of areas with extraordinarily high population concentrations. In each case,
there is a population imbalance between these areas and sparsely populated outlying areas: Mindanao in the Philippines, Sumatra in Indonesia,
and the Amazon basin in Brazil. Population imbalances create a number
of policy problems. They tend to inhibit economic growth because some
of these areas are rich in natural resources that are left untapped for lack
of an adequate local labor force. In addition, the most densely populated
areas are a drain on resources because of the problems associated with
them: high crime rates, public health problems, squatters, pollution.

As a result, in each case national policy has been to attract people away
from the more densely to the more sparsely populated areas. In some
instances, such as in the Philippines and Brazil, these efforts have had the
unintended consequence of creating communal conflict betweeen the
original inhabitants of the underdeveloped areas (e.g., Muslims and
Indians) and the new migrants (Christians and non-Indians).

Urbanization is another population distribution factor that influences
public policy. The proportion of the population living in urban as
opposed to rural areas influences policy by virtue of the fact that urban
residents tend to be more highly dependent upon publicly provided goods
and services than the self-reliant rural inhabitants. The high population
density associated with urbanization generates the need for such services as
full-time professional police and fire protection, traffic control, zoning,
public health, welfare, and recreation. The more highly urbanized a
nation, the more likely it is to have greater resources allocated to providing the above-mentioned goods and services.

Cultural pluralism

A nation's linguistic, racial, religious, and cultural structure is another
demographic variable that may have far reaching policy consequences. Of

particular relevance is the degree of communal diversity within a nation. As Adelman and Morris have noted for developing nations, "these primordial attachments characteristically come into severe conflict with the requirements for effective political integration and, in particular, with the need for more generalized commitments to a relatively impersonal, nation-wide civil order."[7] Communal conflict is, of course, by no means restricted to less developed nations. Racial problems in the United States and South Africa, linguistic conflict in Canada and Belgium, religious strife in Northern Ireland, and efforts by Jews to leave the Soviet Union are but a few of the manifestations of communalism in advanced nations.

Because communalism undermines the political order itself, it demands the attention of policy makers. The range of policy solutions is as diverse as the problem itself. In racial matters the solutions have ranged from a national policy to end racial discrimination and segretation in the United States, to a deliberate policy of racial separation (i.e., apartheid) in South Africa, to the elimination of a racial minority by forced expatriation in the case of the expulsion of 40,000 Asians from Uganda in August 1972.

Linguistic diversity is another condition that requires policy attention. Decisions *must* be made concerning which language or languages are to be used in public schools, governmental agencies, the military, street signs, public documents, and so on. The decision to choose one language over another confers a distinct advantage in education, employment, and every-day life on one group over another. No wonder language policy has been so hotly debated in countries like Canada, South Africa, India, and Malaysia. In terms of policy solutions, many multilingual nations have adopted two or more official languages. Among these are Yugoslavia, Belgium, Czechoslovakia, Afghanistan, the Philippines, Cameroon, Tanzania, and Switzerland. Other countries, such as Malaysia, the Soviet Union, Kenya, and Uganda have established one national language, encouraged its use through educational and employment incentives, but countenanced the continued use of other languages.

Whatever the nature of the problem, whatever the solutions, pluralistic nations face different policy problems than do nations with homogeneous populations. For those countries where diversity does not exist, the policy agenda does not include divisive communally oriented problems. In addition, the ability of these more homogeneous nations to solve public problems is enhanced by the absence of internal conflict that drains national resources and inhibits unified national commitments to public problems.

Quality of human resources

Still another demographic characteristic that affects policy decisions is the quality of human resources of a society. The skill base of a population, typically measured in terms of literacy rates and educational achievement, influences policy in two ways. First, it provides the reservoir of talent upon which decision makers can draw to carry out the tasks of running a modern polity and economy. Clearly, the United States, with 4,253 college students per 100,000 people and a literacy rate of 99 percent, is better equipped for these tasks than Gabon, with 13 college students per 100,000 population and a literacy rate of 30 percent. Second, the level of education and degree of literacy determine whether this policy area requires extraordinary remedial action. Obviously, Gabon, along with scores of other African nations, must devote a greater proportion of resources to modernize effectively.

Ecological factors

The natural environment of nations – their geography, climate, and resources – is also part of the policy context within which they operate. The natural environment provides policy makers with both opportunities and constraints. In some instances, for example, the very nature of an environment dictates what must be done by the public sector. One seemingly frivolous example of environmental determinism is the nearly $2 million per year that Uganda spends on tsetse fly control. This sum is for all practical purposes dictated by the peculiar ecological conditions of Uganda in much the same way that snow removal is mandated in northern latitude countries. Whatever political change may occur, whatever the ideology or personality of the nation's leadership, policy makers in Uganda cannot ignore, without the most callous disregard for the health of their people, the demands dictated by the nature of their climate and natural environment.

Geography can influence policy in other ways. The geographical isolation of the United States during the nineteenth century allowed this country to concentrate its public and private resources on internal expansion and development without diverting a significant proportion of its resources for military purposes. Unlike Europe in the eighteenth and nineteenth centuries, where war-related public debt constituted the single largest item in many budgets, the United States was not similarly burdened. Geographical isolation has played an important, although somewhat different, role in Australia. One author argues, for example, that the stern and unchanging reality of geographical isolation led Australians to rely heavily upon the state as an agent for national development and supplier of a broad range of goods and services.[8]

Finally, the natural resources of a country, the quantity and quality of its agricultural lands, fuel, and nonfuel minerals influence the policy paths traveled by nations. The demonstrated vulnerability of the non-oil-producing nations during the Arab oil boycott of the winter of 1973–4 led

some countries to reassess their foreign policies; spurred national governments to encourage oil exploration, national fuel conservation, and the
search for alternative fuels; and resulted in curtailing various domestic
programs because of increasing balance-of-payments deficits. On the other
hand, such major oil producers as Iran, Kuwait, and Saudi Arabia were
able to undertake massive development and modernization schemes as a
result of their increased earnings from higher oil prices.

The nature and degree of dependency on a particular natural resource
significantly affect what governments can or cannot do. Countries like
Malaysia (rubber and tin), Chile (copper), Ghana (cocoa), Colombia
(coffee), and the Philippines (sugarcane), which are heavily dependent
upon a single export product, find that their ability to provide public
goods and services is closely tied to fluctuations in international market
prices and demand. The more diversified the resource base of a nation,
the less vulnerable it is to market fluctuations.

Economic structure

The relationship between the economic structure of a society and its public
policies has received a good deal of attention in recent years. No one, we
assume, would dispute the close, although not necessarily causal, relationship between a nation's economic structure and its public policies.

This discussion is limited to three areas in which fundamental structural
factors have a demonstrated impact on public policy: level of economic
wealth, predominant economic base, and type of economic system.

Economic wealth

The economic wealth or income of a nation, usually measured in
terms of its gross national product (GNP), has a clear impact on public
policy. In general, the wealth of a nation determines the degree of freedom or constraint imposed on a nation's decision makers in providing
public goods and services. Clearly, in 1974 the governments of
Switzerland ($7,632 per capita GNP), Sweden ($6,808), and the United
States ($6,666) were better able to serve their people than those of Upper
Volta ($80), Rwanda ($76), and Mali ($73). But beyond the obvious and
extraordinarily important point that wealthier nations have more money to
spend than poorer ones lies the fact that they spend money differently.
"Wealthy nations spend more of [their] national income on science and
education than do poor nations and more on highways and on traffic
control."[9] In addition, there is a tendency for the size of the public sector
to be larger in wealthier nations than in poorer ones. "One explanation
for this tendency is that the advanced economies tend to spend relatively
larger amounts upon social welfare, education, and other public services
than does the typical lower income economy."[10] Thus, a nation's

economic wealth influences not only how much, but also in what ways, a government spends the money available to it. It should be noted here that GNP is, strictly speaking, a measure of national income rather than national wealth. Nevertheless, the two are closely related, and GNP conventionally is used in political science as a measure of national wealth. In subsequent chapters the terms national income and national wealth are used interchangeably.

Predominant economic base

Although one can make a number of subtle distinctions among types of economic structures, the most useful and frequently cited is the distinction between industrial and agrarian economies. There is, to be sure, a good deal of coincidence between this variable and some others discussed in this book. For example, industrialized nations also tend to be highly urbanized, to be wealthier, and to have populations with non-traditional cultures. Nevertheless, it is useful for analytical purposes to treat the economic base as if its policy influence acts independently of those other factors.

The most obvious association between economy and policy derives from the simple fact that the nature of the issues, and hence the required policy solutions, are different in the two types of economic structures. Industrialization, for example, is accompanied by increasing complexity of economic organization and life. The development of modern corporations and large-scale industrial enterprises "may generate a new set of basic public services which are of a remedial sort."[11] One simply does not find great policy emphasis on industrial pollution, the use of atomic energy, or unemployment insurance in Laos, Nepal, Yemen, Chad, Dahomey, Malawi, and the other nations in which 80 percent or more of the population is engaged in traditional subsistence agriculture.

A nation's economic base influences not only the content of public policy but also its administration. Generally speaking, industrialized economies are more highly organized, concentrated and, therefore, easier to control for purposes of distributing goods and services, regulating economic activity, and extracting revenues. Furthermore, because industrialized economies are almost exclusively monetized, records of production sales, purchases, and revenues are easier to monitor.

Agrarian economies tend to have widely dispersed and unorganized labor and marketing systems and large nonmonetized sectors. Gunnar Myrdal's description of this type of economy concerns South Asia, but is equally applicable to much of Africa and parts of Latin America.

The non-monetized part of the economy is very large, since it includes a very large share – in many countries by far the largest share – not only of food production but also of the production and consumption of other consumer goods and services, and also a considerable part of total investment, especially in agricultural and house construction.[12]

The dispersed, nonmonetized nature of large segments of traditional agrarian economies makes it much more difficult for governments to distribute goods and services, extract revenues, and regulate economic behavior. Consider, for instance, price control in Ghana. In 1962 and again in 1965, the Ghanaian government passed laws aimed at controlling prices within the country. The laws, however, were not terribly effective. The problem of policy enforcement resides in the fact that in Ghana

the retailing of goods, especially foodstuffs, is not in the hands of a small number of easily controllable supermarkets. Rather it is in the hands of a very great number of petty traders, most buying their commodities on credit and selling in small quantities at locations close to the people throughout the country. Effective price controls, therefore, are not easily imposed.[13]

In sum, both the policy agenda and the administration of public policy are influenced by the nature of a society's economic base.

Type of economic system

It is common to classify economic systems by the origin of the industrial and social services produced in the society. When all or a major proportion of the ownership, production, and distribution of goods and services is in the hands of the public sector, the economy is described as socialist or controlled. Conversely, when the private sector is the major owner and producer of the means of production, the system is described as a capitalist or free market economy. Most economic systems in the world are mixed types. They may be viewed as lying along a left (controlled) to right (free) spectrum, depending upon the degree of public versus private ownership of the means of production. Moving from left to right, we find the Soviet Union (mainly controlled), Great Britain (mixed, leaning left), Canada (mixed, leaning right), and Japan (mainly free).

There are various ways in which the nature of the economy influences policy making. Consider, for example, revenue-raising policies. There are basically three ways in which governments finance their operations: by taxation, by borrowing, and by the application of user fees for public goods and services. Free market economies typically depend heavily upon taxation as their main source of income: In the United States taxation provides about 75 percent of all public revenues.[14] Controlled or planned systems, however, in which there is considerable public ownership of the means of production and provision of services, depend heavily upon user fees or service charges as a source of revenue. Therefore, the need for increased revenues leads to higher taxes in predominantly capitalist systems and to an increase in user fees in socialist systems. In other words, the type of economic system influences the nature of revenue-raising policies.

The type of a nation's economic system also influences the range of solutions available to decision makers in setting economic policy. For example, when the Lockheed Aircraft Corporation faced possible bankruptcy in 1971, the U.S. government provided Lockheed with a loan, thereby allowing the company to survive as a private enterprise. Although there was some discussion of government takeover, this solution had little support in or out of Congress. On the other hand, when the Rolls Royce Company of Great Britain faced bankruptcy in 1971, the Conservative-led British government nationalized the airplane engine division of Rolls Royce. Thus, Rolls Royce joined the telephone, radio and television, airlines, coal, railway, steel, and electricity industries as a public enterprise. What was an unacceptable policy solution in the United States was both acceptable and logical in Great Britain.

The nature of the economic system also influences the policy agenda of a nation. For example, under normal circumstances in the United States the prices of automobiles and cigarettes are set by private market forces (i.e., supply and demand), not by government policy. In France, however, because the largest automobile producer, Renault, is owned by the government and because the government has a monopoly of cigarette manufacturing and sales, the prices for these commodities are part of the policy agenda (i.e., decisions the government must make).

Political structure

In the final analysis all demands for public policy, be they functions of ecology (e.g., tsetse fly control), demography (e.g., more schools), or outbreaks of violence (e.g., more money for police forces), must be processed by the political system. The political structure or institutional context within which decisions are made then becomes another part of the policy milieu, influencing the course and content of public policy. This section completes the analysis of the structural context of public policy by examining its political component.

Formal political organization

Nations are frequently differentiated by their formal political organization. Introductory courses in comparative politics invariably cover the differences between federal and unitary states, presidential and parliamentary forms of government. From a policy perspective, the questions one must ask are: Does the formal structure of government affect the content of public policy? Are parliamentary regimes more effective in providing for the public's welfare than presidential regimes? Are the defense policies of unitary and federal systems different? There has been remarkably little research into the impact of formal political organization on the content of public policy. The available evidence suggests that the formal political organization plays only a minor role in the content or direction of public policy. This is not to suggest, however, that the type of political organization has no influence at all on policy or that it is unimportant. In June 1976, the military leaders of Nigeria decided that when that nation returns to civilian rule (scheduled in 1979) it will adopt a presidential form of government rather than the previous parliamentary one. The reason offered for the switch in formal organization was that the presidential form would provide a more effective means of dealing with public policy problems. The Nigerians feel, rightly or wrongly, that formal organization does matter. Let us look at some of the ways political organization can affect public policy.

The clearest impact derives from the distinction between a central or national government and several subnational governments, such as provinces or states. There were formally 20 federal systems in 1979, although in countries like Burma, Mexico, and the Soviet Union, the subnational units enjoy little real autonomy. In truly federal systems the distribution of power includes a division in the provisions of goods and services. Typically, education, roads, and many social services are primarily locally provided in a federal system. Thus, when one compares national expenditures in federal and unitary states, apparent differences in policy priority appear: National governments in federal systems appear to be less committed than unitary states to education and social welfare. However, the national government budget does not always accurately reflect the level of public commitment to a particular service, especially in federal systems where local units may provide some of the public services.

A more important difference than the apparent composition of the budgets in federal and unitary systems is the administration of policy. In federal systems there tends to be less uniformity in the application and administration of policy owing to decentralization of authority. It is true that national government policy "often stipulates uniformity in execution throughout the country," thus facilitating cross-national comparisons.[15] Unfortunately, such a stipulation does not ensure uniformity in effort or consequence throughout a country. A case in point is the national policy, mandated by the Supreme Court, of public school integration in the United States. Clearly, the (in)ability of the federal government and the (un)willingness of various local governments have resulted in great variation in efforts to implement and enforce racial integration. As a result, in 1973 only 29 percent of the schoolchildren in the North compared with 44 percent in the South were attending desegregated schools – almost two decades after the policy was established.[16]

There have been few studies examining the policy implications of presidential versus parliamentary systems. One might expect that policy making would be easier in a parliamentary system, where there is no separation of power between the legislative and executive branches, than in a presidential system, where the two are separate and may be controlled by different parties. In practice, however, this is not always the case. Parliamentary systems are efficient policy processors only when party discipline can be enforced. Thus, the Italian parliamentary system is a far less efficient policy producer than the Mexican presidential system. The reason for this is that the Mexican Congress has always been dominated by a single disciplined party, the Institutional Revolutionary Party (PRI). The Mexican Congress routinely and invariably approves policy proposals submitted by the president, who is the leader of the PRI. On the other hand, Italy has a highly fragmented and undisciplined party system.

Some direct evidence on the policy impact of "responsible" parliamentary party government and presidential government is contained in a study by Roland J. Pennock.[17] The study examined the differences between Great Britain and America in terms of the ability of decision makers in the two systems to resist pressure from special interest groups. Pennock examined one policy area: agricultural subsidies. His conclusion was that policy makers in the United States, with its system of separation of powers, were no more susceptible to agricultural interest group pressure than their British counterparts operating in a system of "responsible government." Any definitive conclusion concerning the impact of forms of political systems on public policy, however, must await further research.

Type of political regime

The term *political regime* refers to "the underlying goals that members of the system pursue, the norms or rules of the game through which they conduct their political business, and the formal and informal structures of authority that arrange who is to do what in the system."[18] Although several types of regimes have been identified, two of the most commonly used classifications are military versus civilian and authoritarian versus democratic regimes. There is obviously a good deal of overlap between the two classifications: Military regimes are also authoritarian. However, because civilian regimes can be authoritarian or democratic, it is justifiable to deal with them separately. We begin by looking at similarities or differences in public policy that may be a function of the differences between military and civilian regimes.

Intuitively one might expect certain gross policy differences between civilian and military regimes. For example, it is not unreasonable to assume that military regimes have relatively larger military establishments and spend more on defense and defense-related projects than do civilian regimes. Existing evidence on this assumption is unfortunately conflicting. An early (1970) study by Eric Nordlinger comparing military and civilian regimes in non-Western nations found that "the proportion of GNP devoted to defense is almost twice as large in countries overtly ruled by the military as it is in countries with a non-politicized officer corps."[19] However, a 1975 study by McKinlay and Cohan, which includes a sample of developed and less developed countries, differentiates among (1) military regimes, (2) civilian regimes that have experienced military rule, and (3) civilian regimes that have never experienced military rule and concludes "that military rule does not lead to an increase in military expenditures or in the size of the armed forces."[20] Although the change to military rule may not lead to increases in the size of the armed forces or the amount spent on them, McKinlay and Cohan, like Nordlinger, "find that countries that have had military regimes have higher levels of expenditure and larger armies than countries which have not had military regimes, *even though the differences are slight.*"[21] The authors, however, qualify the extent of their agreement with Nordlinger by noting that civilian regimes which have lower levels of military spending actually have higher rates of growth in spending. The evidence, therefore, on the intuitively obvious policy difference between military and civilian regimes remains ambiguous, at least as it relates to military spending and the size of the armed forces.

McKinlay and Cohan do find corroboration, however, for another commonsense expectation about military and civilian rule policy differences. They find that in the area of political rights, military regimes place greater restriction than civilian regimes on legislative and political party activity. In addition, military regimes are more likely than civilian regimes to rule without a constitution and presumably, therefore, without the protection of civil rights usually contained in constitutional documents. Although the evidence appears mixed, there is still reason to expect differences in policy performance between military and civilian regimes.

Because of the overlap between authoritarian and military regimes, one would expect certain performance similarities in a comparison of military–civilian and authoritarian–democratic regimes. Indeed, as "democratic politics can be defined in terms of the effective diffusion and openness of popular participation in politics,"[22] by definition they differ from authoritarian (and military) regimes in terms of extending political rights. But as Alexander Groth notes, the policy implications of democratic compared with authoritarian rule extend beyond the realm of political participation. Among the policy differences that Groth finds distinguish authoritarian and democratic systems are: (1) "indirect and basically regressive taxation characterizes many autocratic systems," whereas taxing in democratic systems is more progressive; (2) economic policy in democratic systems, unlike in authoritarian systems, is made openly, is susceptible to a variety of interest pressures, and is subject to scrutiny and review by public opinion and periodic election; and (3) fascist authoritarian regimes limit the expansion of education, whereas democratic and left-wing authoritarian regimes promote its expansion. Groth's study suggests that on a rather wide range of policy fronts authoritarian and democratic regimes differ in performance.[23]

Policy process variables

Certain features about the way decisions are made in political systems and by whom have taken on a structural (i.e., permanent) quality. As in the case of the other structural factors, the expectation is that national public policy reflects the existence or absence of certain features of the policy process.

One such process variable is policy incrementalism and particularly incremental budgeting. As described by Aaron Wildavsky, the process works in the following manner:

Budgets are almost never actively reviewed as a whole, in the sense of considering at one time the value of all existing programs compared to all possible alternatives. Instead, this year's budget is based on last year's budget, with special attention given to a narrow range of increases or decreases.[24]

For various administrative, fiscal, and political reasons, annual expenditure changes where policy incrementalism prevails are of only marginal or incremental nature. Clearly, expenditure changes of this limited range impose significant restraints upon policy makers. Among other things, incremental expenditure changes inhibit, although need not prevent, major policy changes.

How widely used is incremental policy making? The available evidence shows that it is fairly widespread. Charles Lindblom makes the unsubstantiated claim that it is a common practice among democracies "to change their policies almost entirely through incremental adjustment."[25] On somewhat firmer empirical ground, Wildavsky specifically found incrementalism characteristic of budget making in Britain, France, and Japan, and argues that it is common among rich nations. He also claims that "budgeters in poor nations would like to use incremental methods but they lack the stable (resource) base from which to proceed."[26] Whatever the actual extent of its usage, incremental budgeting is clearly an important part of the policy context in some nations, influencing their public policies and differentiating them from those nations in which it is not used.

Closely related to policy incrementalism is the impact existing policy has on the content and direction of future policy. Decision makers, even those who come to power by revolution, inherit both problems and policies from their predecessors. Inherited policy is a fixed (i.e., structural) part of the policy context within which current policy is made. Just how important this can be in influencing public policy is demonstrated in the discussions of the development of health care policy in Germany, Great Britain, the Soviet Union, and Japan.

The role of the bureaucracy is another structural factor that influences the content and nature of public policy. In the extreme case, as when the military or a colonial power rules, the bureaucracy actually makes policy. In democratic political systems, the bureaucracy is supposed to be responsible and responsive to the elected leadership. Theoretically, its function is simply to implement the policies determined by the popularly elected branches of government. In fact, however, even in democracies, bureaucrats become involved in the policy-making process at several key junctures. First, they are frequently the source of policy initiative; that is to say, they raise issues to be placed on the policy agenda. Second, bureaucrats provide information and advice to those formally empowered to make law. In this way they have a significant influence on the formation and content of policy. Third, bureaucrats administer or implement policy. Because laws are often imprecise or incomplete in detail, bureaucrats have great leeway in interpreting and in a sense making law as they administer it. Whether they directly rule or simply serve those who do rule, bureaucrats help determine public policy.

The impact bureaucrats exert on policy varies, of course, in any one system from agency to agency. Cynthia Enloe found that the political support an agency receives greatly affects the influence it exercises over policy. The influence of the French Ministry of the Environment was enhanced by the fact that it was established in 1971 by a decree from President Georges Pompidou and headed by a prominent fellow Gaullist. Similarly, the Polish Ministry of Regional Planning and Environmental Control was a pet project of Communist Party leader and prime minister, Edward Gierek, and therefore, it too enjoyed favored political and financial support. By way of contrast, when Valéry Giscard d'Estaing succeeded Pompidou as French president, he selected for his environmental minister a man not known to be close to him. Giscard also raised questions about the future efficacy of the ministry when he renamed it the Ministry for the Quality of Life, a title that made its mission less clear.[27] The French and Polish cases illustrate the importance of having both political support and a timely issue. The 1970s saw worldwide interest in ecology-related issues and considerable activity by the general public, environmental interest groups, and the media. This helped determine not only the policy agenda but also the effectiveness of environmental protection agencies.

The degree of public support, the timeliness of an issue, interest group hostility or support, political support of administrators, the financial and manpower resources available to agencies, the nature of relations among agencies – these and other factors all help shape the role bureaucratic agencies play in the policy arena. The end product of the policy process – public policy – in no small measure reflects the role of the bureaucracy and the bureaucratic process.

The impact of culture and ideology on public policy

Political culture may be defined as the set of values, beliefs, expectations, and attitudes concerning what government should do, how government should operate, and what the proper relationship is between the citizen and the state. The term refers to the belief systems of the nation as a whole as well as those held by individuals within the nation.

Political ideology may be viewed as a subset of political culture. A nation's political culture may include a formal ideology consisting of "a closed, comprehensive, logically consistent set of ideas which can subsume all conceivable social issues or questions."[28] Thus, the Chinese political culture includes Marxist-Maoist ideology as well as acceptance of authoritarian leadership, a value typical of traditional China.

In characterizing the political culture of a nation, it is not necessary, nor is it usually assumed, that every individual embraces all the same beliefs, values, and so on. The characterization of Italy, for example, as having an "alienated political culture" does not mean that every Italian feels alienated from the Italian political system. It does mean that the *majority* of Italians are politically alienated, that they lack pride and trust in the political system.[29]

Political culture provides part of the milieu or context within which public policy is made. It involves beliefs and attitudes concerning both the input side of politics (i.e., the nature of political participation and the processes by which decisions are made) and the output side (i.e., what governments can and should do). The following discussion illustrates how differences in political culture help influence variations in policy and policy making among nations.

The first point we wish to make is that "the cultural norms, transmitted across the generations, dictate and regulate which wants a member is expected to solve for himself or in cooperation with others, and which is acceptable in the society for the members to seek to fulfill through political action."[30] In other words, what may be considered worthy or proper in one system, may not be so considered in another. Cynthia Enloe found in her comparative study of pollution policy that concern about the environment is more compatible with the Swedish political culture and the high values Swedes place upon "love of nature" than with either the American or Soviet culture, each of which is more deeply attached to the values of economic and technological progress. Hence the higher priority assigned to environmental protection and the greater seriousness with which the subject has been treated in Sweden compared with the United States and the Soviet Union.

The relationship between cultural values and the elevation of certain public concerns into the policy arena is also illustrated in matters dealing with personal morality and behavior – especially in traditional societies. The high value attached to personal modesty and proper appearance, at least by political elites, has led the government of Singapore to prohibit men from wearing their hair long and the government of Malawi to prohibit women from wearing their skirts short. In the case of Singapore, the government has used various sanctions including expulsion from universities, loss of governmental jobs, and fines in order to ensure compliance. It is difficult to imagine the British, French, or Italian governments taking similar action or the British, French, or Italian people demanding that they do so.

The political culture of a nation determines not only what people value but also how and by whom they expect matters that concern them to be handled. Monitoring and enforcing codes of morality could have been entrusted, in the cases of Singapore and Malawi, to private institutions like the family or religious agencies, rather than to the government. In these two countries, however, as in many others, the political culture supports the active intervention by government in solving problems, regulating behavior, and providing goods and services. Thus, one of the major ways of differentiating among nations concerns the cultural definition of the proper role of government.

The importance of political culture to the definition of the proper role of the state, and the resulting policy differences, are the subjects of a comparative study by Anthony King. The study seeks to explain public policy differences, and particularly variation in the scope of governmental activity, among five Western nations: the United States, Canada, Britain, France, and West Germany. King examines two broad policy areas: public versus private ownership of such industries as communications, transportation, fuel, and finance and the provision of such social services as education, pensions, insurance, medical services, and housing. His major finding is that in every policy area except one – education – the state has played a far less active role in the United States than in any of the other nations. How does one account for this difference? After dismissing explanations involving differences in elite roles, mass behavior, interest group activity, and political institutions, King concludes that "the state plays a more limited role in America than elsewhere because Americans, more than other people, want it to play a limited role. In other words, the most satisfactory explanation is one in terms of Americans' beliefs and

assumptions, especially their beliefs and assumptions about government."[31] King explains the aberrant American commitment to public
education as an attempt to reconcile two contradictory American values:
equality of opportunity and individualism. He argues that in public
education Americans found a way of allowing both values to flourish.
What are the beliefs that distinguish the American culture and, hence,
public policies from those of the other Western nations? King suggests
they can be summarized in such phrases as "free enterprise is more efficient than government; governments should concentrate on encouraging
private initiative and free competition; government is wasteful; governments should not provide people with things they can provide for themselves; too much government endangers liberty; and so on."[32] One need
not agree completely with King's characterization of the American
political culture. The point is to illustrate the potential impact of political
culture on public policy.

The difference between the American value orientation and that of the
other Western nations suggests a rather comprehensive and consistent
system of beliefs, although not nearly as complete and cohesive as, say,
Marxist ideology. Political culture, however, can have a much narrower
and more selective impact on policy. A case in point is population control
policy in parts of Asia. South Asia and Southeast Asia include nations
with political ideologies or value systems ranging from communism to
right-wing authoritarianism. Despite this range, there is remarkable
similarity in the region on the issue of population control policy. This
similarity stems from certain general cultural values that apparently super-
sede political differences.

The region, like so much of the less developed world, suffers from a
rapidly expanding population that retards economic growth and contributes to individual poverty. Yet, with the possible exceptions of India and
Sri Lanka, governments in South Asia and Southeast Asia have moved
slowly, if at all, in implementing population planning programs. The
main reason for this lies in the opposition on the part of the masses to
birth control. This opposition stems from a combination of religious and
traditional values. In terms of religion, the impact of Catholicism in the
Philippines, where 90 percent of the people are Catholic, and to a lesser
extent in the former South Vietnam, has made it difficult for these
governments to undertake birth control programs. Similarly, the desire in
Hindu societies to have male offspring has been an obstacle to birth
control. "A young man does not acquire the status of full manhood
before a son is born to him, and it is believed to be essential for salvation
that a man's skull after his death, be opened by a son. There is then an
urge to have a son, and, in view of high mortality, preferably two or
three."[33] Finally, children in Asia, as in other less developed societies,

have long been viewed as security against the dangers of illness and old age. Large numbers of children appear to offer greater security, as well as evidence of a man's sexual potency. Thus, religious and traditional values combine to make it difficult for South and Southeast Asian governments to implement population control policies.

The case of population planning in India deserves attention because it illustrates the resiliency of traditional values as well as the introduction of cultural and situational factors in the policy process. In April 1976, the Indian government, under the authoritarian regime of Indira Gandhi, embarked upon a vigorous birth control program. The program raised the minimum marriage age and paid people to have themselves voluntarily sterilized. Initial feedback from the program indicated some positive results. Then early in 1977, Mrs. Gandhi decided to call elections. The mandatory, and in some instances forced, sterilization aspects of the program, which were widely unpopular, immediately became a campaign issue. The result was that both the government and the opposition, which swept the election, backed away from support of the program. Family planning centers began disappearing, and the program of incentives was canceled. Traditional values and electoral politics (a situational factor) combined to cause policy change.

Political culture also influences group activity in the policy process and, by extension, the content of policy itself. Here again the work done by Cynthia Enloe on pollution policy is instructive. Enloe contrasts the ineffective or nonexistent role of interest groups in the agitation for and formulation of environmental policy in Mexico and France with the influential role of environmental interest groups in Sweden. In both France and Mexico, interest group participation is generally not viewed as a legitimate or efficacious form of political activity. In contrast, the Swedes, much like the Americans and the British, are "joiners." In France and Mexico, there was little group input into the environmental policy process; in Sweden, there was an active interest. The differences in group behavior resulted in policy differences. "When, as in 1971, air pollution restrictions are imposed in Mexico, they are likely to be the result of presidential initiatives rather than environmental group lobbying, and there are likely to be loopholes for the privileged classes who dominate the nation's politics and discourage broader participation."[34]

In conclusion, political culture shapes public policy in several ways. It helps determine what are to be policy issues and the way with which they are to be dealt. It defines the acceptable role of both government and citizen in the policy process. Whether or not political culture "explains" as much as Anthony King suggests is still open to question. That it explains a good deal of cross-national policy differences and similarities is quite clear.

The impact of environmental factors on public policy

Public policy makers must respond to demands and conditions that ema-
nate from without as well as from within a political system. Since World
War II in particular, increasing international interdependency, fostered by
advanced communications and transportation technology, has accorded to
environmental factors increasing influence in the determination of national public policy. Such influences are not, however, uniform; environmental factors have a differential impact on policy and policy makers in
different nations. As we shall shortly suggest, less developed nations in
particular are more susceptible to extrasystemic influences than are developed nations. This section examines three environmental forces and demonstrates how each influences public policy. The three forces are the
international political climate, cross-national policy diffusion, and international obligations and agreements.

International political climate

One of the clearest examples of how the international political climate
affects public policy concerns defense spending and the size of government. Because national defense is exclusively a public sector and national
government concern, any increases of personnel or spending in this area
are recorded as an expansion of national government activity. "The
growth of government in developed and underdeveloped countries in the
years since World War II is also attributable to a high level of international tension and the accompanying importance of the military and its
technology."[35] This point becomes abundantly clear when defense spending is examined in Chapter 4.

The impact of international tensions on public policy is apparently not
confined to defense policy. There has been a good deal of debate over the
so-called trade-off between defense and other areas of public spending.
The main issue involved has been whether increased defense spending
results in decreased spending for health, education, and other social
services. The evidence, thus far, has been mixed. Bruce Russett found in
the case of the United States that: "Guns do come at the expense of
butter."[36] Similarly, Margaret Hayes found substitutes or trade-offs
between military allocations and those for other areas of public spending
in Brazil.[37] Finally, a study by David Caputo examined health, education,
and defense expenditures in Australia, Sweden, the United Kingdom, and
the United States from 1950 to 1970. His conclusion both confirms and
denies existing evidence on the issue of policy trade-offs or substitutions.
In the case of health expenditures, Caputo found "*that increased defense
spending did not lead to a decrease in health expenditures;* in fact, the

opposite took place."[38] On the other hand, his research confirmed that increases in defense spending lead to decreases in education allocations although the relationship is not statistically significant. Obviously, no definitive conclusion can be reached at this time concerning policy trade-offs. Nevertheless, it appears that at least in some nations, and in some policy areas, defense spending exerts a negative influence on resource allocations in other policy areas.

To return to our original point, international tension appears to have a significant impact on public policy. At a minimum, it results in increases in defense spending, but beyond this there is some evidence to suggest that it produces displacements in other policy areas as well.

The international political climate affects policy in other ways. An example is the nonfiscal policy implications of the cold war on United States policy, particularly in the late 1940s and 1950s. The atmosphere produced by the cold war led in this country to trade and travel restrictions, the McCarran Act, government-endorsed or -sponsored harassment of individuals, and government incursions in the civil rights and liberties of many Americans. Although we are unaware of any systematic comparative studies of similar policy responses to the cold war in other countries, one suspects that the American reaction was by no means unique.

Policy and issue diffusion

Public policy and problem solving are extraordinarily imitative arts. Several students of comparative policy analysis have been "struck by how seldom a really original or revolutionary approach is to be found."[39] Rarely do policy makers embark upon entirely new courses of action; rather, they borrow heavily from an apparently finite, existing repertoire of policy solutions. There is a tendency for policy makers, when faced with a particular problem, to look for an analogous situation in another system and to emulate the solutions used by others. Policy borrowing may be rather specific, as in the case of a British minister who, when introducing the 1965 Rent Bill in Parliament, acknowledged that the government had copied heavily from a similar New York State statute.[40] Or policy imitation may be much broader and more consequential, as in the case of economic policy making in Franco's Spain. On this point Charles Anderson notes:

When one looks back on it all, perhaps the most striking fact is that the Spanish policy transformation was almost exclusively imitative and was not in the least an experimental or creative approach to public problem solving. If the Spanish experience contributed anything to the wisdom of how to conduct modern government, it was the more or less successful transfer of the policy equipment of one culture to another.[41]

The relative lack of originality in public policies apparently cannot be attributed to a lack of ingenuity or creativity on the part of the world's current set of policy makers. Ernest Barker, a historian of political thought, has written:

When we consider the history of the Modern State . . . we cannot but recognize the debt which all States owe to one another. Each country has developed according to its own genius; and each has produced its own fruit. But each has produced . . . some method of public service, which has served as an example to others; and each, in turn, has borrowed from each.[42]

In Part II of this book there is ample demonstration of the degree to which policy borrowing has influenced the development of health care policy.

We might add here that given the frequency of scholarly and technical exchange programs, the general lack of experience and expertise, and the continuing impact of the colonial legacy, one suspects that policy borrowing is particularly prevalent among less developed nations.

Policy diffusion across national boundaries is by no means restricted to borrowing specific solutions for particular problems. It also involves the borrowing of ideals and standards concerning appropriate state behavior and national policy direction. Consider, for example, the standard of state conduct proclaimed in Article 25 of the Universal Declaration of Human Rights, adopted by the U.N. General Assembly in December 1948 and formally accepted by most of the member nations today.

Everyone has the right to a standard of living adequate for the health and well-being of himself and his family, including food, clothing, housing and medical care and necessary social services, and the right to security in the event of unemployment, sickness, disability, widowhood, old age, or other livelihood in circumstances beyond his control.

Although not all states have subscribed to these ideals, either in word or deed, there is widespread intellectual and policy commitment to these and other goals established by United Nations proclamations. Much like a nationally owned airlines system, an openly espoused commitment to social welfare has become one of the hallmarks of modern statehood. Even though many nations are totally incapable of fulfilling these commitments, it has become obligatory to aspire to the premise of a modern welfare state.

Another, more limited illustration of the international diffusion of public policy values is the impact of a book by Lord Beveridge of Great Britain at the close of World War II. The book, entitled *Full Employment in a Free Society*, provided the blueprint for the extended social welfare system in Great Britain after World War II. The impact of the sentiments and ideals stated in the book extended well beyond the United Kingdom. One author writes that the report "served as a guide to social development not only in the United Kingdom but throughout the Western world.''[43]

Thus, we can add to the list of factors that account for differences and similarities in the content of public policy the impact of diffusion and emulation of policy across national boundaries.

International agreements and obligations

The increasing interdependency among the world's nations is nowhere more manifest than in the number and range of international agreements, organizations, and obligations that have developed during the last four decades. The United Nations, its specialized agencies (UNICEF, UNESCO, UNEP, and WHO), and the periodically sponsored international conferences such as the 1972 Stockholm Conference on Man and the Environment, the International Conference on the Law of the Sea in Caracas and the World Population Conference in Bucharest, both in 1974, and the 1975 Mexico City Women's Rights Conference illustrate some of the most frequent but not necessarily binding external policy stimuli. The ability of these agencies and conferences to ensure compliance with decisions is severely limited by the lack of power and sanctions of the United Nations. Thus, it is not unknown for the policy makers of participating nations to ignore international agreements. A case in point is Brazil's opposition at the 1972 Stockholm conference to accepting environmental pollution controls for fear these would interfere with the nation's industrialization. Similarly, Brazil announced at the 1974 World Population Conference that it had no intention of controlling its population and, in fact, planned on expanding it in order to populate the country's interior.[44] Despite the recalcitrant behavior illustrated in the Brazilian case, United Nations–related activities have exerted influence on national decision makers.

A second category of international obligations stems from various international defense, economic, cultural, and technical organizational relationships. There are over 30 such international organizations, among which are the North Atlantic Treaty Organization, the Warsaw Pact, the European Economic Community, the Organization of African Unity, the Latin American Free Trade Association, the Organization of Petroleum Exporting Countries, the Organization of American States, and the Association of Southeast Asian Nations. With varying degrees of comprehensiveness and effectiveness, organizations such as these set export prices on raw materials, eliminate trade and tariff barriers, establish common economic policies, determine with whom member nations may trade, and influence armed forces personnel and defense expenditure levels.

Finally, there are several public and private international financial institutions and agreements that invariably involve policy constraints and implications for the borrowing nation. Here again, the less developed nations are the most frequently affected because they are most heavily dependent upon international monetary assistance. Among the public agencies involved are various regional development banks including the African, Asian, Inter-American, and Islamic development banks. In addition, there is the International Bank for Reconstruction and Development (often called the World Bank), which is a specialized agency of the United Nations. Although there are variations, most of these financial institutions supply loans and provide technical and administrative assistance for development purposes to less developed nations. Eligibility for and approval of the loans, credits, and other forms of assistance are often contingent upon acceptance of certain requirements involving financial and administrative reform, currency revaluation, and tax structure changes by the recipient nation. Hence national economic development policy for many less developed nations is in part at least determined by external forces. An interesting case in point is the impact the World Bank, the International Monetary Fund, and creditor nations had on Ghanaian economic policy, and ultimately on the stability of the political regime, between 1969 and 1972. Ronald Libby persuasively argues that the economic policies imposed on Ghana by these agencies (e.g., devaluation in return for credit assistance) undermined popular support for the democratic regime. The devaluation resulted in an increase in import prices of 92 percent and an overall cost-of-living increase of 14 percent. The devaluation was announced on December 27, 1971, and the military staged a successful coup on January 13, 1972.[45]

Private financial institutions and multinational corporations, too, can exert influence on national economic and political policy through financial assistance. For example, the *New York Times* reported on August 4, 1976, that a consortium of United States banks was "making strict economic and political demands in exchange for badly needed additional loans" to the Peruvian government. As a result of the pressure, the Peruvian government devalued its currency, raised gasoline prices, removed subsidies from basic food products, and promised to reduce public spending. Two years later, in May 1978, the Peruvian government was again forced to raise prices on gasoline, wheat products, milk, and cooking oil in an effort to persuade foreign banks to restructure Peru's massive foreign debt. The price increases led to widespread violence and caused the Peruvian regime to institute martial law. In both 1976 and 1978, an environmental factor imposed itself on the Peruvian national policy scene, constraining policy makers from taking certain courses of action and compelling them to take others. The Peruvian and Ghanaian examples are by no means unique and illustrate the general vulnerability of less developed nations to environmental pressures.

Conclusion

Variations in the content and direction of public policy among nations are the result of a multitude of factors. This chapter lays the basis for an understanding of cross-national policy differences and similarities by organizing those factors into four general categories: situational, structural, cultural, and environmental variables. We stressed at the outset, and feel compelled to reiterate here, that rarely can the variations in the content of policy among nations be explained by a single factor. Public policy results from the interaction of several factors, all of which must ultimately lead to a political decision – in some cases, a decision not to decide – by an authoritative political actor. Politics, in the final analysis, always prevails.

In the remainder of this book the organizing scheme is applied to the comparative analysis of distributive public policies. Chapter 4 looks at the causes and content of public spending in 132 nations. In Chapters 5 through 8 the scheme is applied to an examination of the development of health care policy in four nation-states.

4

Comparing policy priorities

One need not be excessively materialistic or cynical to recognize that, in terms of governmental activity, money does indeed "make the world go 'round." There is little, if anything, that does not require an expenditure of funds. "No matter how idealistic and presumably non-material a policy might be, sooner or later an entry will have to be made in a public budget to implement that policy."[1] Public expenditures provide one of the most obvious and important statements of the political goals and priorities of a nation.

The purpose of this chapter is threefold. First, it compares the relative priorities, as measured by public expenditures, assigned to three major service areas: defense, education, and health. These three areas were chosen because they are among the most important, and costly, of the services provided by governments today. Second, it tries to explain the variation in spending among nations in terms of the factors outlined in Chapter 3 (Table 3-1). The analysis demonstrates, among other things, that situational and environmental factors are apparently more important in explaining defense spending than various structural or cultural factors, that level of economic development is among the most important factors in accounting for levels of education and health spending, and that no matter what descriptive or statistical generalizations one makes, multi-nation aggregate data analysis is useful only when accompanied by a discussion of specific cases. Lastly, the chapter examines certain service and performance indicators of these three policy areas in order to determine what, if any, is the relationship between expenditure and output and performance. The major conclusion reached is that, in general, expenditure is a poor predictor of output and performance.

Before the analysis can proceed, however, the reader must be apprised of the limitations inherent in using expenditure and aggregate data as measures of public policy. In presenting this discussion, we are doing more than simply fulfilling an academic obligation to inform the reader of the quality of the evidence being presented. Beyond this requirement lies the fact that public expenditure and such aggregate measures as infant mortality and school-age population rates are the public policy measures most frequently cited in academic and journalistic accounts. Thus, this discussion is presented as a general statement on interpreting and evaluating public expenditure and aggregate data wherever they appear.

What budgets and aggregate data can and cannot tell us

In this chapter we compare, explain, and evaluate similarities and differences among nations in regard to public policies, outputs, and impacts. To do this, we examine such indicators of policy as public expenditures and a whole range of impact variables (e.g., literacy, life expectancy, mortality rates). As one might expect, the value of our conclusions is limited by the quality of the data used. Unfortunately, there is perhaps greater reason to be concerned about the quality of the data available to comparative policy analysts than about the data available to those in other fields. This concern is well founded with regard to data from Third World countries – where limited material and technical resources make data collection erratic, incomplete, and frequently unreliable – and communist nations – where political ideology often influences collection and (the lack of) data reporting. Any comparative study that includes Third World or communist nations faces severe handicaps. Two brief examples illustrate this point: (1) almost all cross-national policy comparisons are hampered by severely limited data for countries such as Albania, Cuba, the People's Republic of China, North Korea, and North Vietnam; (2) data for Third World countries, although generally more readily available, are often contradictory and unreliable. For example, three different sources consulted gave the amount spent on defense in Bolivia in 1974 as 786.7 million pesos (*U.N. Statistical Yearbook: 1976*), 820 million pesos (Ruth Sivard, *World Military and Social Expenditures: 1977*), and 831.1 million pesos (*The Europa Yearbook: 1977*). Such discrepancies occur frequently enough to cause serious problems for comparative analysis.

As the last example suggests, those students of comparative policy who rely heavily upon aggregate data analysis are going to be most troubled by problems of reliability and validity. In addition to those already mentioned, these problems include (1) lack of comparability of policy measures (e.g., in some countries national defense expenditure includes money spent for a national, i.e., internal, police force; in other countries it does not); (2) falsification or deception in the presentation of political, social, and economic indicators (e.g., incidents of communal violence between Malays and Chinese in Malaysia often go unreported or untabulated for fear of the potential repercussions from their publicity); (3) various unsystematic errors and "peculiarities" in data collection (e.g., until the 1970 U.S. Census, Spanish-speaking and Spanish-surnamed persons were counted among the "white" population, thus rendering any analysis of this group impossible); and (4) "hidden" or unreported expenditures. To these should be added a fifth technical problem: cross-national variation in the "price-cost" of goods and services. As Alexander Groth pointedly asks: "Does $100 million buy the same quantity and quality of school buildings in India as it does in Japan?"[2] Obviously, it does not.

The severity of these problems varies from country to country and according to policy area. As noted in Chapter 1, data from Communist bloc and less developed countries are generally the most unreliable. Actually, there has been some improvement in data collection in recent years among less developed countries, owing in large part to the demands by regional and international development agencies for more detailed and accurate information before loans and assistance are granted. In addition, annual United Nations–sponsored surveys have encouraged and facilitated more consistent and reliable data collection throughout the world. Despite these advances, problems remain. We have tried to minimize these by cross-checking the information with at least one and, in many instances, two or more additional sources. This does not guarantee data accuracy and reliability, but it does improve their chances.

The accuracy of budgetary allocations as a measure of societal commitment to a particular policy and of aggregate data as measures of policy impact is further jeopardized by yet another problem. Typically, most aggregate level cross-national policy studies examine *national* government policy efforts and accomplishments. One of the dangers in taking a national level policy perspective, as we do here, is that it may ignore alternative public and private sources for satisfying essential human needs. Before we can compare and evaluate the performance of a national government in providing for those needs, we must determine the degree of responsibility assumed by, granted to, and expected of that government. Among the appropriate questions that must be asked in this regard are: Is the national government the sole supplier of political goods and services or are there subnational units that also have some responsibility? What is the ratio of responsibility between national and subnational authorities? What about the private sector? To what extent are fraternal, charitable, and/or religious organizations expected to provide various goods and services? In addition, what role do social institutions, such as the extended family in traditional societies, or modern financial arrangements, such as private health and retirement programs, assume in the satisfaction of human wants and needs? In the area of defense, national expenditures represent for all practical purposes the total societal commitment, although as Pryor notes, "this has not always been true, e.g., during the Italian renaissance private armies of mercenaries played an important role; and in the 1920s and 30s in Germany, private armies had an important influence."[3]

Health and education expenditures provide a more uncertain situation. In truly federal systems, such as the United States and West Germany, the national government provides a relatively small contribution to health and/or education. In most unitary countries (e.g., Spain, the United Kingdom, France), the central government assumes the major burden. There are, to be sure, exceptions in both cases: Austria and Mexico are federal systems in which the central government assumes extraordinarily high financial obligations for social spending. On the other hand, South Africa is a unitary state in which educational expenditures are legally a provincial responsibility. Despite these exceptions, the unitary–federal dichotomy is generally the most accurate predictor of jurisdictional responsibility. As the majority of the world's nations are unitary, we can be reasonably confident that national level expenditures reflect a significant proportion of the financial commitment to health and education. Nevertheless, to ensure comparability and accuracy in reflecting the total public commitment to these policy areas, we have included health and welfare expenditures for all levels of government. Once again, we stress that in most cases the central government is the major, and often the exclusive, contributor.

With regard to public versus private responsibility for education, it is instructive to examine the results of a somewhat dated (1967), but still relevant, study by UNESCO. The organization surveyed the proportion of total educational expenditures assumed by the private sector in 20 non-communist nations. The study found that private expenditures for education (as a percentage of total expenditures for education) ranged from 15 percent in Malawi to 70 percent in Kenya.[4] Given the difference in public and private financial responsibility between the two countries just mentioned, it would be misleading and unjustified to suggest that the people of Kenya do not enjoy the same educational advantages as those of Malawi simply because the Kenyan government spends only 9.7 percent of its budget on education, while the government of Malawi spends 15.2 percent. Presumably, the Kenyan government does not or need not allocate a greater proportion of its resources for education given the private sector contribution in this area.

In sum, then, before we can render any normative or empirical judgment about the commitment on the part of a national political regime to the education (or the health and welfare) of its citizens, we must take into account both local government and private sector responsibility.

A second problem in comparing *national* level public policies is the danger of concealing significant *intranational* policy variations and thereby weakening the validity of cross-national comparisons and evaluations. The aggregate data approach is again especially vulnerable in this regard because policy data are usually given in terms of national averages. Such

averages may be quite misleading when used for comparative purposes
because intranational policy differences may be greater than average international differences. For example, the average infant mortality rate in the
United States (a policy impact measure) is 16.5 deaths per 1,000 live
births. However, a recent study revealed that in a predominantly black
section of Chicago the rate was 44.6 deaths per 1,000 live births – a rate
higher than that in many nations in the world, including Singapore,
Cyprus, Kuwait, and Jamaica. Similarly, it would be inaccurate to infer
from expenditure or performance data anything about the distribution of
health and educational finances or goods and services within any country.
We cannot assume that, because the governments of Ghana and Bolivia
spend the same amount per person ($3) on health, all the citizens in both
countries are receiving equal or equitable health care. In fact, one study
on the availability of government physicians in Ghana found there was 1
physician per 6,000 people in the Greater Accra region but only 1
physician per 100,000 people in the rural areas.[5] As little comparative
research has been done on the equity or equality of resource distribution,
we can do little more than alert the reader to the problem.

A second inferential problem involves the relationship among expenditures, public services, and performance. Public expenditures are demonstrations of purpose and intent, not measures of quality or accomplishment. More money neither represents nor ensures higher quality education
or health services; it does not ensure that people are better educated or
healthier. In fact, one comparative study of health and education policies
in Malaysia and Turkey found that higher levels of expenditure did not
result in higher levels of service (e.g., more doctors or teachers per person)
or actual improvements in the health or education of the people (e.g.,
decreased mortality rates or increased school enrollment).[6] In the field of
public spending *more* does not necessarily mean *better*. Despite this
important qualification, levels of public spending are important policy
measures in that they reflect different policy goals and/or public needs. It
is important to a people, and important for a student to know, if a nation
spends more money on guns or butter. For this reason alone expenditure
policy demands our attention.

There is one final limitation to the expenditure data of which the reader
should be made aware. The data presented here are, in the main, for a
single year: 1973. It would have been extraordinarily difficult, and sometimes impossible, to get comparable time-series data for as large a number
of nations as is examined. The analysis in this chapter is cross-sectional (or
more simply cross-national) at one point in time. What are the implications of this limitation? The most important is that we are unable to
measure and explain expenditures over time. Because such change is frequently associated with situational factors (e.g., wars, economic depres-

Table 4-1. *Defense spending as a percentage of gross national product: selected countries, 1966 and 1973*

Country	1966	1973
Libya	1.4	1.6
Tunisia	1.8	1.4
Burma	6.4	6.2
Cambodia	6.3	14.8
Malaysia	4.1	4.1
New Zealand	2.3	1.7
Ethiopia	2.8	2.4
South Africa	2.9	2.3
Argentina	1.5	1.9
Venezuela	2.2	1.8

Sources: Data for 1973 from Ruth Legel Sivard, *World Military and Social Expenditures: 1976* (Leesburg, Va.: WMSE Publications, 1976); data for 1966 from *Japan: Analytical Bibliography* (Washington, D.C.: Department of the Army, 1972).

sion) the analysis is not as sensitive to the impact of events on policy as a longitudinal study. However, we emphasize that using data for only one year is not as severe a limitation as it first may appear. Because public expenditure changes incrementally in most countries, there is actually close correspondence in absolute expenditure levels from one year to the next. More importantly, there is remarkable consistency over the years in proportional budgetary allocations within nations. Consider a comparison of defense spending as a proportion of gross national product (GNP) in 10 quite diverse nations between 1966 and 1973 (Table 4-1). As one can clearly see, only in the case of Cambodia did the passage of 7 years result in any significant change in defense spending. The increase in defense spending in Cambodia from 6.3 percent of the GNP in 1966 to 14.8 percent in 1973 is, of course, attributable to that country's direct involvement in the Indochina War after 1972.

Because we are primarily concerned in this chapter with policy priorities as reflected in relative resource allocations, the fact that the data are for a single point in time should not detract significantly from our claim of presenting an accurate representation of the relative policy priorities of most nations. Barring major crises, the relative policy priorities of most nations in 1973 should bear a close resemblance to what one will find in 1983 and perhaps beyond.

One final methodological point. The data analysis to follow is of a rudimentary nature: simple correlations and descriptive statistics. The decision to keep the analysis simple reflects the desire to provide a readable introduction to the aggregate data approach to comparative policy analysis. It is certainly not our intention definitively to resolve the issues raised in earlier chapters concerning the primacy of political or socioeconomic factors in gross policy patterns. Such an undertaking would require more elaborate data analysis techniques. We are content to leave that task to others and simply provide the reader with a relatively uncomplicated, but meaningful, introductory overview.

Defense policy: spending and output

In 1973 the world's nations, combined, spent more money ($244 billion) (American billion) for defense than for any other area of public policy. On an individual basis, one-third of the nations studied here (44 of 127) allocated a larger proportion of their national incomes for defense than for either education or health care. The overwhelming majority of these nations (30) were poorer countries of the Third and Fourth Worlds – nations with per capita GNPs of under $500. All Middle East countries except Cyprus and Kuwait and all Far East countries except Japan, Malaysia, and the Philippines, spent more on defense than on education or health. Among the more advanced nations spending more on defense than education or health were the United States, Czechoslovakia, East Germany, and the USSR.

Despite the worldwide trend toward generally high levels of defense spending, there is considerable cross-national variation in the relative emphasis placed upon this policy area. At the top of the list is Israel, which allocated over one-third of its total national income (37.6 percent) to defense; at the bottom of the list is Panama, which spent less than 1 percent (0.1 percent) of its GNP on defense (see Appendix 1). How does one account for such differences in national policy priorities? The explanation in the case of Israel and Panama is quite obvious. Since becoming independent in 1948, Israel has fought its Arab neighbors on three occasions: 1948–9, 1967, and 1973. Since independence, Israel's overriding public policy concern has been survival in an international environment characterized by constant hostility. Panama, on the other hand, has not been significantly affected by an international conflict since it broke away from Colombia in 1903. But most importantly, Panama and its most valuable national asset, the Panama Canal, enjoy the protection of the American defense umbrella. Apparently without enemies and protected by the military might of the world's most powerful nation, Panama, with a population of 1.5 million people, spent only $2 million on defense in 1973, or $1 per person. Surrounded by enemies and without any formal defense alliance, Israel, with a population of just over 3 million, spent more than $3.5 *billion* (American billion) for defense in 1973 or $1,137 per person.

Not all cross-national military policy differences can be explained so easily. Take, for example, Austria and Sweden. Both are similar in size of population, geographical location, and political structure: parliamentary forms of government led by socialist-oriented regimes. Furthermore, both are neutralist nations. Neither has been at war since the end of World War II (and in the case of Sweden, since 1814), and neither nation appears to be threatened by external or internal enemies. Despite these important similarities, Sweden in 1973 spent 3.5 percent of its GNP on defense and ranked 45th among the 127 nations, whereas Austria spent only 0.9 percent and ranked 115th. How does one explain the difference between two relatively small African nations like 24th-ranked Chad and 121st-ranked Malawi? How does one explain the similarity in level of spending between 14th-ranked Iran and 15th-ranked Laos? Before answering these specific questions, let us begin a systematic analysis of some of the situational, structural, cultural, and environmental differences and similarities among these 127 nations to see if we can explain at least some of the variation in policy priorities in the area of military expenditures.

National income and military spending

A main conclusion of many policy studies based on aggregate data has been that public spending is closely associated with economic wealth. Recall, for example, that Cutright found that the higher the level of economic development of a nation, the more generous its social welfare program. Does a similar relationship exist between national wealth and military spending? The answer is an emphatic no. The data for the 127 nations studied here indicate that in the area of military spending the statistical relationship between per capita GNP and the percentage of the GNP allocated to military spending is −0.04. In other words, for all practical purposes no statistically significant relationship exists between a nation's wealth and the percentage of its GNP it spends for defense. In fact, an examination of specific cases (Table 4–2) reveals that some of the world's largest military spenders are among the world's poorest nations. To emphasize this point, we have divided the nations into four economic "worlds": First World countries are those in which per capita GNP is $1,000 or more; Second World countries, $999 to $500; Third World countries, $499 to $100; Fourth World countries, under $100. When we averaged the percentage of GNP spent on defense for each "world," we found that the First World spent 3.9 percent, the Second World 3.9 percent, the Third World 4.0 percent, and the Fourth World 5.0 percent, confirming the picture that frequently those least able are most likely to spend at high levels on defense. On an individual basis we see that the more glaring examples of this pattern are Egypt, the Yemen People's

Table 4–2. *National income and military spending: selected countries, 1973*

Percent GNP spent on defense	First World	Second World	Third World	Fourth World
10 or more	Israel Saudi Arabia USSR	Iraq	Egypt Yemen People's Republic South Vietnam Syria North Korea	North Vietnam Cambodia
5.0–9.9	United States Portugal East Germany Singapore United Kingdom	Albania Iran Taiwan Mongolia Cuba	China Nigeria Equatorial Guinea	Laos Pakistan Burma Somalia Chad
2.0–4.9	Greece Yugoslavia France Sweden Australia	Turkey Malaysia Peru Lebanon Uruguay	Sudan Congo Zaire Zambia India	Yeman Arab Republic Indonesia Rwanda Mali Ethiopia
1.0–1.9	New Zealand Finland Switzerland Venezuela Libya	Algeria Dominican Republic Nicaragua Ivory Coast	Rhodesia Paraguay Honduras Ghana Tunisia	Afghanistan Upper Volta Bangladesh
Less than 1.0	Japan Austria Luxembourg Trinidad-Tobago	Panama Mexico Costa Rica Jamaica	Sri Lanka Sierra Leone Guatemala Malawi Mauritius	Nepal

Correlation = −0.04; significant at 0.287 level. All correlations in Chapter 4 are Pearson's correlation coefficients.

Note: In this and subsequent tables in Chapter 4, we have selected certain nations for illustrative purposes. The nations were chosen for one or more of the following reasons: (1) they are specifically mentioned or discussed in the text, (2) they represent a diversity in rank or type of country, (3) we thought they might be of particular interest to the reader (e.g., United States, China, United Kingdom, USSR). Where only one, two, or three nations appear in a particular cell, it is because they were the only ones out of all the nations that fell into that group. We strongly urge the reader to examine, and analyze, the complete listing of nations in Appendixes 1 through 3.

Republic, North and South Vietnam, Cambodia, Syria, Laos, and Pakistan. Conversely, those nations that could easily afford to spend more – Japan, Austria, Luxembourg, Finland, and New Zealand – tend to be the least inclined to allocate substantial portions of their national wealth to the military. As we shall soon see, in these and other nations various political factors, not the ability to pay, have resulted in lower levels of defense spending.

Military regimes and military spending

In Chapter 3 we discuss the fact that there is conflicting evidence concerning the impact of military regimes on public policy. Here we ask the straightforward question: Do military regimes spend more on defense than civilian regimes? The answer, at least for 1973, is no. In 1973 there were 21 nations directly ruled by military regimes. However, the data indicate only 3 of these appear among the top 25 nations ranked according to military spending: Syria (ranked number 6), Burma (20), and Somalia (21). Only 7 military regimes – Syria, Burma, Somalia, Nigeria (28), Sudan (31), the Congo (35), and Peru (40) – appear within the top one-third leading defense spenders. Military regimes do not appear to be particularly extravagant or parsimonious in allocating resources for military purposes. In actuality, military regimes tend to cluster around two moderate levels of spending: 8 of the 21 nations spent between 2.0 and 2.6 percent of their GNPs on defense; 6 spent between 1.3 and 1.7 percent. Finally, it should be noted that, on the average in 1973, military regimes spent a smaller proportion of their national incomes on defense (3.3 percent) than civilian regimes (4.1 percent).

Regime type and military spending

It is commonly asserted by Marxist theorists and political leaders that socialist regimes are more committed to socially useful policies, whereas the expansionist, imperialist, and militarist capitalist countries are more concerned with producing weapons of war. Based upon this assertion, one would expect socialist regimes to spend less than nonsocialist regimes on defense. Previous research on this question, using only a limited number of cases, has found this assertion to be unfounded.[7] We, however, have data on almost every nation in existence in 1973 and, therefore, should be in a better position to examine the question: Do socialist or communist nations spend less of their available resources on defense than nonsocialist nations?

Following the lead of Anderson, Von der Mehden, and Young, we have classified all the nations into four categories according to the orientation of the regime in power in 1973:

1. Communist nations or those with regimes that have formally adopted Marxism-Leninism as the operating philosophy and model of state (e.g., USSR, China, North Korea, Cuba).
2. Militant or radical socialist nations or those with regimes that

are not totally committed to the communist model as such but
that favor a single, monolithic socialist party and a "total
reorientation of economic and social institutions under state
auspices" (e.g., Algeria, Tanzania, Burma).

3. Moderate reformist socialist nations in which the regime operates in a democratic, pluralistic environment and favors some
degree of state ownership of the means of production and the
provision of social services. Nationalization of industry and
state-provided social services are viewed, however, as one of
several policy strategies, and a substantial private sector continues to operate (e.g., Sweden, Kenya, Singapore).

4. Nonsocialist countries in which regimes subscribing to socialist
principles have played no significant role in the policy process
(e.g., United States, Greece, the Philippines).[8]

For purposes of analysis we have divided the four categories into two:
militant socialist and communist (referred to in the tables as *radical
socialist*) and reform socialist and nonsocialist (referred to in the tables as
nonsocialist). The justification for combining communist and militant
socialist regimes into a single category lies not only in their similar economic orientation but, more importantly, in their authoritarian nature.
The relatively small number of reform socialist regimes did not seem to
warrant separate tabular or analytical presentation. Furthermore, no significant statistical analysis was possible given the few countries involved.
Hence, these regimes are included in the nonsocialist category.

Upon analysis, the data suggest that, if anything, militant socialist/
communist regimes are more likely to spend a higher proportion of their
resources on defense than reformist/nonsocialist regimes. Of the top one-
third defense spenders, 40 percent (17 nations) were led by militant
socialist/communist governments, although such regimes constituted only
21 percent of the world's nations in 1973 (see Appendix 1). The average
level of defense spending, as a percentage of GNP, for nonsocialist
regimes was 3.4 percent; the average for the 27 radical socialist nations was
6.7 percent.

A strong socialist commitment does not, of course, guarantee a high
level of defense spending: Sri Lanka, Romania, and Algeria had militant
socialist regimes in 1973; yet they spent less than 2 percent of their GNPs
on defense (Table 4–3). Nevertheless, there appears to be a tendency for
high levels of military spending among socialist states.

International politics and political events

Despite the aggregate tendencies noted above – that radical socialist
regimes are inclined toward higher military spending – an examination of

Table 4–3. *Regime type and military spending: selected countries, 1973*

Percent GNP spent on defense	Radical socialist	Nonsocialist
10 or more	Yemen People's Republic North Vietnam North Korea USSR	South Vietnam Jordan Cambodia Saudi Arabia
5.0–9.9	Albania China Mongolia Burma	Iran Laos Taiwan Pakistan
2.0–4.9	Congo Yugoslavia Czechoslovakia Guinea	Sudan Turkey Greece Malaysia
1.0–1.9	Romania Algeria Libya	Switzerland Cameroon Kuwait Philippines
Less than 1.0	Sri Lanka	Jamaica Nepal Costa Rica Mauritius

Table 4–3 leads one to wonder whether, in fact, it is regime type or ideology or some other factor that explains differences in military spending. Obviously, ideology has little to do with the fact that 4th-ranked communist North Vietnam and 5th-ranked noncommunist South Vietnam, or 16th-ranked China and 17th-ranked Taiwan, committed similarly large proportions of their national wealth to the military. In addition, only the most committed capitalist could seriously suggest that ideology is responsible for the high levels of military spending by the reformist socialist regimes in Israel and Egypt.

It does not take an expert in international politics to recognize some all too familiar names among the world's top military spenders. The war in Indochina provided us with the nations ranked 4th (North Vietnam), 5th (South Vietnam), 8th (Cambodia), 15th (Laos), and 22nd (United States). The on-going Arab–Israeli conflict contributes numbers 1 (Israel), 2 (Egypt), 6 (Syria), 7 (Jordan), and 9 (Saudi Arabia).

Regional rivalries and conflicts also contribute to high levels of defense spending. In this category are Iraq (10) and Iran (14), Yemen People's

Republic (3) and Yemen Arab Republic (33), Turkey (32) and Greece (34), and Pakistan (19) and India (54). Lastly, we find a group of nations in which international tension and/or conflict (it used to be called the cold war) contributes to proportionately high levels of defense spending. Included are North Korea (11), USSR (12), China (16), Taiwan (17), Cuba (25), East Germany (26), and the United Kingdom (30).

Conversely, those nations that spend relatively little on defense (i.e., less than 1 percent of their GNPs), are generally those not normally associated with major international power politics or regional rivalries. One reads little of the arms race, military alerts, or battle field reports from Mauritius (126), Trinidad and Tobago (125), Jamaica (124), Nepal (122), Malawi (121), Luxembourg (117), or Austria (115). Clearly, relative freedom from international political entanglements and regional rivalries helps keep military spending down.

The impact of the international political environment on military spending manifests itself throughout the ranks of nations, not simply among those at the extreme poles. It is beyond the scope of this study to account for the spending levels of all 127 nations for which data are available, but we can offer some additional examples to illustrate the point. In his study of government spending in Canada, Richard Bird makes the following observation:

The most important explanation of the minute and diminishing significance of defense expenditures in Canada appears . . . to be in Canada's relationship with the United States, for if there is a foreign military threat to Canada's security, it may be assumed to be deterred primarily by the existence of U.S. military strength . . . In short, Canada, like most other NATO countries (except where military expenditures are distorted, as in the case of Portugal, by the pursuit of old-fashioned colonial objectives) is in a real sense resting in the shade of the American defense umbrella.[9]

We cannot say with certainty that nations like West Germany, the Netherlands, and Belgium would be spending more of their national incomes on defense if they were not NATO members. However, at least in the case of Canada and Portugal, Bird's comments appear appropriate and complimentary to our own findings. For example, Canada ranked 73rd among 127 nations and spent only 2 percent of its GNP on defense in 1973. This was down from 4.2 percent in 1960 and 3.0 percent in 1965. Bird's observation about Portugal's "distorted" level of defense spending is corroborated by our data. Portugal, which in 1973 still maintained colonies in Africa (Angola, Mozambique, and Portuguese Guinea) and Asia (Macao and Portuguese Timor), spent 5.6 percent of its GNP on defense and ranked 23rd in the world – ahead of all other NATO nations except the United States, which ranked 22nd and spent 6.1 percent. The costs of colonialism were apparently high for Portugal.

Another politically related factor that appears to contribute to relatively high levels of defense spending involves internal political conflict resulting from communal or ideologically oriented insurgency or from separatist or national liberation movements. Nations affected by such conflict in 1973 were Chad (24), Equatorial Guinea (29), Malaysia (36), Zaire (38), Indonesia (47), Thailand (58), and Ethiopia (65). In each case, the evidence suggests that military spending was in part related to the need to maintain internal order and the existing regime.

We began the discussion of military spending by asking what factors might account for the similarities and differences among nations. Among the specific nations mentioned, for illustrative purposes, were Chad (24) and Malawi (121), Iran (14) and Laos (15), and Sweden (45) and Austria (115). We believe the situational factors discussed above are the major determinants of military spending: war in the case of Laos, regional conflict in the case of Iran, preserving order in the religiously polarized society of Chad, and the relative absence of internal and external conflict in Malawi. But what about the comparison of Sweden and Austria? Should not neutralist, culturally homogeneous, and politically stable Sweden spend less on defense than it does: roughly the amount of neutralist, culturally homogeneous, and politically stable Austria? We believe the difference can be attributed to the international political status and historical experience of the two countries.

As part of the agreement to end the four-power occupation in 1955, Austria, upon the urging of the Soviet Union, proclaimed its permanent neutrality. This position is internationally recognized and, in a real sense, guaranteed by the major powers. Therefore, Austria's position in the world community is that of an accepted neutral whose international status is further legitimized by major power backing. On the other hand, "Sweden, though it shuns alliances and pursues a policy of neutrality in the event of war, does not enjoy such legally recognized status."[10] Sweden, therefore, much like Switzerland, relies in large measure on military preparedness rather than international recognition of neutrality. The result, of course, is a necessarily higher commitment than Austria's to defense.

The major conclusion of this section is that national and international political events and conditions (i.e., situational factors) appear to be generally more important than national income, regime type, or ideology in determining levels of military spending. In the case of Sweden and Austria, more permanent or structural factors (i.e., international political status) help account for levels of military spending.

Service and performance

In Chapter 1 we distinguish among *policy* (statements of purpose), *output* or service (what is actually done), and *impact* or performance (what is actually accomplished), and suggest that policy studies should include all three dimensions. Therefore, we conclude the discussion of military policy by examining the relationship among the intentions of a government, its efforts, and its accomplishments.

The measure of policy output chosen is the number of people per soldier in each nation. This is admittedly a rather crude measure of output because there is no certainty that the higher the ratio of soldiers to population (i.e., the fewer the number of people each soldier is theoretically responsible for defending), the more effectively protected is the population. For example, the soldier/population ratio in North and South Vietnam was virtually identical in 1973 (see Appendix 1) – 1:39 in North Vietnam; 1:35 in South Vietnam. Yet most observers agree that the North Vietnamese army was far superior to its southern counterpart. In addition, the more modernized a nation's armed forces, the lower the soldier/population requirement. In a traditional war, one soldier in a tank is probably more effective than one infantryman with a rifle. Despite these qualifications, the population/soldier ratio does provide a reasonably reliable and uniform standard for comparing military policy output.

What is the relationship between military spending and the level of defense provided by national governments? To test the relationship between the two policy dimensions, we computed correlations between the level of defense spending and the number of soldiers per population. The results of the computation indicate a marginally negative relationship between policy and service. The correlation was –0.11, suggesting that little, if any, relationship exists between how much a nation spends and the soldier/population ratio.

On the surface, measuring policy outcome in the area of defense appears relatively easy. The purpose of a military establishment is to defend a nation. To the extent that a nation's military deters others from attacking or, if attacked, successfully defends the nation, it is performing well. That sounds simple, but in practice it is not. To begin, there is the problem of what to measure. Do we count the number of times a country has been invaded? The number of international wars in which it has been involved? The number of wars it has won or lost? The duration of the conflicts in which it has been involved? The number of battle deaths and casualties? Should we measure only international conflicts or include civil wars, insurgency movements, and large-scale civil strife as well? Based upon existing studies there appears to be little agreement on these questions.[11]

In addition to the definitional problem, there are inferential problems.

Can we infer or assume that a nation has not been involved in any armed interstate conflict because of the perceived or actual strength of its military? As suggested above, military preparedness may be responsible for Sweden's ability to avoid involvement in an international war for over 150 years. However, it is unlikely that the perceived or actual strength of the armies of Trinidad-Tobago, Liberia, or Nepal has been responsible for keeping these nations out of war.

For all these reasons, we have decided to omit any measure of military performance.

Educational policy: spending, output, and performance

In 1974, for the first time in decades, total world expenditures for education exceeded military expenditures: $280 billion compared with $270 billion (American billions). On an individual basis, 85 of the 132 nations studied here (64 percent) spent more of their GNP on education than on defense or health. Although world military expenditures again exceeded education spending in 1975 ($324 billion compared with $300 billion), one can expect the latter to keep pace with, if not exceed, the former in future years. In fact, since the end of World War II, educational expenditures in most nations have been the fastest growing area of public spending. There are several explanations for this phenomenon.

First, educational spending tends to follow demographic trends. Thus, as Ruth Sivard notes: "Education needs, unlike military are directly related to population growth. Every year an additional 25 million children must be absorbed into school systems. Since 1960, it is estimated, the world population between the ages of 5 and 19 has increased by 320 million."[12] Demography alone, however, cannot explain increasing absolute or relative expenditure commitments to education. Despite the categorical imperative suggested by Sivard that "25 million children *must* be absorbed into school systems," viewed historically no such imperative automatically can be assumed. After all, throughout human history, including the beginnings of the twentieth century, most of mankind remained uneducated and illiterate. Population expansion did not and need not always lead to increasing educational expenditures.

The increasing priority assigned by policy makers to education can in large measure be attributed to the skills and attitudinal changes associated with the processes of political modernization and industrialization. It is unclear whether the expansion of education necessarily precedes or succeeds the introduction of modernization and industrialization, but there is little doubt that the two are closely related.

Fulfilling the educational requirements of a society need not, however, have been the responsibility of the public sector. It was only after adoption of the welfare-oriented state ideology around the turn of the century among the early industrializers, and more recently among the less developed nations, that the state became responsible for providing education. The role of the state as the primary provider of educational services is in a real sense the logical extension of the role assumed by the state in the area of economic activity. The relationship among economic growth, educational policy, and state activity is nicely illustrated in the case of France. According to André Garcia: "Throughout the 19th century, France, like the United Kingdom, achieved its industrial expansion with an almost totally illiterate population; today, with [industrial] expansion as one of its responsibilities, the State is concerned with training the executives and technicians necessary for an economy in full expansion."[13]

Still another factor that has led to the relative and absolute growth of educational expenditures, particularly since the end of World War II, is the universal popular demand for education. This demand derives from humanistic, democratic, and economic motives.[14] So widespread have such demands become that there are those who argue popular pressure for education, and not the requirements of economic development, are the primary cause for the expansion of educational expenditures in recent years.

It is unnecessary, and probably impossible, to pinpoint a single explanation for the rapid rise in educational spending in the last few decades. Undoubtedly, demographic, economic, and political factors all have played important roles. The task is to examine and explain some of the similarities and differences among nations in terms of how much they spend on education and with what results.

Educational spending: an overview

Before we examine individual national variation in educational spending, an important general observation about the overall level of spending in this area is in order. An examination of the data for 1973 reveals that there was less difference among nations in levels of spending for education than for defense (see Appendix 2). In the case of military spending, the difference between the nation that allocated the largest proportion of its national resources to defense, Israel, and the one that allocated the least, Panama, is enormous: 37.6 percent compared with 0.1 percent. Even if one eliminates the extraordinary case of Israel, the difference is still considerable: 18.8 percent for 2nd-ranked Egypt compared with 0.1 percent for Panama. The range of relative spending in education is considerably narrower: Canada ranks first, with 8.5 percent of its GNP devoted to education; Haiti ranks last, with 0.7 percent. How does one account for this overall major difference between policy areas?

The answer, we suggest, lies in the fact that a nation's educational needs and its policy responses are more likely to reflect structural factors –

levels of economic wealth or age group distribution – than situational variables. In the case of defense policy, we have seen that situational factors – international tension, war, and internal conflict – have an important impact on military spending. This was particularly obvious among the largest defense spenders. Because education spending tends to respond to more predictable and consistent demands, which are common to all nations, cross-national variation is likely to be less than in the area of defense spending, where situational factors have a more selective impact and produce more extreme variations.

Although international differences in spending for education are not as striking as those for military spending, enough variation exists to warrant explanation. We can proceed, as before, by testing alternative explanations for cross-national similarities and differences in policy, service, and performance.

Regime type and educational spending

We begin the analysis by examining the relationship between regime type and public spending for education. Do radical socialist / communist and nonsocialist, or military and civilian, regimes assign significantly different priorities to education?

In terms of military versus civilian regimes, this apparently is not the case. Table 4-4 shows that military regimes are scattered throughout all levels of spending. The military regimes of Malagasy, Libya, and the Congo rank among the top nations in education spending; the military regimes in Upper Volta, Somalia, and Nigeria rank among the lowest spenders. On the average, in 1973, military regimes spent 3.7 percent of their GNPs on education; civilian regimes 3.9 percent. The difference is not particularly significant.

Are educational needs neglected by military regimes because resources are diverted to finance military projects? Because we are not dealing with time-series data, we cannot directly answer this question. The answer requires examining regimes that have moved from military to civilian control, or the reverse, to see if there has been a shift in relative emphasis in public spending.[15] We can point out, however, that in only 5 of the 21 military regimes did the military budget exceed the education or health budget. Those nations are Syria, Burma, Somalia, Nigeria, and Sudan. Some military regimes actually spent considerably more on education than on defense. Oustanding examples are Libya and Malagasy, which each spent 6.8 percent of its GNP on education and only 1.7 and 1.4 percent, respectively, on defense. It does not appear that funding for education necessarily suffers from military rule.

On the other hand, regime ideology does appear to have an impact on education policy. On the average, radical socialist regimes (including

Table 4–4. *Regime type and educational spending: selected countries, 1973*

Percent GNP spent on education	Military	Civilian	Radical socialist	Nonsocialist
6.0–8.5	Malagasy[a]	Canada	Algeria	Canada
	Libya	Denmark	USSR	Denmark
	Congo	Ivory Coast	Libya	Netherlands
		USSR	Congo	Ivory Coast
4.0–5.9	Sudan	United Kingdom	Guinea	France
	Dahomey[b]	United States	Cuba	United States
	Bolivia	Japan	East Germany	Italy
		Yugoslavia	Mongolia	Ireland
2.0–3.9	Peru	China	North Vietnam	Peru
	Syria	Iran	Tanzania	Ghana
	Burma	Thailand	Hungary	Kuwait
	Upper Volta	Argentina	Romania	Spain
Less than 2.0	Somalia	India	None	Greece
	Nigeria	Laos		Pakistan
		Afghanistan		South Africa
		Haiti		Nepal

[a]Since 1975, Malagasy has been called Madagascar.
[b]Since 1975, Dahomey has been called Benin.

communist regimes) spent a larger proportion of their national incomes (4.4 percent) than nonsocialist or reformist regimes (3.8 percent) on education. There are two possible explanations for this trend. The first is that by definition the state in the socialist society provides a larger proportion of goods and services, including education, than it does in nonsocialist regimes. In all the communist countries, and in many strongly socialist ones, public spending represents virtually the entire societal commitment to formal education. In nonsocialist countries, however, the private sector assumes varying degrees of responsibility for education, thus reducing the need and/or incentive for higher levels of public spending.

The second explanation is more problematical. It is that socialism involves a stronger commitment to egalitarian, socially beneficial enterprises, such as education, than is found in nonsocialist systems. This is, of course, an ideological argument that cannot be successfully tested by our data. It is true that in 1973 socialist regimes, on the average, spent more on education than nonsocialist regimes. It is also true that only 3 of the 27 radical socialist regimes appeared among the one-third of the nations that spent least on education. Despite such evidence, we can neither confirm nor deny that this represents a higher level of humanitarianism, egalitarianism, or social commitment than is displayed by nonsocialist regimes.

Table 4-5. *National income and educational spending: selected countries, 1973*

Percent GNP spent on education	First World	Second World	Third World	Fourth World
6.0–8.5	Canada Sweden Denmark Netherlands USSR	Algeria Ivory Coast	Malagasy Zambia Tunisia Congo Yemen People's Republic	None
4.0–5.9	United Kingdom France United States Japan Saudi Arabia	Costa Rica Malaysia Cuba Iraq Panama	Guyana Swaziland Kenya Egypt Bolivia	Lesotho Botswana
2.0–3.9	Israel Bulgaria Singapore Argentina Spain	Peru Taiwan Iran Albania Chile	China Ecuador Sri Lanka Rhodesia Uganda	Burma Rwanda Indonesia Ethiopia Burundi
Less than 2.0	Greece Portugal South Africa	Dominican Republic	Nigeria Paraguay India Haiti	Somalia Bangladesh Pakistan Afghanistan Nepal

Correlation = 0.42; significant at 0.001 level.

National income and educational spending

In the introduction to this section we suggest that government spending on education is likely to reflect relatively stable factors such as national income. The explanation for this predicted relationship seems fairly obvious. "The poorer countries cannot be expected to spend as much on education as the countries at the top of the rank-order. Their small income per head is earned, as a rule, by producing the bare necessities of life."[16] Public education, beyond the primary level, is a luxury many poorer nations cannot afford.

The logic of this explanation is apparently corroborated by our data (Table 4-5). In aggregate terms the statistical correlation between per capita GNP and educational spending was a moderate 0.42. The aggregate relationship between national income and educational spending is further underscored when we examine the average level of spending among nations according to their level of economic development. The relationship is descriptively linear: In 1973, First World countries spent, on the average, 4.6 percent of their GNPs on education; Second World countries, 4.1 percent; Third World countries, 3.7 percent; and Fourth World countries, 2.6 percent.

Examination of the individual countries reinforces this picture. Of the 10 nations that spent most on education, 6 (Canada, Sweden, Denmark, Netherlands, USSR, and Libya) are First World countries. The data support the notion that spending for education is closely related to the level of national income.

Despite the overall or aggregate trend, there are deviant nations – nations one would expect to have higher or lower levels of spending on education given the resource level of the society. It is beyond the scope of this study to examine and explain all such deviations. We would be remiss, however, if we did not point out at least some of these anomalies and suggest explanations for their occurrence.

First is the apparent incongruity between the relative affluence of such countries as Argentina, Spain, Greece, Portugal, and South Africa and their relatively low public commitment to education. The most obvious explanation for this situation is the important role private, church-run schools play in these nations, with the exception of South Africa. In Argentina, for example, private educational expenditures account for just under 50 percent of the total spent on education; in Greece the figure is about 40 percent. In these and in other countries, particularly those with large Catholic populations, the relatively low level of *public* expenditures is a function of important private sector activity. In the case of South Africa, the apparently low public commitment is a result of the white minority government's neglect of educational opportunities and public spending for the overwhelming black majority. This neglect is reflected in the fact that although literacy among whites is 98 percent, it is only 35 percent among nonwhites.

At the opposite end of the spectrum, how does one explain the rather substantial investment in education by Third World countries like Malagasy, Zambia, the Congo, Yemen People's Republic, and Tunisia? One explanation is that these poor nations view education as an invest-ment, a way to ensure economic development and modernization. This view is reinforced by the imitative nature of policy, particularly in poorer nations.

In modern times, most nations tend to formulate their economic, social, and political goals by comparing themselves with other countries . . . For example, *educational goals* in many countries are based on the idea that the most backward regions should, in the future, be brought to the present average standard, or that the general average should be brought up to the standard of the presently most advanced regions.[17]

Another explanation for high spending in many poor countries relates to the demographic structure of these nations. It is to this point that we now turn.

Demographic structure and educational spending

As suggested earlier, demographic structure plays an important role in defining the educational needs of a nation. Of particular significance is the age structure of a nation's population. The larger the proportion of people 15 years of age or under, the greater the need for educational facilities. Because of high birth rates and decreasing mortality rates, the age structure among poorer nations is substantially younger than in rich nations: About 50 percent of the population in developing countries, compared with about 25 percent in developed countries, is 15 years old or younger.

The youthfulness of their people and the resulting demand for education have undoubtedly contributed to increasingly higher expenditures in this area. Returning to those Third World nations that ranked high on educational spending in 1973, we find that the proportion of young people ranged from 41 percent in the Congo to 46 percent in Malagasy. It seems safe to conclude that population pressure plays some role in setting national policy priorities. This conclusion is reinforced by the moderate (0.44) aggregate statistical relationship between the proportion of school-age population (5 to 15 years old) and the percentage of GNP spent on education in 132 nations.

The relationship between age structure and educational spending, outlined above, does not apply in all cases. In 1973, Somalia, Bangladesh, Pakistan, Laos, Yemen Arab Republic, Afghanistan, and Nepal had populations in which at least 42 percent of the people were 15 years old or under; yet they were among the lowest educational spenders.

The fact that demographic structure appears to influence public spending in some nations, but not in others, raises an issue mentioned in Chapter 3 and is worth reemphasizing here. Rarely in the study of public policy can one find a single factor that totally explains cross-national policy differences and similarities. Public policy is the end product of a process involving many factors, including the ideological and cultural traditions of a nation, the needs and resources of the society, and the very way in which the policy process operates. And in the final analysis, policy is made by people – men and women with unique personalities, political biases, and intellectual capacities. How does one explain the difference in policy emphasis between Nigeria, which spent only 1.9 percent of its GNP on education, and Malagasy, which spent 6.8 percent? Both nations in 1973 were relatively poor ($177 per capita GNP for Nigeria, $173 for Malagasy), had youthful populations (45 to 46 percent under 15 years of age), and were led by military regimes without any particularly socialist bias. Perhaps General Gowon of Nigeria was less firmly committed to education than General Ramanantsoa of Malagasy. Only an in-depth study of the policy process in each country can answer this question with certainty. The contribution that multinational comparative policy analysis can make is to point out general relationships among gross structural, cultural, environmental, and situational factors and suggest how these contribute to the overall policy-making process.

Educational service and performance

We conclude the discussion of educational policy by briefly examining educational output and accomplishment. What is the relationship between public spending for education and output and accomplishment? Can we expect a high correlation between spending and the proportion of the school-age population actually attending school (an output measure) or the rate of literacy (a performance measure)?

A statistical analysis of the aggregate picture for 1973 reveals a positive but relatively weak relationship between spending and the proportion of the school-age population actually attending school (0.30) and between spending and the rate of literacy (0.27). To be sure, in a number of specific instances the relationship among policy, output, and impact is congruous. Countries such as Canada, Sweden, Denmark, and the Netherlands committed relatively high levels of resources to education, had large proportions of their school-age population in school, and had virtually eliminated illiteracy. At the other end of the spectrum, countries such as the Yemen Arab Republic, Afghanistan, Nepal, and Haiti spent relatively little with corresponding results.

Some countries made significant commitments to education but had not by 1973 experienced results commensurate with that effort. Outstanding examples are Algeria, the Ivory Coast, and Malagasy. In contrast are countries such as Argentina, Spain, and Greece, which provided relatively little in the way of public support for education but still had substantial proportions of their young people in school and low rates of illiteracy (see Appendix 2).

The explanation for these seeming incongruities are rather obvious. In Argentina, Spain, and Greece a substantial portion of educational spending came from the private sector. In these and other countries where there is substantial private education, the relationship between *public* policy and educational achievement is not necessarily congruous. In Algeria, the Ivory Coast, Malagasy, and other developing nations there is apparently a lag between the financial investment made by the public sector and the effort to get a larger proportion of young people in schools and to witness results in the form of increases in literacy. Clearly, we can expect an increasing correspondence among poor nations relative to public policy, output, and performance in the future.

In closing, we draw the reader's attention to the range of differences the data in Appendix 2 display and the human implications of these statistics. In 1973, in a typical First World nation, between 60 and 85 percent of the school-age population actually was in school, and the overall rate of literacy among the population exceeded 90 percent. In a typical Third or Fourth World country, 10 or 20 percent of the school-age population was actually enrolled in school, and only 5 to 15 percent of the people could read or write.

Health policy: spending, output, and performance

In 1973 only 3 governments out of 132 (those in the Dominican Republic, New Zealand, and West Germany) spent more on health than on either defense needs or education (see Appendix 3). Despite the relatively low public priority attached to health policy, there is no other area of public policy that brings home so dramatically and in such human terms the differences among nations. Consider a comparison of Denmark and Ethiopia. A child born in Ethiopia in 1973 could, if it was not among the 181 of every 1,000 children to die before its first birthday, expect to live 38 years. During that time, if the child became ill, it *might* be attended by a qualified physician who, theoretically, was responsible for 73,749 other people as well. A Danish child born on the same day would have a much better chance of surviving its first year (only 13 per 1,000 die in infancy) and could expect to live almost twice as long (74 years) as the Ethiopian child. If the Danish child became ill, it *would* be cared for by a qualified physician who, theoretically, was responsible for only 591 persons. Needless to say, these figures do not come close to capturing the human implications of being born Danish or Ethiopian, the pleasure or pain, satiation or hunger, happiness or sorrow. What about health policy in these two countries? In 1973 Denmark allocated 4.4 percent of its national wealth, or $243 per person, to health care; the Ethiopian government allocated 0.8 percent of its GNP, or $1 per person. How does one account for this difference? Let us examine some of the possible explanations for the differences in health policy among nations.

Regime type and health spending

As in education, cross-national differences in health priorities in 1973 were not as great as differences in military spending. Differences between

Table 4-6. *Regime type and health spending: selected countries, 1973*

Percent GNP spent on health	Military	Civilian	Radical socialist	Nonsocialist
4.0–6.5	None	Sweden Canada Netherlands United Kingdom	None	New Zealand West Germany Zaire Denmark
2.0–3.9	Libya	Panama USSR United States Cuba	Poland Czechoslovakia Chile Libya	Luxembourg Japan Venezuela Ireland
1.0–1.9	Bolivia Dahomey Somalia Peru	Portugal Australia Morocco Italy	Romania Sri Lanka Congo Burma	Nicaragua Gambia Turkey Spain
Less than 1.0	Ecuador Syria Nigeria Brazil	Lebanon Mexico South Africa Pakistan	Iraq North Vietnam Syria North Korea	Colombia South Vietnam South Korea Indonesia

regime types in the relative priority assigned to health care tended to be small on an absolute scale but, in one instance, rather significant on a proportional or relative basis (Table 4–6).

Rather surprisingly, we did not find a significant difference between radical socialist and nonsocialist regimes in health spending. Radical socialist regimes allocated 1.8 percent of their GNPs, compared with 1.7 percent for nonsocialist regimes. Given the generally higher levels of public compared with private sector activity in socialist regimes, we expected to find a difference similar to that found in the area of education. One possible explanation for the lack of significant difference between socialist and nonsocialist regimes may be purely technical. In some nations with state-run national health insurance programs, part of the funding comes from fees charged to patients. As a rule, government spending does not reflect these fees and, therefore, tends to underestimate the public commitment to health care. One example of this situation is Norway, which had a reform socialist-oriented government and a national health program and yet ranked 89th in the world in 1973, spending only 1.1 percent of its GNP on health. This actually represented only about 40 to 50 percent of Norway's total public spending on health care.

In comparing the average level of spending between military and civilian regimes, we did find statistically significant differences. For example, on the average, civilian regimes spent 1.9 percent of their GNPs on health, compared with 1.1 percent for military regimes. Although this represents an absolute difference of only 0.8 percent, it indicates that, in aggregate, civilian regimes spent about 30 percent more than military regimes. This difference, based upon a standard significance test, is statistically significant.

Do these differences confirm the Western democratic bias that civilian regimes are more concerned with the health needs of their citizens than are authoritarian military regimes? Much as we would like to conclude that this is the case, additional evidence suggests that another, more important factor is at work: national income.

National income and health spending

The relationship between national income and health spending can be introduced and illustrated best by comparing the average levels of spending for each of the four economic worlds referred to earlier. In doing this, we found that, as in the case of education, a linear pattern exists between general levels of national income and health spending. Specifically, the pattern is as follows: First World countries averaged 2.6 percent of their GNPs on health care; Second World countries, 1.6 percent; Third World countries, 1.3 percent; and Fourth World countries 0.9 percent. The overall aggregate statistical relationship between per capita GNP and public expenditures for health was a strong 0.61.

Looking beyond the aggregate pattern, an examination of the data underscores the close relationship between national income and spending for health, especially among the highest and lowest spending nations. In 1973, 20 of the top 25 health spenders were First World nations, 3 were Second World nations, and just 2 (Zaire and Zambia) were Third World nations. Conversely, 20 of the lowest 25 health spenders were from the Third or Fourth World; only 2 (South Africa and Israel) were First World nations (Table 4-7). Clearly, the level of national income in Denmark (a First World nation), Ethiopia (a Fourth World nation), and most other nations plays a major role in determining how much of its nation's wealth a government can allocate to serve the health needs of its people.

Returning to the differences in health spending between military and civilian regimes, we find a high percentage of military-led countries are Third and Fourth World countries. We suggest that it is not civilian rule, but rather a nation's wealth, that accounts for its ability to serve its people's health needs. Thus, among the world's leading health spenders

Table 4-7. *National income and health spending: selected countries, 1973*

Percent GNP spent on health	First World	Second World	Third World	Fourth World
4.0–6.5	Sweden Canada New Zealand West Germany United Kingdom	None	Zaire	None
2.0–3.9	Japan USSR United States Hungary Ireland	Panama Taiwan Costa Rica Chile Cuba	Zambia Swaziland Guyana Egypt Tunisia	Lesotho Botswana Yemen Arab Republic
1.0–1.9	Portugal Australia Saudi Arabia Greece Norway	Nicaragua Malaysia Ivory Coast Algeria Iran	Sri Lanka Congo Guatemala Tanzania Uganda	Somalia Mali Chad Burma Rwanda
Less than 1.0	Argentina Israel South Africa	Iraq Lebanon Mexico Brazil	Colombia India Ecuador Philippines Nigeria	Upper Volta Nepal Bangladesh Indonesia Pakistan

Correlation = 0.61; significant at 0.001 level.

are Sweden, Canada, and New Zealand, as well as the USSR, Czechoslovakia, and East Germany. Like education, health care remains a luxury for many of the world's poorest people.

We conclude the analysis of the determinants of health care spending by noting moderately strong aggregate statistical relationships between percentage of GNP spent on health and urbanization (0.48) and industrialization (0.53). In the case of urbanization, there is an assumption that the more urbanized a society, the higher the level of health care spending. Two explanations for this relationship are (1) urbanization and the health problems associated with living in areas of high population density create a greater *need* for health facilities, and (2) there is apparently a greater *demand* by urban dwellers for modern professional health care. Rural people, particularly in traditional societies, tend to rely more heavily upon traditional forms of medical care (e.g., medicine men) than do their more sophisticated urban cousins. The moderate (0.48) aggregate statistical relationship suggests there is some validity to the argument.

With regard to industrialization, we suggest that this is probably a surrogate measure for national wealth. It is generally the case that the more industrialized a nation, the wealthier it is. Although we do not deny that industrialization or, indeed, urbanization produces certain conditions that increase health care problems, needs, and demands, we maintain that the public sector response to these needs is, in large measure, determined by the ability to finance public programs.

Health service and performance

The examples of Denmark and Ethiopia referred to above might lead one to expect a close relationship among the amount a nation spends on health (policy), the number of people per physician (output), and the infant mortality and life expectancy rates (performance). In 1973, Denmark ranked among the world's leaders on health spending (7th), had a good population/physician ratio, and had low infant mortality and high life expectancy rates. Ethiopia, on the other hand, consistently ranked low on policy (110th), output (132nd), and performance (125th on infant mortality and 126th on life expectancy).

In fact, however, the aggregate relationship for all 132 nations between health spending and population per physician is negative (-0.27). The relationship between spending and performance is mixed: It is moderately negative with regard to infant mortality (-0.40) and moderately positive with regard to life expectancy (0.49). How can one explain these mixed and intuitively unexpected relationships? It seems reasonable to expect that the more a nation spends on health care, the greater the number of physicians, the lower the infant mortality rate, and the longer the life expectancy in the society will be. But several factors intervene between policy effort, as measured by money spent, and output and achievement in medical care.

First, there are varoius idiosyncratic factors. Consider, for example, the case of Sweden, which ranks first in public spending for health but 22nd in population/physican ratio. The explanation for this apparently incongruous relationship is that Swedes tend to use hospitals more readily than people in other countries. The reason for this is that hospital care in Sweden is free, while there is a charge for general practitioner care. Sweden, therefore, has a higher rate of hospital utilization and commensurately fewer physicians because institutionalized or in-patient medical care does not require as many physicians. In addition, many countries, particularly Eastern European nations, Japan, and many less developed countries, rely heavily upon clinics rather than one-physician offices to provide primary medical care. In these cases, too, the physician/population

ratio need not be as high as in those countries where solo general practitioner services prevail.

Second, in several countries the private sector provides a substantial
proportion of medical services available in the society. Thus, relatively low
levels of *public* spending may occur in nations with relatively good
physician/population ratios. Relevant cases here are Spain, which ranked
99th in spending but 24th in population per physician; Greece, which
ranked 87th in spending, but 11th in population per physician; and
Iceland, which ranked 74th and 20th on the two indicators.

In terms of the impact public spending has on the health status of a
people, several points should be emphasized to explain why, as in the case
of the negative correlation between health spending and infant mortality
rate (–0.40), there does not appear to be a positive relationship between
policy effort and accomplishment.

First, there exists a time lag between public investment in health and
improvement in infant mortality and life expectancy rates. Countries like
Zaire, Zambia, and Swaziland will have to wait years before their public
health investment pays off.

Second, there is a whole series of social, cultural, and demographic
factors prevalent in developing nations that interrupt the nexus between
health policy and performance. Included among these factors are continued reliance on traditional rather than modern medical services; the
concentration of qualified medical personnel in urban areas, rather than in
rural areas where a majority of the people live; climatic conditions in
which communicable diseases tend to be more prevalent and more difficult to control; and the lack of potentially qualified persons to enter
medical and public health professions. These are among the factors that
intervene between the desire to improve life and the ability to do so.

Third, there is again the issue of the contribution by the private sector
to the overall health status of a nation. For example, in Israel, where
about 70 percent of health care is privately financed, there is an obvious
incongruity between public expenditures (Israel ranked 118th) and health
performance (Israel ranked 23rd in infant mortality and 20th in life expectancy). For reasons discussed above, a similarly incongruous situation exists
in Norway, which ranked 89th in health spending but 1st in life expectancy and 4th in infant mortality.

There is one final point we wish to emphasize with regard to the
relationship between health policy effort and the health status of a people.
Trite as it may sound, money cannot buy good health for individuals or
for a nation – at least not directly. Without proper nutrition, adequate
sanitary facilities, and mass health education programs, substantial expenditure of money has little impact on improving health. Presumably the
incongruity between relatively high levels of spending in Zaire, Zambia,

and Swaziland, for example, and the continued high infant mortality and low life expectancy rates has a good deal to do with the generally low standard of living in these countries. Health care policy provides an excellent illustration of the interaction of several factors in explaining public policy output and performance.

Conclusion

This chapter examines three areas of distributive public policy – spending for defense, education, and health – and tries to account for relative differences and similarities in levels of public spending among nations. In the area of defense the major conclusion is that political conditions, particularly those involving the presence or absence of conflict, largely explain how much of its national income a nation devotes to defending itself. Other factors, such as regime type and ideology, have little (or moderate in the case of socialist regimes) impact on defense policy. In aggregate statistical terms, there appears to be only a moderate relationship between national income and defense spending.

In the areas of education and health, however, national income plays an overriding role: Wealthier nations spend more than poorer nations in both policy areas. This conclusion can hardly be viewed with optimism by the 70 percent of the world's people living in developing countries. Given the limited prospects and generally slow progress in economic development, these nations, left to their own devices, appear condemned to low levels of education and health spending for the foreseeable future. On a more sanguine note, the data show that there are exceptions to this overall aggregate trend. Countries such as Zambia, Zaire, Malagasy, and the Ivory Coast have broken rank and, in the areas of education and/or health policy, are spending more than what would be predicted for them. One would hope that farsighted leadership has played some role in these countries.

There is also deviation from the general pattern among countries in which the private sector continues to play an important role in providing health and educational services. Here too, however, national wealth clearly plays a significant role: There must be a sufficiently large private professional class to offer these services and a reasonably large class of people who can afford to purchase them. Such a situation prevails in Spain, Greece, or Argentina; it does not in Ethiopia or Haiti.

The relationship between how much nations spend on defense, education, and health and their accomplishments in these areas is also examined. Without exception, spending is a poor predictor of accomplishment or performance. The role of the private sector, along with a lag between resources and commitment and improvements in education and health contribute, in a number of countries, to a relatively weak relationship among policy, output, and performance.

The analysis in this chapter illustrates how aggregate data analysis, as an instrument in the study of comparative public policy, can be strengthened. It is useful, to be sure, to know that national wealth influences public policy. It is more useful and, we feel, more interesting to identify those countries in which aggregate trends do not hold. Such cases offer the student of comparative policy analysis both academically interesting and socially useful opportunities.

The analysis also draws attention to some of the major weaknesses of multination comparative policy studies. Without a truly encyclopedic knowledge of the personalities, events, structures, culture, and environmental influences on public policy, it is impossible fully to understand or explain the policy activities and accomplishments of 132 nations. Although we are able to disaggregate the data and "peek into" some of the cells, there surely must be some interest in knowing more about why specific governments do what they do. The case studies in Part II are intended to satisfy that interest by examining in greater detail one of the three policy areas discussed in this chapter: health care.

Part II

National health care policy in four nations

Introduction to Part II

State participation in the regulation and/or provision of medical care has a long tradition. Probably the earliest, and certainly the most consistent, form of involvement has been the licensing of medical practitioners. Indian kings, as early as 1500 B.C., required all new medical graduates to demonstrate their professional competence before royal assent to practice was granted. Ostensibly, these and other regulations were intended to protect the public from incompetent and unscrupulous physicians. In practice, these regulations have had the effect of limiting the number of physicians in a society and thereby improving the physicians' social and economic position.

State responsibility in the actual provision, as opposed to the regulation, of medical care had its origins in the sixteenth century. Publicly financed medical care at that time was, however, limited to impoverished elements in society. Thus, under the Elizabethan Poor Laws, local authorities assumed, or more accurately had imposed upon them, the responsibility for the health care needs of paupers within their jurisdiction.

For the most part, collective responsibility and concern for the health care needs of the mass of the working population were provided by private rather than public institutions. Craft guilds and, later on, mutual aid or friendly societies offered some degree of collective security through health relief funds. Under these arrangements, a worker contributed a set sum to a fund, which he could then draw upon in the event of illness or disability.

Not until the nineteenth century, and the advent of industrialization and urbanization, did the health care of the working class increasingly become the concern of the public sector. Initially, as we have seen in Chapter 2, this involved various public health and sanitary measures. Public health boards, commissions, and departments became part of the local, and in some instances national, administrative structure of most modern nations and many colonial states. Public health care policy was not, however, particularly innovative. To a considerable degree it was merely an extension, although an important one, of the "medical police" or regulatory function that states had been performing, in some cases, for centuries.

The innovative, almost revolutionary, aspect of nineteenth-century health care policy came with the introduction of social insurance. This concept involved the state directly in ensuring the delivery of medical care to the working class and minimizing the financial problems associated with the loss of work owing to sickness or disability. Social insurance, in its various forms, is a hallmark of the modern positive state, and health insurance has become the cornerstone of national health care policy in a majority of those nations that have adopted public health care systems.

There are few modern governments which fail to provide some form of national health care, and few governments of developing nations do not aspire to do so. The state provides health care in so many nations today in large part because such care is demanded and expected. The notion that health care is a *right* to which all citizens are entitled has gained widespread popular acceptance, if not formal government implementation. Today, an essential feature of the general-welfare state in most modern nations is acceptance of the principles that ill health is not a private, but a public, misfortune; that care of the sick is not a private, but a public, responsibility; and that the quality and availability of health care should be based upon citizenship, not social status.

Despite the widespread acceptance of these principles, health care remains a policy area of extraordinary importance and political concern. In the United States in the late 1970s, for example, the issue seems to be when and what kind of national health system the nation will have. In countries such as Great Britain, Sweden, and West Germany, to name a few, the issue is reassessment of national health systems in light of several decades of experience. In many of the less developed countries, the questions are whether they can afford such expensive programs and, if so, which model is the most appropriate. For all these nations, the experiences of others provide a fundamental source of information upon which governments and citizens will make judgments about the nature, content, and direction of health care policy in the decades to come.

In this part of the book we examine the health care systems of four modern nations: Germany, Great Britain, the Soviet Union, and Japan. It is hoped that the case studies will be informative, in the most literal sense of the word: that they will provide knowledge and understanding of health care programs with which most readers have little, if any, acquaintance.

A second and related purpose is to provide a basis for assessing the value, relevance, and performance of these four health care systems. In this regard, each case should be viewed both as an account of a specific national experience and as a general model of, or approach to, providing national health care.

A third purpose is to identify what have been and continue to be the major issues in health care policy. In each country discussed, different factors influenced the timing, nature, content, and scope of the health policy. Despite these differences, the issues each nation faced have been remarkably similar. Although we have chosen to treat the development of health care policy in Germany, Great Britain, the Soviet Union, and Japan as separate studies, the reader is alerted to several recurring themes common to the development of health care in all these nations. Particular attention should be paid to how each nation dealt with some of the following issues:

1. Who should provide health care? Is this exclusively a state function, or should the state and the private sector collaborate? In the Soviet Union the decision was in favor of total state responsibility. In Great Britain during the twentieth century there has been an evolution from a mixed system to one in which the state plays the predominant role. In Japan and Germany there is a mixture of private and public responsibility.

2. Who should receive state-sponsored health care? Should it be universal or available only to a selected portion of the population? Initially, in each of the nations discussed here, priority was placed on providing publicly supported care to the industrial working class. In each case, however, coverage was gradually extended to the entire population, although in the Soviet Union industrial workers continue to occupy a favored position in the system.

3. Should state-sponsored health care be comprehensive and include routine as well as major medical care? On this issue the tendency has been toward more comprehensive coverage in each country.

4. How is the medical system to be financed: by contributory insurance, general taxation, and/or cost sharing? The general trend in each of the countries has been away from reliance upon individual insurance contributions and cost sharing toward general taxation, although this has varied in degree from one country to the next.

5. Who should operate and administer a national health care program: the government, private insurance carriers, fraternal organizations? Here, too, there have been different approaches,

but the trend over the years has been toward increasing state administrative control.

6. What are the role and status of the medical profession in a national health system? In the Soviet case, physicians have never exercised any significant control over health care policy or enjoyed much professional autonomy. In Great Britain and Germany, and in Japan to an even greater degree, physicians have maintained a good deal of professional autonomy, clinical freedom, and policy influence.

These are among the most important issues each nation must consider in formulating a national health care policy.

The final purpose of these case studies is to explain *why* each of the nations chose the particular health care system it did. The following chapters examine each of the issues raised above – the nature and degree of state and private sector participation, the extent of medical coverage, the type of financing, the locus of administrative control, and the role of the medical profession – and try to account for the policies of each system in terms of the scheme described in Chapter 3. It is suggested, for example, that situational factors played the dominant role in placing health care on the policy agenda in each nation and, in part, influenced the content of that policy. In addition, the case studies illustrate the importance of policy diffusion, particularly at the early stages of health care policy development, in each of the nations. They also show how political culture and ideology have affected issues of finance and coverage of state-sponsored health care. For example, the decision by the British Labour Party in 1946 to change from a limited, contributory health insurance system to a universal health service, financed primarily by general taxation, was very much a function of the socialist inclinations of the Labour Party leadership. In each case study, a common set of health care issues is examined and the responses to these issues are explained in terms of a common analytical framework: the accounting scheme. Although the development of health care policy in Germany, Great Britain, the Soviet Union, and Japan is presented as four separate case studies, the issues involved and the explanations for the policies chosen are analyzed using a common measure, making implicit, and in some instances explicit, comparisons possible.

Because current policy is often rooted in the past, and particularly in past policy experiences, the analysis in each case is historical in perspective. We examine both current and past health care policies in each country and the impact that situational, cultural, structural, and environmental factors have had on these policies.

Selecting cases

We conclude this introduction to Part II with some comments about the reasons for selecting these four nations. Comparative research necessarily involves a sampling or selection procedure. The researcher chooses, from a given universe (e.g., all nation-states), a manageable number of cases to study. These case studies provide data or generate, confirm, or reject hypotheses about the relationships among variables.[1]

The sampling procedure is, or should be, governed by theoretically defensible considerations.[2] Inevitably, however, practical and pragmatic factors also influence the sampling process – for example, limitations in the researcher's time, resources, and expertise. In our case, several factors guided the selection of health care policies in Germany, Great Britain, the Soviet Union, and Japan for detailed study.

First, we were committed, for reasons noted above, to a historical perspective. Therefore, we chose nations that had long-established national health care systems. This afforded us the opportunity to examine and explain the circumstances under which national health care programs were adopted and the reasons for changes in those programs. In addition, we felt it necessary to compare nations over roughly the same period of time, in terms of both duration and historical equivalency. All too often comparative research has involved comparing, for example, the policies of Nazi Germany or Stalinist Russia with those of contemporary America or Great Britain. We reject such comparisons as being ahistorical and basically invalid.

Second, we wanted to test certain generalizations or assumptions concerning the impact of situational factors on public policy making. Of particular interest were the policy consequences of war (in the form of "displacement" and an "inspection process") and of regime change. The impact of situational factors is most likely to be revealed in a longitudinal study.

Third, given the convincing evidence concerning the impact of aggregate level socioeconomic factors on social policy, we felt it necessary to hold some of these variables constant so that we could better account for the similarities and differences among systems. We thus decided to choose from among the *relatively* more populous and affluent, highly literate, modern, industrial nations. We recognize, of course, the considerable difference between a nation with a population of 56 million persons (Great Britain) and one of 252 million persons (the Soviet Union). Nevertheless, it seems to us that this difference in scale or magnitude is of less consequence than, for example, the difference between nations of 8 million (Sweden) and 56 million people. Similarly, although the difference between a per capita GNP of $2,789 (the Soviet Union) and a per capita

GNP of $6,201 (West Germany) is substantial, it is less significant than, say, the difference between per capita GNPs of $145 (Haiti) and $2,789.

Having ensured relative comparability in terms of length of health care policy experience and level of socioeconomic development, we then turned to selecting nations that differed in certain intuitively and demonstrably important respects. We were particularly interested in examining and comparing the impact of political ideology and culture on health care policy. It seemed essential, therefore, to include a variety of regime types and ideological systems. In addition, some geographical and cultural variety was considered, if not essential, desirable. Including an Asian, African, or Latin American country offered the opportunity to examine the policy consequences of a non-Western cultural system, as well as to fill an enormous gap in the literature. A communist nation recommended itself for similar reasons.

Given the above requirements, the sampling process was relatively easy. There are only 15 nations in existence today that have had a long enough experience with some form of national health care program to meet our longevity requirement. Each of these is among the first generation of nations to adopt a national policy. These nations are Germany (1883), Austria (1888), Hungary (1891), Luxembourg (1901), Norway (1909), Great Britain (1911), Russia and Romania (1912), Bulgaria (1918), Czechoslovakia and Portugal (1919), Poland (1920), Japan and Greece (1922), and Chile (1924). From this group, one nation self-selected: Germany. Germany was the first nation to adopt a national health insurance program. As such, it exercised enormous influence over other first-generation nations as well as many more recent adopters.

Japan too was a relatively easy choice. It was the first Asian nation to adopt a national system and was one of the few non-Western nations that met our other criteria.

The British and Soviet health care models have received enormous international attention and, in the case of the Soviet system, emulation. Both provide more extensive state participation than either the German or the Japanese system. Nevertheless, each represents a different model or approach to the provision of medical care. The Soviet Union and Great Britain were chosen from the list of eligible nations on the basis of the variety they offered in policy approach and political system, as well as the general interest they have provoked.

It is clear that in the future more and more people throughout the world will have their health care needs provided, in whole or part, by the state. Because health care policy, like most policy, reflects the unique features of each society, no two systems will be identical. Nevertheless, as we emphasized before, to a remarkable extent nation-states share similar problems and adopt similar solutions. Therefore, we can expect that the historical experiences and public policy responses of some nations have been or will be repeated by others. The reader may judge for himself which of the systems, if any, is the most worthy of emulation.

5

Germany: the pioneer
in national health care

Rarely, if ever, in modern history has a single piece of legislation had such a profound worldwide impact as the German Sickness Insurance Law of 1883 – the cornerstone of German health care policy for almost one century.[1] Chapter 6 describes the extent of that impact on Lloyd George and his assistants in preparing the British National Health Insurance Act of 1911. While British policy makers took inspiration from the German model, the British medical profession fueled its members' fears and mounted its attack on the proposed national health insurance plan with accounts of the plight of its German colleagues. Professional medical publications, such as the *British Medical Journal* and *Lancet,* regularly carried stories of how poorly the German medical profession had fared under national sickness insurance.[2] In the United States too, the medical profession and the general public periodically were warned: Don't Copy Germany's Mistakes.[3]

The irony of all this attention is that, at least initially, German health care policy had greater political impact, and was deemed more important, outside Germany than within. Of the three major pieces of social welfare legislation introduced by Chancellor Otto von Bismarck in the 1880s – sickness insurance (1883), accident insurance (1884), and invalidity and old-age insurance (1889) – the health care bill caused the least controversy and was of the least interest to Bismarck.

Despite its "inconspicuous start,"[4] the sickness insurance program shortly became a major concern of German policy makers and interest groups. The original law has been amended hundreds of times and has been often surrounded by controversy. This chapter examines this pioneering effort – "a leap into the dark," as Bismarck once called it – tracing the social and political conditions, as well as the personal motivation, that prompted its introduction. The major changes in the original scheme and German national health care policy in general also are examined. The chapter concludes with a description and evaluation of the current system.

In terms of the accounting scheme, we see the interplay of situational,

structural, and cultural factors, and the relatively minimal role of environmental factors, in the formation and development of German health care
policy. Of these, situational factors loom particularly large.

Before we turn to a discussion of the origins of the sickness insurance
law, it is necessary to alert the reader to a shortcoming in the approach
followed in this and subsequent chapters. Case studies that focus on a
single policy distort political reality. Rarely are policy makers preoccupied
with a single issue. The policy agenda typically includes several issues that
compete for the time, attention, and resources of the policy makers and
the general public. The Sickness Insurance Law of 1883 was one part – and
the least important from Bismarck's perspective – of a social reform
program. Indeed, one could argue that the health measure was adopted as
readily as it was because it was less "radical" than Bismarck's other
reforms. The existence of several issues on the policy agenda influences the
saliency, timing, content, and likelihood of acceptance of a particular
policy decision.

Unfortunately, a longitudinal study of even a single policy issue cannot
do justice to the interaction and consequence of competing or supporting
policy issues. Our focus here is on health care policy. We remind the
reader that decisions affecting health care policy did not occur in a
vacuum.

Origins of national sickness insurance

Structural changes

In accounting for the development of national health care policy in Germany in the latter part of the nineteenth century, one must distinguish
between (1) general and long-term socioeconomic conditions and (2) the
more immediate political and personal motivation of Bismarck. With
regard to the former, we have outlined already the story of European
industrialization and its social, economic, and political consequences. The
case of Germany differs little from the situation in other industrializing
nations. Although industrialization began somewhat later in Germany
than in Britain, France, or the United States, once begun it proceeded
rapidly. The German takeoff period of sustained economic growth is
generally placed between the 1850s and the 1870s. The magnitude and
velocity of the process can be seen in certain key economic areas. Growth
in the German railway system, both a requirement and measure of
industrialization, is one such area. In 1850 there were 3,720 miles of rail-
road tracks in Germany; by 1880 there were 21,018 miles of track. Production in the key industrial areas of coal and iron also demonstrates this

Table 5-1. *Population growth of major German cities, 1850-80 (in thousands)*

City	1850	1880	Percent increase
Berlin	419	1,122	168
Bremen	53	112	111
Cologne	97	145	49
Dortmund	11	67	509
Dresden	97	221	128
Düsseldorf	27	95	252
Essen	9	57	533
Frankfurt-am-Main	65	137	111
Hamburg	132	290	120
Hannover	29	123	324
Leipzig	63	149	137
Munich	110	230	109
Nuremberg	54	100	85
Stuttgart	47	117	149

Source: B. R. Mitchell, *European Historical Statistics* (New York: Columbia University Press, 1975), pp. 76–8.

growth. The output of the Ruhr hard coal mining industry increased from about 2 million tons in 1850 to over 22 million tons in 1880. Pig iron production rose from 208,000 tons to 2.7 million tons over the same period.[5] Finally, employment in the machinery industry rose from 51,000 workers in 1861 to 356,000 in 1882.[6]

Predictably, industrialization was accompanied by substantial demographic changes. The most profound of these were the urbanization and proletarianization of the population. In 1867 there were 2 million factory workers; in 1882 there were 6 million. Overall, the working class increased from one-fifth of the population in 1870 to one-fourth in 1882 and one-third in 1901.[7] The urban population grew from 28 percent in 1858 to 47 percent of 1890. More important than the overall rate of urbanization was the rapid growth of major industrial and financial centers. Table 5-1 records the phenomenal growth of major cities during Germany's economic takeoff period. Clapham colorfully describes it as "a whole nation rushing to town."[8]

The growth of the cities was largely the result of rural migration, particularly from Prussia. The movement of peasants and agricultural workers was the result of such conditions as the weakening of traditional social ties in the wake of the revolutionary ferment of 1848, low agricultural wages, increasingly uneconomical small landholdings, demand for labor at deceptively attractive wages, German unification, and perhaps most importantly, the extension of the railway system, which facilitated the rush to the towns. For many who sought a better life in the cities and towns, the experience was somewhat less than exhilarating. Many found "oppressive working conditions, low wages, long hours of work, ruthless exploitation of children and women and other abuses, all of which were typical of the economic and social conditions of wage earners in the early stages of industrialization."[9]

Rural migrants were not the only ones adversely affected by urbanization and industrialization. The mechanization of traditional craft industries (e.g., cutlery, cabinetmaking, clockmaking, textiles) either eliminated or drastically reduced the need for independent skilled craftsmen. Even in the industries where hand skills were still required, craftsmen found themselves laboring under new, more impersonal, often unsafe industrial conditions.

In addition to the radically different workplace conditions, the newly emerging German proletariat faced considerable social and economic insecurity. Traditional protective mechanisms, such as a paternal landlord, guild societies, or local welfare institutions, were either unavailable or inadequate to provide assistance during times of need. Public health problems caused by rapid urbanization and unsafe workplaces increased such occasions. For the worker, one possible, indeed logical, source of assistance at such times was the state itself. We have already seen that the Prussian state traditionally had performed social welfare functions as part of its Christian-paternal mandate. Therefore, one might expect the state to have responded to the social insecurity created by industrialization. And, as we shall see below, to a certain extent it did. However, the overall effort was limited by the dominance of laissez-faire thinking at the time. The period from 1850 to the 1870s was not only a time of accelerated industrialization, it was also "the heyday of German Liberalism."[10] German Liberals counseled the virtues of economic freedom and socioeconomic self-help. "Work and save. Let your own need be the stimulus, and the enjoyments of those better-off the incentive that gives you the drive to increase your will power to take the first steps on the road to salvation from economic distress."[11]

The German working class apparently was not particularly impressed by such exhortations. However, some self-help workingmen's organizations did develop in the 1850s, and a number of industrial employers offered private health and accident insurance to employees. For example, in 1856 Krupp industries, one of Germany's greatest industrial enterprises, introduced compulsory health insurance for its employees with the company paying one-half of the premium.[12] But neither these nor the scattered instances of state assistance could meet the ever-increasing needs of the German working class.

The argument that the workingman was his own source of salvation was heard from other quarters as well. In the early 1860s the message was frequently repeated by Ferdinand Lassalle, a major figure in the German socialist movement. Lassalle argued that only through their own efforts could workers achieve economic and social freedom. He believed that exploitation of the workers would end only when they acquired the means of production. Specifically, he envisioned the establishment of worker-owned cooperatives, established with capital provided by the state. As a practical matter, the workers would first have to acquire universal suffrage in order to influence the state. German socialism, whose birth is generally associated with the ideas and efforts of Lassalle, was to have a profound impact on social policy making for the rest of German history – with the exception of the Nazi period.

The history of the German socialist movement is an interesting, but complex, subject.[13] It would take us too far afield even to attempt to do it justice. Suffice it here to note that on August 7, 1869, in Eisenach, the Social Democratic Workers' Party (later called the Social Democratic Party) was founded by Wilhelm Liebknecht and August Bebel, two men who had disassociated themselves from the followers of Lassalle.[14] Between 1869 and 1875, the socialist movement was racked by feuding between rival factions. In May 1875, the major groups, including the followers of Karl Marx and Friedrich Engels as well as of Lassalle, reconciled their differences at a convention in Gotha and issued a party program. The Gotha Program committed the socialists to work ''with every legal means for a free state and socialist society.'' Specifically, the party sought greater political and personal freedom and improved working conditions for the laboring class.

Support for the Social Democrats grew rapidly, although erratically for reasons explained below, between 1871 and 1890 (Table 5–2). By the election of 1877, when it received nearly 0.5 million votes, the conservative regime of Chancellor Bismarck began taking the socialists much more seriously. Bismarck correctly perceived a rising, and potentially threatening, tide of working-class discontent implicit in the electoral returns.

Regime reaction

The negative phase

In 1878 two attempts were made on the life of Kaiser Wilhelm I. Although neither assailant had socialist connections, Bismarck used the attacks as a pretext for punishing the German socialist movement. After the first unsuccessful attempt on May 11, Bismarck proposed an anti-socialist bill, only to have it rejected by the Reichstag. When a second assailant (on June 2) succeeded in severely wounding the aged emperor,

Table 5-2. *Growth in support for the German Social Democrats; 1871-90*

Election year	Social Democratic vote	Percent of vote	Reichstag seats[a]
1871	124,655	3.0	2
1874	351,952	6.8	9
1877	493,288	9.1	12
1878	437,158	7.6	9
1881	311,961	6.1	12
1884	549,990	9.7	24
1887	763,128	10.1	11
1890	1,427,298	19.7	35

[a] Under the system of electoral representation in effect during the period, the less populous rural areas were overrepresented in the Reichstag, and the urban areas, in which the Social Democrats were strongest, were underrepresented. Thus, the number of Reichstag seats does not accurately reflect the growing strength of the socialists.
Source: William D. P. Bliss and Rudolph M. Binder (eds.), *The New Encyclopedia of Social Reform* (New York: Arno Press, 1970), p. 1141.

Bismarck had the Reichstag dissolved, called new elections, and campaigned for his antisocialist bill. The Social Democrats suffered a moderate setback in the 1878 elections, experiencing the first electoral decline since the founding of the empire in 1871 (Table 5-2). The newly elected parliament passed the Act Against the Aims of Social Democracy Dangerous to the Commonwealth, which went into effect in October 1878.

The law prohibited "the formation or existence of organizations which seek by social democratic, socialistic or communistic movements to subvert the present State and society."[15] The police were empowered to prohibit or dissolve socialist meetings, organizations, and publications, as well as to restrict the freedom of movement and choice of domicile of those identified as Socialists or Communists. The law did not prohibit Social Democratic members of parliament from holding their seats, nor did it interfere with parliamentary elections or debates. The initial impact of the Anti-Socialist Law was considerable. Hundreds of persons were either imprisoned or forced to leave their homes, 150 periodicals were forced to cease publication, and hundreds of books and pamphlets were confiscated. In addition, Social Democratic reverses in the 1878 Reichstag election were followed by a further decline in 1881 – from about 437,000 votes in 1878 to about 312,000 in 1881.

Despite this obvious setback, the Anti-Socialist Law ultimately was a failure. Although the law took a heavy organizational toll, the Social

Democratic Party survived its onslaught, and by 1884 party support began
a period of sustained growth.

The positive phase

The Anti-Socialist Law was renewed in 1880, 1884, and 1886.
Thus Bismarck did not completely abandon the negative dimension of his
attack. Yet he recognized as a matter of political expediency and personal
conviction that some positive measures were necessary to win support of
the rapidly growing and potentially powerful working class. It was the
desire to assure industrial working-class allegiance to the empire and to
preserve a system to which he was so firmly committed that prompted
Bismarck's social reform program. Bismarck is reported to have told one
admirer of his efforts that the purpose of the reform was "to bribe the
working classes, or, if you like, to win them over to regard the State as a
social institution existing for their sake and interested in their welfare."[16]

The reform program was launched in the spring of 1881 with the introduction of the Accident Insurance Bill. In a series of imperial and ministerial messages during 1881, Bismarck, directly or through the emperor,
provided the rationale for social insurance. We quote two of these statements at length, for they reveal, with remarkable candor and clarity, the
motivation and reasoning of their author. A Memorandum of Explanation
(*Begrundung*) to the first Accident Insurance Bill, dated March 8, 1881,
noted:

That the State should interest itself to a greater degree than hitherto in those of its
members who need assistance, is not only a duty of *humanity and Christianity* – by
which State institutions should be permeated – but a duty of *State-preserving
policy*, whose aim should be to cultivate the conception – and that, too, amongst
the nonpropertied classes, which form at once the most numerous and the least
instructed part of the population – *that the State is not merely a necessary but a
beneficent institution.* These classes must . . . be led to regard the State not as an
institution contrived for the protection of the better classes of society, but as one
serving their own needs and interests. The apprehension that a Socialistic element
might be introduced into legislation if this end were followed should not check us.
So far as that may be the case it will not be an innovation but the further development of the modern State idea, the result of Christian ethics, according to which
the State should discharge, besides the defensive duty of protecting existing rights,
the positive duty of promoting the welfare of all its members, and especially, those
who are weak and in need of help, by means of judicious institutions and the
employment of those resources of the community which are at its disposal.[17]

Bismarck's social reform package was announced on November 17,
1881, in an imperial message to the Reichstag. The emperor referred not
only to the Accident Insurance Bill, which already had been submitted,
but also to proposals for health and disability and old-age insurance. The
message stated:

The remedy of social ills cannot be exclusively achieved through the repression of

Social Democratic excesses but must at the same time envisage constructive measures for the improvement of the workers' welfare. We regard it Our Imperial duty again to charge the Reichstag with the task and We should review with greater satisfaction the successes with which God has visibly blessed Our reign if We could one day be certain to have left Our Fatherland new and permanent guarantees for its internal peace and to those in need that greater security and more generous assistance to which they are entitled.[18]

These official pronouncements provide an interesting picture of the motives behind the reform program. There is, first, recognition that negative, repressive measures alone would not defeat the Social Democrats or woo away their working-class supporters. State action of a positive nature was needed to convince the proletariat of the beneficence of the regime, to secure their support, and thereby, to preserve the Reich. Such a policy would be natural in a paternalistic system based on Christian morality and a concern for humanity. The phrases Bismarck most frequently used to describe the reform program were "state socialism" and "practical Christianity on legislative display."

Thus, through the welfare reforms of the 1880s the concept of the "positive state" was formally introduced in Germany – and, by way of policy example, in much of the rest of the world. That its original purpose was the maintenance of an authoritarian, conservative regime does not detract, in our view, from the incalculable contribution it made to the development of the positive state ideology of the twentieth century.

The Sickness Insurance Bill

We turn now from the general issue of social reform to the specific one of sickness insurance. As noted earlier, of the three "state-preserving" reform measures, sickness insurance was the least controversial.

The relatively undramatic and uncontentious birth of this extraordinary legislation can be accounted for by two main factors: (1) it was not particularly radical in the context of existing German social policy, and (2) the provisions of the law offended few.

Health care had long been a matter of public concern in the German states. As early as 1623, the Prussian government had begun setting doctors' fees. More importantly, prior to 1883 the state already was involved in certain compulsory insurance schemes. These generally were limited to critical industries and involved state oversight or regulation.[19] Particularly noteworthy were the long-established miners' relief funds in Prussia (*Knappschaftkassen*). In 1854 a law made the organization of such funds *compulsory* for all mine workers. Benefits included free medical aid, pensions, funeral benefits, and aid to widows and orphans. The insurance was financed by equal contributions from miners and employers and was administered by an executive committee composed of an equal number of both parties. In 1876, 264,000 persons were enrolled in these funds.

Prussia took the lead in other industrial insurance programs as well. In 1845 and 1849 laws were enacted empowering local authorities to require journeymen in handicraft industries and, later, factories to insure their workers against illness. In addition, the above-mentioned 1854 law required the establishment of sick relief societies in certain industries and provided for local administration, compulsory membership, and employer contributions. In 1874 there were 5,000 industrial relief societies in Prussia with 800,000 members.

Whereas Prussia often took the initiative, other German states adopted similar, although generally more limited, measures. In the South German states of Bavaria, Würtemberg, and Baden local authorities were empowered to charge unmarried workers and domestic servants a weekly premium in return for medical care.

In addition to the state-supported or state-encouraged sickness insurance programs, there were voluntary programs run by private insurance companies, trade unions, craft guilds, and industrial employers. In 1876, with Germany unified under the kaiser, the government enacted a health insurance law that sought to regulate these private insurance funds. The intention of the law was to eliminate certain abuses and to encourage voluntary insurance programs for workers. In addition, the law gave local governments the option to make health insurance compulsory on a local basis. The law was not particularly successful. Few local governments exercised the option, and private voluntary efforts developed slowly.

Despite the failure of the 1876 law, by 1883 when the Sickness Insurance Law was passed, Germany had both organizational and experiential bases for a system of compulsory sickness insurance. Although innovative in terms of its national scope, the 1883 law was by no means a radical policy departure for the German state.

A second reason for the comparatively calm acceptance of the Sickness Insurance Bill was that it threatened few of the powerful ideas or institutions in Germany. The bill envisioned a relatively minor administrative and financial role for the national government. Administration was to be decentralized, using, whenever possible, existing public and private institutions. In addition, the program would be privately, not publicly, financed. These provisions contrasted significantly with those of Bismarck's earliest effort at social insurance: the first (and unsuccessful) Accident Insurance Bill of 1881. The Accident Insurance Bill proposed a powerful and highly centralized Imperial Insurance Office, excluded private insurance organizations, and involved a state subsidy.[20] The bill was attacked from all positions on the German political spectrum. The trade unions and Social Democrats feared the "bribe" might work and reduce their support among the workers. The Center and Right opposed both the centralizing tendency inherent in the proposed Imperial Insurance Office, as well as the government subsidy. As a result, the first Accident Insurance Bill was rejected by the Reichstag.

The Sickness Insurance Bill omitted many objectionable features, including a state subsidy, while at the same time incorporating many existing insurance carriers. As a result, it was much more acceptable to parliament than the accident insurance proposal. From Bismarck's perspective, however, the bill did not hold the political promise of his other reforms. "Bismarck apparently had less interest in health insurance because its assistance to the worker was of a short-term nature and would not be effective in creating ties to the state."[21]

On May 31, 1883, the Reichstag approved the Sickness Insurance Bill by a vote of 216 to 99. The Social Democrats voted against the measure. The bill became law on June 15, 1883, but its operation was postponed until December 1, 1884, so that a companion accident insurance law could be passed.

Interest groups and the Sickness Insurance Bill

Before we examine the Sickness Insurance Law, it is worth noting here the role played by groups with an apparent interest in the program. What role did the medical profession, workers, employers, and existing insurance carriers play? The answer is almost none. Imperial Germany was an authoritarian system in which public policy was largely a product of imperial, ministerial, and bureaucratic design. It was not a pluralistic democracy in which diverse groups competed for power and influence over policy. Policy initiative flowed from above, although, as we have seen, it could be in response to demands or pressures from below. The Reichstag, which Bismarck generally held in contempt, could influence, as in the case of the Accident Insurance Bill, the course of legislation. It was not, however, an independent, competing source of power.

Interest groups, of the sort found in Western democracies today, either did not exist or were relatively new and politically impotent. A case in point is the medical profession. One would expect a high degree of interest and activity on the part of physicians. Yet, there was virtually none. Henry Sigerist, one of the earliest students of comparative health policy, reported that in researching the origins of the sickness insurance bill

we looked up the leading journals of the period and also consulted dozens of autobiographies of contemporary physicians. It was rather surprising to find that with very few exceptions neither the journals nor the biographies mention sickness insurance . . . The medical profession was not consulted when the bills were in the making and apparently did not care to be consulted.[22]

How does one explain the lack of interest on the part of the medical profession? One explanation is that physicians were poorly organized. German doctors did not have an independent, nationwide professional association to represent their interests until 1900. There were various local medical societies whose main concern was to protect the public image of the profession and to police professional standards. Membership was voluntary, and not all physicians chose to join the associations. In 1873 the *Aerztevereinbund* ("Union of Medical Societies") was founded in Leipzig. Although the purpose of the union included "the furtherance of medical science and art, as well as of the material interests of the profession," there is no evidence that the union sought influence in the drafting of the insurance law or took any official position on the issue.[23]

A second factor explaining the absence of medical interest is that physicians apparently did not believe the law would have much impact on their lives. Originally, it was to cover only a very small and poor segment of the working population. And the majority of the physicians had little contact with this group. The poor generally went unattended or received care in charity institutions. The typical worker consulted a physician only in times of great need. On the limited occasions when they did treat the poor, physicians often did so without payment. Furthermore, many of the existing insurance companies offered their members only cash and funeral benefits, not medical care. In short, the working poor and the medical profession had little contact at the time in Germany.[24] Hence, physicians did not see the new law as a threat to their economic interests or the nature of medical practice. If anything, the introduction of compulsory sickness insurance might provide a new source of income. These two factors, in addition to the generally unfavorable political environment for interest group activity, resulted in no visible impact, and no desire for any, by the medical profession on the Health Insurance Bill.

A similar lack of interest and activity characterized the behavior of other groups. Employers, for example, did not view the law as making extraordinary demands upon them, particularly as some already were contributing to voluntary schemes. The bill, as we shall see shortly, compulsorily insured only the poorest of the industrial wage earners and required a relatively small contribution. In addition, many employers agreed with Bismarck's political goal of defusing worker discontent by reform measures. Sickness insurance particularly recommended itself, for it appeared to have the additional virtue of increasing worker productivity.

Perhaps the most vocal, but by no means effective, opposition came from the Social Democrats. In part this opposition stemmed from the belief that the measure did not deal with the most critical needs of the workers: improved working conditions, better wages, property ownership.

In addition, there was the fear that Bismarck's "bribe" just might work and thereby weaken support for the party.

In short, none of the groups that one might expect to be either keenly interested or politically influential had much impact on the legislation. Such indolence and/or impotence eventually changed.

The Sickness Insurance Law (1883)

The original Sickness Insurance Bill requires our attention for two reasons. The first and most important is that it has been the basis of German national health care policy for almost one century. Unlike England and Russia, which moved from health insurance to health service systems, Germany has maintained contributory insurance as the basis of its health policy. Second, the bill was assiduously studied and highly influential in the development of health insurance schemes in other countries. Thus, an examination of the German insurance law provides the basis for understanding and explaining the development of health care policy in other nations.

Eligibility

The Sickness Insurance Law came into effect in December 1884. It provided for compulsory participation by all industrial wage earners (i.e., manual laborers) in factories, ironworks, mines, shipbuilding yards, and similar workplaces. There was no income limit for this poorest, and presumably most politically dangerous, segment of the working class. Almost immediately (in 1885), coverage was extended to workers in commercial enterprises and, in 1886, to some farm workers as well. An income limit for salaried employees in both commerce and industry was set at 2,000 marks (approximately $500). The law did not cover self-employed persons, dependents, or those earning above the income limit in commerce and industry. Even with the extension of coverage in 1885 and 1886, the proportion of the population covered during these early years remained quite low: 10.5 percent in 1886 and 14.3 percent in 1890.

Financing

The program was financed by joint employee and employer contribution – the state, contrary to Bismarck's original intention, made no contribution. Workers were to pay two-thirds and employers one-third of the premium. The total contribution was limited by law to a maximum of between 3 and 6 percent (depending on the type of fund) of the worker's daily wage although in practice most paid less. At the turn of the century the premium ranged from 3 to 30 cents per week or $5 to $17 per year.[25]

Benefits

The premise underlying the Sickness Insurance Law was that vulnerable segments of the population should, when taken ill, have access to medical assistance and that they and their dependents should receive income maintenance during periods of illness. Under the original law, the worker was entitled to four types of benefits: medical, cash, maternity, and funeral.

The medical benefit provided free routine medical and dental care at home or in a physician's office, prescribed medicines, and incidental treatment for up to 13 weeks. Where hospitalization was necessary, the patient was entitled to free complete medical care and accommodations in a third-class room (i.e., multibed ward) for up to 26 weeks.

The law also provided a maternity benefit in the form of free medical attention and a lump sum cash benefit for 3 weeks after confinement.

Finally, the law provided a cash funeral benefit for a deceased worker's family, ranging from 20 to 40 times the basic daily wage of the worker.

Administration

At the administrative heart of the sickness insurance system, then and now, are the insurance funds. For both practical and political reasons, Bismarck chose to use existing organizations wherever possible to administer the provisions of the law. As a practical matter, it made sense to use the existing insurance institutions described earlier. These institutions had the experience of administering insurance programs and would save the government the time and money of having to establish an elaborate bureaucratic apparatus.

It also made good political sense. The trade unions and guilds, in particular, were jealous of their position as providers of insurance for their members. Thus, of the six types of "sickness funds" (*Krankenkassen*) recognized as legal insurance carriers in 1883, four were based upon existing organizations: building trade, miners, guild, and industrial sickness funds.

Where no organizations existed, the law provided for the establishment of two new types of funds. One was the local or "district funds" (*Ortskrankenkassen*), which were established on a territorial basis by a municipality for one or more trades within its jurisdiction. The second type of new fund was modeled after the South German system of parochial or communal insurance. This too was a territorially based fund and required local, usually rural, authorities to insure any eligible persons not covered by other insurance funds. In practice, as more persons were brought into the insurance system, the two new territorial funds became the largest carriers. Thus, by 1905, 59 percent of all the insured belonged to either a local or a rural sickness fund. In any event, the decentralized nature of the insurance system, so strongly supported by the political Right and Center, was realized. In 1885, there were 18,942 sickness funds.

The insurance funds were granted legal status by the government and given considerable administrative autonomy. The law specified minimum benefits and maximum contributions only. It left each individual sickness fund considerable discretion to set specific benefit and contribution levels. The wealthier funds could provide larger cash benefits than the law required, longer periods of coverage, and extra benefits (e.g., false teeth, health resorts, care for dependents).

The insurance funds were governed by an executive committee chosen by a general assembly of workers and employers. Representation reflected the rate of contribution: Workers had two-thirds of the votes in the general assembly; employers had one-third. The executive committee of each fund negotiated contracts with physicians to provide medical care for the members. The physician received payment directly from the insurance fund. The basis or type of remuneration depended upon the specific sickness fund. The most commonly used was a capitation fee, whereby the fund paid a lump sum for each of its members. This total sum was divided among the physicians who worked for the sickness fund. Where the fund was large enough, and many were not, the patient could choose from a panel of physicians working for a particular fund.

In sum, the management of the sickness insurance program, in virtually all its aspects, was assigned by law to the several thousand sickness funds throughout Germany. Administratively, the funds were under the supervision of the local authorities in the form of insurance offices. Ultimate authority for the supervision of the system and the arbitration of disputes rested with the administratively weak Imperial Insurance Office.

Operation

In practice, the operation of the insurance system was remarkably simple. A worker was automatically insured upon entering employment in an industry or occupation in which insurance was compulsory. The worker had no choice with regard to the specific sickness fund in which he was enrolled. He was assigned automatically to the fund in the place where he worked or lived. The employer paid the entire premium directly to the sickness fund for each insured worker and deducted the worker's share from his wages.

When taken ill, the worker went for treatment to a physician contracted by the particular fund. If the illness lasted longer than 3 days, and was certified as legitimate by the physician, the worker became eligible for a cash benefit, which the fund administered.

Conclusion

If election returns are any indication, Bismarck's attempts to undermine Social Democratic support by "bribing" the working class with social insurance did not work. Following reversals in the Reichstag elections of 1878 and 1881, Social Democratic support again grew among the voters. Between 1884 (the year in which the Sickness Insurance Law went into effect) and 1890 (the year Bismarck was removed from office), Social Democratic support rose from 549,990 votes (9.7 percent of the total) to 1,427,298 votes (or 19.7 percent of the total). However, it could be argued, and indeed was in later years, that these reforms bought social peace for Germany. In a 1911 report to the Royal Commission on University Education in London, Dr. Friedrich von Muller of the University of Munich, described the considerable financial costs of the German insurance program. But he went on to ask: "Should we not characterise it as expenses paid for the prevention of social war?"[26] Regardless of its real or imagined political impact, sickness insurance had become an integral part of German social policy. We can now examine how it progressed following its rather modest beginning.

The development of German national health care policy until 1933

The tranquil beginning of the sickness insurance system contrasted sharply with the volatility of its development. Sickness insurance eventually became one of the most hotly debated issues in German domestic policy. With the benefit of hindsight, one of the social scientist's most precious tools, it is easy to see the inevitability of such conflict. The sheer number of the sickness funds (18,942 in 1885 and 23,354 in 1910), differences in their administrative competence and honesty, and variation in benefits, procedures, and contributions were destined to be sources of discontent among various interested parties. In addition, there was the anomalous position of the medical profession. Although critical to its operation, doctors were not an integral part of the program's decision-making structure. It is inconceivable that the system could develop without some redefinition of the role of the physician.

Superimposed upon the problems inherent in the original scheme was the fact that in the first three decades of the twentieth century Germany suffered through a world war, unprecedented inflation, and a disastrous depression. This section examines the development of the sickness insurance system and related health policy issues from roughly 1900 to 1933. Three interrelated themes are developed: (1) although the health insurance system began rather modestly, it proceeded to expand rather ambitiously; (2) this expansion finally stirred the medical profession to action; and (3) both these developments were influenced heavily by the catastrophic events of World War I, the inflation of the early 1920s, and the Great Depression.

Expansion and administrative rationalization of the sickness insurance system

From a limited program for a small portion of the new industrial working class, the sickness insurance program developed into a far more ambitious and encompassing system. Development proceeded along two lines: (1) eligibility was extended to new categories of persons, and (2) benefits were increased. Neither development was linear. War and economic dislocation imposed limitations and caused some retrenchment. But the general trend of enlarging the insurable population and expanding benefits was unmistakable.

Expansion of the insurable population was accomplished in two ways. The first was to extend coverage beyond manual industrial laborers. Between 1885 and 1932 the following groups were brought under compulsory sickness insurance: all agricultural workers (1886 and 1911); transportation workers and salaried employees in offices and industrial enterprises (1903); domestic servants, persons engaged in home industries, and certain groups of professionals (1911); and seamen (1927). In all instances, except for manual industrial workers and domestic servants, an income limit was imposed. The general trend, in these early and subsequent years, and the second major method of extending coverage, was gradually to increase the income limit. For example, from January 1885 to 1904 the ceiling for nonmanual workers was set at 2,000 marks (roughly $500) per year; in 1914 it was raised to 2,500 marks; in 1925 to 2,700 marks; and in 1927 to 3,600 marks. All these changes had the effect of increasing the proportion of the population covered by sickness insurance and broadening its class structure. Whereas in 1885, just under 10 percent of the population (4.7 million people) was insured, by 1932 over one-third of the population (approximately 20 million people) was covered by sickness insurance.

Another area of insurance expansion involved workers' dependents. Prior to World War II, the dependents of insured persons were not compulsorily covered by sickness insurance; this was an optional benefit. Here too, the trend was toward including a larger segment of the population. In 1914, 37 percent of the sickness funds provided some benefit for dependents; by 1925 the proportion had increased to over 85 percent.

In addition, but of lesser importance than the extension of coverage, was an expansion of mandatory benefits. The most important of these was to extend both the medical and cash benefits from 13 to 26 weeks of coverage. The expansionary period of the German sickness insurance system came to a halt between 1929 and 1930, when the worldwide Depression hit Germany. With widespread unemployment (1.4 million in 1929, 3.1 million in 1930, and 6 million in 1932), the contributions to and income of the various insurance schemes declined precipitously. In 1929 total contributions to the health funds were about 2.2 million marks; by 1932, they had declined to 1.3 million marks. The German government responded to the crisis by issuing the Emergency Decree of 1930. The action was intended to stabilize the economic position of the system by increasing revenues and decreasing demands. With this in mind, the emergency legislation imposed a nominal fee, 50 pfennigs (12 cents), for medical care in the form of a doctor's certificate (*Krankenschein*), which the patient purchased from the fund and presented to the physician. It also reduced, or in some instance eliminated, cash benefits and limited "additional" benefits. Although expenditures and demands upon the system (along with revenue) declined, this reduction was partially offset by making insurance coverage for dependents obligatory. This change was in response to deprivation suffered during the Depression. The obligatory extension of coverage to dependents did not have a dramatic impact on the system because about 85 percent of the funds already were voluntarily offering some coverage.

In addition to the expansion of coverage and extension of benefits, the pre–World War II development of German sickness insurance was characterized by administrative rationalization. The number of sickness funds had increased from approximately 19,000 in 1885 to over 23,000 in 1910. Many were small and inefficient. In 1911 the Reichstag passed the Reich Insurance Code, which, among other things, led to the dissolution of more than half of the existing funds. The parochial and building trade funds, which accounted for more than one-third of the funds at the time, were the most heavily hit by the reorganization.[27] In their place the law provided for "general local funds" and "rural" funds, both of which covered a larger geographical area and more workers than the former parochial funds. The effect of the law was dramatic. In 1910 there were over 23,000 funds. By 1914, when the law went into effect, there were 10,000 funds.

The decline in the number of insurance funds did not stop with the 1911 consolidation legislation. In the period following World War I (1918–23) Germany suffered from ruinous inflation, high unemployment, and industrial strife. Although wages rose, they did so much more slowly than prices. The value and purchasing power of the German mark began declining: In 1914 the exchange rate was 8.9 marks to $1 U.S. Inflation reached unparalleled proportions in 1923: In November of that year it cost 4.2 *billion* marks (American billion) to purchase $1 U.S. It was a time when Germans literally needed wheelbarrows of money to purchase goods.

It was also a time when politicians and others began discussing the possibility of completely dismantling the entire insurance system. However, neither the political nor economic climate would allow such drastic measures. Instead, the government responded by trying to shore up the hard-hit insurance system. In 1924 an amendment to the Reich Insurance Code imposed upon the funds more stringent standards of solvency and closer government supervision. The result was that by 1929 the number of sickness funds had declined to 7,418. In addition to the organizational changes, the government, in October 1923, imposed certain cost-saving measures. These included limiting sickness benefits and requiring patients to pay 10 percent of all medication fees.[28]

As the above examples suggest, economic factors of a situational nature clearly influenced the course of insurance development during the first three decades of the twentieth century. There were, however, important political factors, of both situational and structural nature, which helped determine the development, and particularly the expansion, of the system. The war itself had led to a number of changes in the sickness insurance system. The War Law of August 1914 placed limitations on contributions (4.5 percent of gross pay) as well as on the types of services that could be offered by the sickness funds.

The defeat of Germany in World War I resulted in the abdication of Kaiser Wilhelm I, the dissolution of the monarchy, and the establishment of the Weimar Republic in 1919. The Social Democratic Party (SPD), then the largest political party in Germany, reversed its earlier position and became committed to extending social services, not as a matter of state paternalism but as a political right. The democratic and positive state impulses of the republic were canonized in the 1919 Weimar Constitution, which guaranteed not only a panoply of democratic rights but also a comprehensive insurance system. Under the Social Democrats, who played a prominent role in 9 of the 21 national governments from 1919 to 1933 and constituted the largest political party in the Reichstag throughout the period, the expansion of the sickness insurance system described above took place. The impact the Social Democrats exerted on the system was not limited to national policy making. It will be remembered that individual funds were administered by executive committees chosen by worker-dominated general assemblies or local authorities. These administrative bodies tended to be controlled by the SPD and its supporters and, therefore, exerted considerable influence over the day-to-day operation of the funds.

Although the sickness insurance program represented an ideological commitment for some, others in the administration saw it as a territory to be protected for its own sake. George Sulzbach, admittedly no admirer of the German sickness insurance system, argues that "the influences that made for the expansion of social insurance were not all on the ideological side. Much of the driving power behind the movement was furnished by the insurance bureaucracy which had gradually developed into a formidable organization.''[29] Though the assertion is undocumented, it is so consistent with our knowledge of bureaucratic behavior as to demand acceptance.

In conclusion, then, two forces were at work during the period from 1919 to 1932 influencing the course of health care policy. The first were the political forces, particularly the SPD and health insurance bureaucrats, who, for a variety of reasons, favored extension of the system. Except for the period of relative economic prosperity (roughly 1924–9), these expansionary forces were constrained by the second factor: economic realities of inflation and the Depression.

These gross political and economic factors were not, however, the only ones influencing health care policy during the time. Partly in response to various political and economic circumstances, and partly in response to their own professional interests, the medical profession belatedly became one of the most active participants in the health care policy process. We turn now to that story.

The medical profession and health care policy after Bismarck

We argued earlier that the initial lack of interest on the part of the medical profession in regard to sickness insurance was a function of two factors: (1) ineffective professional organization and (2) the judgment that the program would not critically affect the doctors' pecuniary or professional interests. It was not long before both conditions changed. It shortly became obvious that many physicians would have some degree of contact with the roughly 4.7 million persons covered initially by the new law. In the fall of 1884, at the twelfth annual meeting of the German Doctors' Association in Eisenach, the physicians called for a remuneration system based on a fee for each service performed. For the next decade or so, there were scattered and largely ineffective attempts – including strikes – by the doctors to influence the administration of the law and particularly the issues of the type of remuneration and free choice of doctor.[30]

The turning point for the German medical profession came in 1900, with the founding of the Association of German Doctors for the Protection of Their Economic Interests – known also as the Leipziger Verband and, later, the Hartmann-Bund after its founder Dr. Gustav Hartmann. The association developed out of the frustrations and impotence of the physicians in their dealings with both the government and the sickness funds. The factor that precipitated formation of the Leipziger Verband was the failure of the various local physicians' associations to persuade the Reichstag to amend the Sickness Insurance Law in a way that would improve the negotiating position of the doctors vis-à-vis the sickness funds. In an article in a professional journal, *Aerztliches Vereinblatt,* a Dr. Warmiensis called upon the physicians to stop work on January 1, 1900, and press their demands on the Reichstag. In a written response to this plea in the same issue of the journal, Dr. Hartmann asked his colleagues to organize into a national level association.[31] Dr. Hartmann indicated the nature of the problems and the frustration of the physicians in his letter. First, he condemned the various *Land*-sanctioned medical associations, which he charged were "absolutely useless" when it came to protecting the material interests of the doctors. "For that reason we require an organization in which neither the state or any sort of supervisory body can say anything." He also condemned government officials for failing to consult with or even listen to the physicians during deliberations on the sickness insurance legislation. Finally, he attacked the insurance companies, which had ignored the pleas, presentations, and threats of the doctors. In the end Hartmann declared that only self-help would accomplish the doctors' goals. And in a play on the words of Marx and Engels, Hartmann urged: "All doctors of the various German states unite yourselves."[32]

Support for Hartmann's organization grew rapidly – from 8,000 members in 1903 to 23,900 in 1911. In 1903 the German Association of Medical Societies and the Leipziger Verband reached an agreement to join forces. Until it was disbanded by the Nazis, the Hartmann-Bund – as it was called after 1923 – was at the forefront of the doctors' struggle.

The most critical years of the struggle were 1903 to 1914 and 1918 to 1923. The major protagonists were the doctors, the insurance companies, and the government. The primary issues were (1) the level and basis of remuneration – the doctors favored an increase in fees and a fee for each service performed, whereas the funds wanted a low capitation fee; (2) "free choice of doctors" – the doctors wanted the insurance patient to choose any physician he wished, whereas the funds wanted to limit choice to fund doctors; (3) the size of the insurable population – the medical profession wanted to limit public insurance in order to maximize their private practice, whereas the funds favored expansion of the system. The first two issues generally pitted the doctors against the insurance funds; the third issue involved the doctors and the government. The battle lines had been drawn by the original law. The act of 1883 empowered the sickness funds to determine the basis of remuneration and to contract physicians for service in the insurance system. On the other hand, the definition of the compulsorily insured population, in terms either of occupational categories or of income levels, was set by law. The conflict between the doctors and the sickness funds was extraordinarily bitter. Aside from the importance of the issues involved, this bitterness was exacerbated by the ideological and class differences between the two groups. We have already seen that most of the sickness funds were controlled by workers and SPD members or loyalists. Although there were some socialist supporters within the medical profession, the majority was openly hostile to the SPD. The fact that the profession found itself, in the early years of the sickness insurance program, at a distinct disadvantage vis-à-vis the well-organized and well-administered sickness funds clearly irritated the physicians' social as well as professional sensibilities.

Between 1903 and 1911 the doctors battled both the government and the insurance funds over the issues of free choice and fees. The Leipziger Verband established a strike fund and on several occasions used strikes or boycotts to press its demands. What the physicians clearly wanted was some statutory uniformity throughout Germany to govern relations between the funds and the physicians. In 1911 the physicians were presented with just such an opportunity.

In 1910 and 1911 the Reichstag considered the earlier mentioned Reich Insurance Code. It was intended to codify the various laws on social insurance, extend coverage, and reorganize some of the administrative apparatus. In a memorandum accompanying the bill, the government recognized the conflict between the physicians and insurance funds and acknowledged that it was time for government action.

It is lamentable that for many years keen dissensions have occurred between the doctors and the sickness insurance authorities, resulting in many places in bitter disputes and a state of open conflict. Disputes of this kind, however, are often prejudicial to the proper medical care of the sick and lead to serious public injury. The abuses have reached such proportions that legal measures were emphatically called for in the most various quarters as the only practicable course, and in fact it is no longer possible for the legislative bodies to evade the duty of seeking a remedy.[33]

Having acknowledged the problem, however, the government stopped short of the solution preferred by the doctors: statutory guidelines on the issues of remuneration and free choice of physicians. These issues were properly an area of negotiation between the interested parties. Ultimately, the law included a provision that, wherever possible, members of sickness societies should be provided with a choice of at least two doctors. In addition, the law extended coverage by increasing the income limit from 2,000 to 2,500 marks and by including new occupational categories: for example, domestic servants and persons employed in home industries.

The law, as one might imagine, was not enthusiastically received by the medical profession. Because various provisions of the law dealing with the sickness insurance system were not scheduled to take effect until January 1, 1914, the doctors resolved in a general meeting of the Doctors' Association in Stuttgart in June 1911 to withhold medical assistance, through sickness insurance, to any person with an income over 2,000 marks.[34] In the years following the passage of the law, but prior to its implementation, the doctors again turned their attention to the insurance societies. Negotiations between the doctors and individual insurance societies over the issues of remuneration and free choice proceeded slowly and inconclusively in the remainder of 1911 and during 1912. However, as the date of implementation approached, the level of activity increased. This was prompted by the fact that the law included a reorganization of the insurance societies. As noted earlier, their number was drastically reduced by eliminating smaller funds and creating larger general local insurance societies. The doctors were preparing for contract negotiations with the new societies. They wanted to use the opportunity to establish the basic principles of free choice, an "equitable" fee schedule, and recognition of the German Federation of Medical Societies and the Leipziger Verband as the bargaining agents for the physicians. The doctors, in the absence of legislative uniformity, were intent upon negotiating uniform contractual provisions with the societies. The insurance funds, however, were just as committed to bargaining with individual doctors or groups of doctors on the local level.

On October 26, 1913, the German Federation of Medical Societies and the Leipziger Verband held an extraordinary meeting in Berlin and, on a motion by Dr. Hartmann, voted overwhelmingly (454 to 4) "not to enter any compact with any insurance society from this date onward, and unconditionally to decline to carry out contracted medical attendance on old as well as new insured members of the societies." The doctors went on to assure the public that its well-being would not be ignored. People would be treated, but "without the intermediation of the managers of the insurance societies."[35]

By late November 1913, with the prospect of utter chaos in the sickness insurance system becoming more likely, representatives of the national and state governments entered the dispute as mediators between the two parties. In mid-December, with no solution in sight, representatives of the medical faculties of German universities met with the Reich secretary of home affairs and various Prussian state ministers and urged the government to try and reach a fair settlement. The professors promised to use their influence to get the physicians to accept a reasonable settlement. This intervention apparently worked. On Christmas Day 1913 the Berlin Agreement was announced. A key provision of the agreement established district committees in each insurance area consisting of an equal number of doctors and insurance society representatives and an impartial chairman. These committees would draw up contracts, prepare a list of doctors who would constitute the local panel (and thereby provide some choice of physicians), and arbitrate disputes between the doctors and insurance societies. With regard to remuneration, the contracts had to provide a specific rate, but the agreement did not specify the method of remuneration; this would be negotiated by the doctor and the insurance funds. Finally, the Leipziger Verband was recognized as the spokesman for the doctors.[36]

The Berlin Agreement, which governed relations between doctors and the insurance societies for 10 years, brought relative peace to the system. The expiration of the agreement in December 1923 was accompanied by a new wave of physician discontent over many of the unresolved issues. The difference in 1923 was the disastrous inflation described earlier. As a result, the government was not content merely to play the role of arbitrator as it had done in 1913. Instead, it acted forcefully and dictated changes in the system. These were proclaimed in the Emergency Decree for Physicians and Sickness Funds, which became part of the Insurance Code.[37] One of the most important parts of the decree provided for federal regulation of insurance contracts. The amended code provided for the Federal Committee of Doctors and Sickness Funds composed of an equal number of doctors, insurance fund representatives, and neutral third parties. The purpose of the committee was "that of drawing up guiding principles to ensure uniformity and appropriateness in the agreements between funds and doctors."[38] For the remainder of the Weimar Republic, the doctors and insurance societies coexisted in an atmosphere of uneasy peace.

In conclusion, the first three decades of the twentieth century witnessed a fundamental change in the relationship between the medical profession and the sickness insurance system. By 1900 the medical profession had come to realize that national sickness insurance would have a considerable impact on both its economic and professional interests. In that year, over 10 million people (17.6 percent of the population) were covered by compulsory sickness insurance. For the next three decades the doctors fought a losing battle against the expansion of the system. By 1932, almost 19 million people were compulsorily covered, and a large number were voluntarily insured. Prior to 1914, about 80 percent of the medical profession's income came from private practice. Writing in 1931, an American observer of the German system noted that "today the average physician and specialist cannot live without *Krankenkasse* [sickness fund] patients."[39] With the formation of the Leipziger Verband in 1900, the doctors became increasingly aggressive and successful in protecting their interests. The forces of war (which led to a government-sponsored acceleration of medical education and an oversupply of doctors) and economic inflation and then depression (which hit the German middle class, the backbone of private medical practice, especially hard), combined to limit the advances the profession could make during these decades. The rise of

Adolf Hitler and the Nazis was yet another in a series of political and economic traumas effecting German life in general and the medical profession and sickness insurance system in particular. We turn now to that sordid story.

Health care policy under the Nazis

Health care – like all areas of German social, political, and economic policy – was refashioned in the hands of the Nazis to serve the political aims of the regime. Health care policy was of particular interest to the Nazis for two main reasons. First and foremost it was an essential tool in achieving the regime's policy of racial purification and national invigoration. Second, because the *Krankenkassen* were bastions of Social Democratic support, the Nazis were determined to eliminate their influence in the health delivery system.

The latter goal was quickly accomplished. In July 1934 the Nazis instituted an administrative reorganization of the sickness insurance system. Although the basic structure of the system was maintained, important (and typically Nazi) innovations were introduced. Under the law, the practice of self-administration of the insurance funds was abolished. In its place, the law introduced the *Führer* or leadership principle, whereby a single person appointed by an appropriate Reich official exercised the power formerly held by the worker-dominated executive committees. Under the law, the leader, typically a loyal Nazi Party member and permanent government employee, was "advised" by a committee consisting of an equal number of employees and employers as well as physicians and local government representatives. However, by 1939 these advisory committees had been discontinued. Thus, the Nazis were able to eliminate the dominant role of labor unions and Social Democrats in the administration of the sickness insurance system.

The position of doctors was also changed under the Nazis. The medical profession was assigned the role of promoting national strength and fecundity and racial purity. These obligations were explicitly set forth in the 1937 Law for the Regulation of German Physicians. Doctors were directed to encourage procreation and discourage contraception and abortion among the "desirable" Aryan population. The Nazis were convinced that a rapid and sustained increase in population, particularly in light of the declining birth rate following World War I, was necessary for achieving national strength. Physicians – along with an army of nurses, midwives, and public health officials – were entrusted with the task of increasing Germany's birth rate. In addition, various incentives – including family allowances, preferential allocations of public housing to large families, and marriage loans – were used to encourage large families.

A second and equally important role assigned to physicians was the purification and improvement of the German racial stock.

This implied the elimination of individuals who, if they should produce offspring, might spoil the "racial" qualities of future generations of Germans. Such individuals were to be sterilized; a woman pregnant with a child of "undesirable" stock was liable to compulsory abortion; persons who were dangerous to the "race" were to be prohibited from marrying; persons who showed symptoms of an "unhealthy" state of mind, such as opposition to the State, were selected for segregation and isolation from the German "race."[40]

"Segregation" and "isolation" meant either prison or, more usually, a concentration camp. In this area, Himmler's Interior Ministry, and particularly the section on genetic and racial matters, was the main policy-making agency.

The role envisioned for physicians by the Nazis clearly required some fundamental changes in the doctors' professional and ethical procedures. The Law for the Regulation of German Physicians (1937), mentioned above, absolved the physicians from the obligation of maintaining confidentiality between doctor and patient. Revelation was not unethical if made "in the fulfillment of a legitimate, moral duty in the interests of any objective that is felt to be socially desirable or if a menace to public welfare is the predominant consideration."[41]

In essence, the Nazis redefined the role of the physician under the Third Reich. Aside from his traditional obligation to heal the sick, the German doctor became part of the political apparatus of the state.

The Nazis were able to enlist the support of the medical profession with remarkable ease. Some physicians genuinely believed in and supported the racist policies of the Nazis. As early as the latter part of the nineteenth century, elements within the medical profession had adopted the philosophical position that some people were of less value than others and that it was economically and scientifically wasteful to render all possible medical assistance to all persons. For most of the medical profession, economics rather than philosophy determined the reaction to the Nazis. In the 1930s the medical profession was in the midst of a severe economic crisis. Physicians, like most middle- and upper-class Germans, had to contend with a loss of income and status during the Depression. In addition, however, their position was made more difficult by an existing and ever-expanding oversupply of doctors. As early as 1927, it was estimated that Germany, with 45,000 doctors, had 5,000 more than it needed. Yet the medical schools, operating under democratic principles, kept admitting more and more students, most of whom saw professional training as the last resort for improving their financial and social positions.

Nazi policy appeared to offer salvation to the medical profession. As we have seen, the Nazis effectively neutralized the doctors' main nemesis, the sickness funds. Other policies too were geared toward ensuring support of the profession. However, a price had to be paid. That price took the form of reorganizing the medical profession itself. In 1933, the government dissolved the Hartmann-Bund and all other medical associations. In their place, the Nazis created a national level professional body, the *Reichsärztekammer* ("Reich Doctors' Chamber"). This body defined conditions and requirements pertaining to every aspect of medical practice. Membership in the Doctors' Chamber was a requirement for medical practice. The head of the chamber was the *Reichsärzteführer*, Dr. Leonardo Conti, an early supporter of Adolf Hitler. Within the Doctors' Chamber were several organizations including the Association of Sickness Insurance Physicians of Germany (KVD). The KVD was empowered to admit physicians to insurance practice, discipline them for any infraction associated with insurance practice, and handle all contractural and financial arrangements between the doctors and insurance funds. The physicians were paid directly by the KVD, which received money from the funds. In short, the new arrangement virtually ended all direct contact between the two hostile groups.

Other Nazi policies too were enthusiastically supported by the economically depressed medical community.

The Nazi programme offered an almost devilish panacea for the woes of the profession, and in particular, for their younger members. Their "solution" of the economic crisis promised new avenues of "employment" for doctors and patients alike; their planning for education promised to divert the surplus of students into other channels; their programme of eugenic measures promised a quick rise of the birth rate and thus an expansion of every existing practice . . . and their pseudo-evolutionary-scientific approach to all wider social problems almost made the medical profession the centre of the whole future structure of the State.[42]

One other Nazi policy won at least the acquiescence, and in many instances the active support, of the medical profession: the removal of Jewish doctors from medical practice. A combination of anti-Semitism and economics governed the profession's position. Starting in 1933, the Nazis began forcing Jewish doctors out of practice; between 1933 and 1937 the number of Jewish doctors declined from 6,480 to 4,220.

On September 30, 1938, an amendment to the Nuremberg racial laws revoked the licenses of all Jewish physicians. From that date onward, Jewish doctors were not permitted to attend any patient of German (Aryan) blood. A small number of doctors were issued special permits to treat Jewish patients, including those covered by sickness insurance. These physicians could not use the title "doctor" (*Aerzt*), but were called "treaters of the sick" (*Krankenbehandler*). In addition, they were required to stamp on each letterhead or prescription the words Eligible to Treat Jews Only.

Given the former economic plight of the medical profession and the strong anti-Semitism that permeated all German society, the Nazi policy toward Jewish doctors was endorsed and encouraged by all but a few courageous members of the profession. The purge of Jewish doctors along with the other actions taken by the Nazis, mentioned above, ensured widespread support for the regime among the medical profession.

The impact of Nazi policy on health care

It is difficult to evaluate dispassionately and objectively the impact of Nazi policy on the German health care system. The prostitution of the medical profession in enforcing the regime's racist policies, including medical "experiments" on concentration camp inmates, are as indefensible as they were barbaric. All other points are trivial in comparison. Despite this, a few additional evaluative comments can be made.

The purge of Jewish physicians caused an almost immediate shortage of physicians in certain major cities where Jews had made up a significant proportion of the medical community. With the beginning of World War II in September 1939, and the military mobilization of about one-third of the medical profession, the shortage became acute. Several steps were taken to meet the problem, including shortening the time required to obtain a medical degree, increasing medical school enrollments, and requiring all physicians in private practice to accept sickness insurance patients.

The wartime expansion of the medical profession did not, however, result in improved health care for the ordinary citizen. Despite the regime's initial intentions, the majority of new physicians did not enter private practice but were channeled toward either the military or various branches of the Nazi Party. In addition, many physicians used their medical skills either in the concentration camps or in implementing the sterilization program. "All this meant that as far as access to doctors was concerned the ordinary *Krankenkasse* patient (protected under the health-insurance scheme) found himself pushed to the end of a queue – a situation which in effect corresponded to a deliberate Nazi design."[43]

Beyond the immediate consequences of its activities, Nazi health care policy had certain long-term implications for health care and health care policy in the post-World War II era: (1) the system of health insurance survived and thus continued to provide the foundation of German health care policy; (2) the Nazis eliminated direct contact between doctors and insurance funds; and (3) by 1943–4, virtually every civilian doctor had had some experience with health insurance patients, whereas prior to the Nazi period 10 percent still practiced outside the system. These factors have provided part of the basis for setting health care policy since 1945. We

Table 5-3. *Development of the German sickness insurance system; 1885-1976*

Year	Number of insured (in millions)[a]	Percent of population insured[b]	Income limit (DM)	Number of insurance funds
1885	4.7	10	2,000	18,942
1911	10.0	21.5	2,000	22,000
1914	16.0	23.0	2,500	13,500
1932	18.7	30.0	3,600	6,600
1951	20.0	48.1	4,500	1,992
1955	22.7	50.0	6,000	2,072
1960	27.1	85	7,920	2,028
1965	28.7	87	10,800	1,972
1970	30.6	88	14,400[c]	1,827
1976	33.5	90	27,900	1,425

[a]Does not include dependents.
[b]Includes dependents.
[c]Since January 1, 1971, the income limit has been automatically adjusted annually to wage and salary changes.
Sources: *Soziale Sicherung,* (Bonn: Der Bundesminister für Arbeit und Sozialordnung, 1977) pp. 181-185; W. H. Dawson, *Social Insurance in Germany 1883-1911* (London: Unwin, 1912).

complete our analysis of the German system by examining that period now.

Health care policy in the Federal Republic

The development of health care policy in the Federal Republic of Germany since 1945 is testimony to the resiliency, some might say obduracy, of preexisting public policy. Despite the severe societal dislocations attending nazism, World War II, the total defeat of Germany, postwar inflation, tripartite, Allied occupation (in the western portion of Germany), and the establishment of a new, democratic political system, the principles underlying German health care policy have remained basically unchanged. Prewar trends, including in some instances Nazi trends, in the evolution of the system continued: The proportion of the population compulsorily insured increased; benefits were expanded; and the number of insurance funds decreased. Table 5-3 records the historical changes in the health insurance system.

From a historical perspective, the most important development has been the change from a limited, class-based insurance system to a virtually universal system. By 1977, 92 percent of the population was covered by the national sickness insurance program. Although important changes have

taken place since 1945, these have been essentially philosophical and substantive reaffirmations of the existing system. There have been some – the
Association of Socialist Doctors in particular – who have championed the
cause of a national health service similar to the British system. Most observers, however, see little prospect of fundamental changes.

There are several reasons for the resiliency of the system. One, and perhaps the most important, has been alluded to already: The longer a program is in existence, the more difficult it is to change. The reasons for this
are obvious. Different interests tend to develop important stakes in the
existence of the program. In the German case, the insurance funds, the
bureaucrats in the Ministry of Labor and Social Affairs, labor unions, and
even the medical profession, all have developed a strong interest in maintaining the status quo. Aside from whatever it means for the health of the
German people, the insurance system means jobs and income for a large
and permanent public and private bureaucracy. In 1970 the insurance
funds alone employed 77,000 people.

Longevity, and the concomitant development of entrenched interests, is
a necessary but not sufficient explanation of the durability of the German
health insurance system. A second, and related, factor is the high level of
approval for the program from the various actors. This is discussed later in
connection with our evaluation of the system. Suffice it here to say that
there has long been widespread popular support for the program. In addition, the doctors, who were probably the most vigorous, if somewhat
belated, opponents of the sickness insurance system, now acknowledge its
virtues – one of which is that most noninstitution-based doctors derive 80
percent of their rather impressive incomes from health insurance practice.

A third factor, explaining the absence of fundamental, as opposed to
incremental and evolutionary, change involves the nature of political
events since the end of World War II in Germany. Two factors are particularly relevant: (1) in the first decade following the end of the war, a time
when one might have expected fundamental policy change, political and
economic circumstances precluded major policy innovations; and (2)
following the end of the Allied occupation of Germany in 1955, the
nation was governed by a political party that envisioned a rather modest
role for the state in the areas of social and economic policy. Let us
elaborate on each of these points.

As argued earlier in this book, an "inspection process" often accom-
panies participation in a major war and frequently leads to fundamental
change in public policy. In the case of Germany, political and economic
circumstances precluded any fundamental examination of health care
policy. In the early years of the occupation, both Allied and German
officials were preoccupied with the most rudimentary and pressing health
care issues: preventing epidemics, providing basic health care, and so on.

Once these immediate needs had been met, systematic policy evaluation and revision were further postponed because of the nature of the Allied occupation. Initially, Germany was governed by the four-power (United States, British, French, and Soviet) Allied Control Council, located in Berlin, which was expected to provide uniform policy direction for the entire country. In practice, it did not work that way. Conflict between the Soviets on the one hand, and the Americans, British, and French on the other, resulted in the ultimate dissolution of the council (in June 1948) and the tripartite administration of the Western portion of Germany. In each of the three Western zones the respective Allied governments pursued different approaches to health care reform. The British set up a central labor office to suggest reforms; the United States empowered *Länder* (state) councils to reform the system; and the French set up regionally based unified insurance companies.[44] In each case, the reforms built upon the principle, and in many instances the actual structure, of the prewar sickness insurance system.

Between 1949 and 1955 Germany prepared for the end of the Allied occupation and the establishment of an independent, democratic form of government. Beginning with the Basic Law of 1949, the Federal Republic moved toward reestablishing its social security system. One of the most significant steps in this direction was the Law of Self-Administration and Changes in the Area of Social Insurance of February 22, 1951. This law essentially restored the social insurance system to its pre-1933 status.[45]

The first stage, then, in the postwar development of German health insurance essentially involved the restoration and de-nazification of the pre-1933 system. Restoration of the previous system rather than major policy innovation was dictated by the need for rapid action to meet pressing health care problems and by both Allied and German satisfaction with the preexisting system.

The second factor that helped determine the incremental course of postwar health care policy is that for its first 17 years the Federal Republic was governed by the conservative-oriented Christian Democratic Union (CDU) and its Bavarian affiliate, the Christian Social Union (CSU). From the first parliamentary election in 1949 until 1966, when it entered into the Grand Coalition with the Social Democrats, the CDU/CSU controlled the government; and until 1969 it held the chancellorship. The doctrine that guided CDU policy was the neoliberal notion of the social market economy. Basically conservative in outlook, it was "not the kind of doctrine that is likely to inspire an aggressive social program."[46] This is not to suggest that the CDU was opposed to state provision of social services. Such a position would be incompatible with nearly a century of German public policy and the expectations of the German people. What the CDU did oppose was the notion of a comprehensive welfare state. Social policy under the Christian Democrats, therefore, was geared to improving established social programs, not introducing new ones.

Intuitively one might expect a more aggressive social policy from the Socialists. Although the SPD, first within the Grand Coalition (1966–9) and then on its own, did sponsor several important changes in health care policy, all these were accomplished within the framework of the existing insurance system. In fact, with the exception of certain fringe elements within the party and among its supporters, at no time in recent years has the SPD questioned the underlying principle of German health care policy: a contributory insurance system. Operating within a basically two-party, pluralistic democratic system and faced with a program that has widespread support and a long history, the SPD, like its political rival, has shaped its health care policy in terms of the sickness insurance system.

Substantive changes in health care policy since 1955

Despite the incremental nature of health care policy change in the Federal Republic in the postwar period, several substantively and ideologically important changes have been introduced or attempted. With the end of the Allied occupation and the beginning of economic and political stability, the dominant CDU attempted to reform the program. These efforts, from roughly 1955 to 1965, were characterized by considerable "social conflict."[47]

The basis of the conflict was a proposed reform made public in October 1958 by the federal minister of labor and social affairs. The direction of the reform had been adumbrated in a speech by Chancellor Adenauer to the newly elected Bundestag 1 year earlier (October 29, 1957). Adenauer said, in part:

Social reforms will be continued. This means a correction of the faults of the present legislation as well as a recasting of health insurance . . . the Federal Government is resolved to promote by all means the idea of self-help and private initiative, and to prevent a slipping into a total welfare state which would sooner or later destroy well-being and prosperity.[48]

In February 1958 the new minister of labor and social affairs, Theodor Blank, spelled out the "faults" of the present legislation and "the idea of self-help." The system was being overburdened by "trivial cases." In order to free the doctors from these and allow them to concentrate on the more serious illnesses, a system of cost sharing for the insured was proposed. Cost sharing would discourage frivolous use of the system, allow for better payment of physicians, and "strengthen the feeling of responsibility of the insured toward the whole community of the insured."[49]

On October 24, 1958, the government presented its entire reform package. It included the following proposals:[50]

1. Preventive medical and dental examinations financed by sickness insurance.
2. Payment of cash benefits for the duration of an illness, but not to exceed 78 weeks – the existing limit was 6 weeks.
3. Hospital care for an unlimited time.
4. Dependents would receive all benefits – with the exception of direct cash payments – on the same basis as insured persons.
5. Cost sharing for physician and hospital care as well as prescribed medicines. The cost would be adjusted to income and family circumstances.
6. Physicians would be paid on a fee-for-service, rather than capitation, basis.
7. Establishment of a medical advisory service to monitor fraudulent claims and ensure proper health service.
8. Limiting the number and category of persons eligible for compulsory insurance to that group of people currently covered. For example, the income limit would be maintained at DM 7,920 per year.

The proposals clearly were intended to provide something for everyone. The first four proposals were consumer-oriented, promising improved and expanded medical services. The fee-for-service proposal was certain to find favor with the medical profession, as was the income ceiling, which would halt the erosion of private practice. Cost sharing and income ceiling were at the heart of the CDU/CSU effort to limit unnecessary and trivial demands and, thereby, reduce the costs of the program. Some of the anticipated income and savings would be needed to offset expected cost increases resulting from proposed expanded benefits. The cost sharing proposal was favored by employers' groups, who generally echoed the position taken by CDU leadership on the issue.

It is not necessary to detail extensively the lengthy and often bitter debate that followed the reform proposals. The government submitted a draft bill in December 1958 that specified its cost sharing plans (e.g., DM 1.50 for each doctor's visit, to be paid directly to the physician, and DM 1 to 3 for medicines). With the proposal made sufficiently specific, various interest groups began responding – and in generally negative fashion. While the doctors favored some form of cost sharing (which they hoped would lead to a higher fee schedule), they opposed the plan to have them collect the fee. This, they argued, would only add to the avalanche of paperwork already required of them. The unions, the sickness funds, and the SPD opposed cost sharing completely, as well as the provision limiting expansion of the eligible population.

In the course of the debate, which proceeded on and off for almost 2 years, various other provisions were added in an effort to attract wider support. Nevertheless, cost sharing remained the key and most controversial provision. With opposition to the provision from doctors, unions, sickness funds, and the SPD, hopes for passage of the entire package dimmed. Following months of rancorous debate, threats of a doctors' strike, and widespread public opposition, the government, in February 1961, finally abandoned the reform bill. Between 1961 and 1965 the CDU continued to push for health insurance reform. The decade of social conflict ended, however, without a fundamental change in the German health insurance system.

In the decade or so following defeat of the CDU-sponsored reform bill, the health insurance system was amended on several occasions. The frequency and nature of these revisions reflect the increased influence of the SPD. In 1969 the Socialists formed a Grand Coalition with the CDU/CSU. In that year the SPD sponsored the Continual Payment of Wages Law, which went into effect on January 1, 1970. This law guaranteed a blue-collar worker full wages for the first 6 weeks of an illness that caused him to miss work. Up until that time, only salaried, white-collar employees enjoyed this benefit; wage earners were granted a certain percentage of their wages. This measure, which the SPD had championed since 1955, eliminated one of the few remaining class-based differences in the insurance system. At the same time, the income ceiling was raised to DM 14,400 per year.

In April 1970, an experts commission was established for the purpose of recommending further changes in the sickness insurance system. The commission was headed by a professor of medicine and consisted of representatives of organized labor, the medical profession, employers, and scholars. It prepared a series of recommendations for the minister of labor and social affairs from 1970 until 1976. The recommendations, most of which were adopted, were wide ranging, covering both the substance and the administration of the insurance system. Among the proposals ultimately adopted were the following:[51]

1. Independent farmers and their dependents (1972) and all students not covered by family insurance (1975) became compulsorily insured.
2. Since July 1, 1971, periodic medical examinations for children below the age of 5, and annual early cancer detection for men (from age 45) and women (from age 30), have been financed by health insurance.
3. Since December 1975, various birth control services, including medical counseling, legal abortion, and sterilization, have been brought under sickness insurance.
4. Coverage was extended in July 1975 to disabled and handicapped persons.

5. All existing health insurance laws were codified.

The substantive changes introduced in recent years, particularly under SPD governments, have subtly changed the nature of the health insurance system. With the inclusion of independent farmers and students, the continued increase in the income limit, and the elimination of the difference in cash benefits betweeen blue-collar and white-collar workers, the German health insurance system has lost most of its class-based nature. In addition, the nature of the benefits, which now go beyond simply curing illness and include important preventive measures as well as "nonillness medicine" (e.g., contraception, abortion), reflects an important philosophical, as well as substantive, change in the system. Although Germany, through all its political incarnations, has remained remarkably true to the Bismarckian system, it has clearly adapted that system to the requirements of a modern democratic society.

The sickness insurance system today

It is useful at this point to describe the current (about 1978) sickness insurance system. This provides the reader with an opportunity to compare the changes from the original law in terms of substance, administration, and, implicitly, the political assumptions guiding health care policy.

Eligibility and coverage

All wage and salary workers and self-employed persons earning (in 1977) less than DM 30,600 (about $15,300) and their dependents are automatically and compulsorily insured. Those earning above the statutory ceiling, which is adjusted annually, may join the system voluntarily. Pensioners and persons receiving unemployment benefits are also compulsorily insured.

Financing

In terms of financing, the current system has remained basically faithful to the original law. Employers and employees each contribute an equal share to the system, which in 1977 averaged 5.7 percent of the worker's monthly earnings. Pensioners' contributions are paid by their pension funds, and the premium for unemployed persons is paid by the unemployment insurance system.

State contributions to the system are minimal. They include (1) a set payment to the sickness fund of DM 400 for each maternity case, (2) a supplementary contribution to the miners' insurance scheme, (3) indirect contributions to pensioners' insurance through partially financing the pensioners' insurance program, and (4) a subsidy to the funds of small (less than 20 employees) companies.[52]

Finally, some minor cost sharing has been introduced. Since July 1, 1977, a minimum payment of DM 1 has been imposed for all pharmaceutical supplies. In addition, various appliances (e.g., eyeglasses, artificial limbs, hearing aids, and dentures) are subject to cost sharing, although these fees are waived for various needy groups.

Benefits

The German sickness insurance system provides comprehensive and extensive medical care coverage and cash benefits for over 62 million (in 1974) persons. The medical benefits include general practitioner, specialist, and dental care; pharmaceuticals and other health care appliances (with some cost sharing); hospitalization for an unlimited duration; complete maternity care; and annual preventive health examinations. There are few limits on the frequency or duration of use. It should be noted here that most hospitals in Germany are privately owned and operated.

Cash benefits include the following:

1. A sickness allowance if an illness results in the loss of wages or salary. This is paid by the employer for the first 6 weeks of an illness and after that by the sickness fund.
2. A household allowance in the event hospitalization is required. This covers normal household expenses including rent.
3. A lump sum maternity payment for dependent women and a variable sum, based on earnings, for working women.
4. A lump sum grant for funeral expenses.

Administration

The principle of decentralization and autonomous administration provided for in 1883 has been maintained, although in considerably simplified form. In 1977 there were 1,425 sickness funds compared with almost 19,000 in 1885.

The funds are subject to administrative supervision by the Federal Ministry of Labor and Social Affairs and the respective *länder* (state) ministries of work and social welfare. They are self-governing corporations managed by elected representatives (executive committees) chosen, in equal numbers, by employers and employees.[53] In practice, there has been little active worker participation in either the delegate assembly or the executive committee. Representatives generally have been nominated by trade unions and accepted by the workers. The funds have considerable administrative autonomy. They must adhere to certain maximum contribution and benefit standards set by the federal and *länder* governments, but beyond this they are permitted to offer members additional benefits.

Table 5-4. *Membership in German sickness funds, 1976*

Type of fund	Number of funds	Total Membership (in thousands)	Percent of all members in this type
Local funds	307	16,070	48
Land funds	19	924	3
Company funds	921	4,207	13
Trade association funds	161	1,595	5
Seamen's Fund	1	67	0.2
Miner's Special Fund	1	1,057	3
Substitute funds			
Blue-collar workers	8	372	1
White-collar workers	7	9,143	27
Total	1,425	33,435	100.2[a]

[a]Exceeds 100% because of rounding.
Source: Soziale Sicherung, 188.

There are seven types of insurance funds. Table 5-4 lists the number and absolute and relative membership of each. As the table indicates the largest proportion of insured persons belongs to general or local sickness funds: 48 percent. The white-collar substitute funds have the second largest proportion and have been the fastest growing: Membership in these funds has grown from 1.8 million in 1950 to 9.1 million in 1976. This growth in part reflects the inclusion of a larger proportion of white-collar workers in the insurance program.

Physicians and health insurance in postwar Germany

The postwar period has seen a gradual improvement in the relationship between the medical profession and the various components of the health insurance system, particularly the insurance funds. The improved atmosphere is largely a function of various changes that have occurred in the system and that have been beneficial to the physician. One of the most important of these occurred in 1960 when a federal constitution court ruled that the practice of sickness funds limiting the number of physicians authorized for insurance practice was unconstitutional.[54] With this decision, virtually all qualified physicians became eligible for insurance practice, thus finally establishing freedom of choice. It is estimated that 98 percent of physicians treat insurance patients.[55]

A second factor accounting for the declining animosity between the two former antagonists is the total elimination of direct contact between the practicing physician and the insurance fund. The insurance law now provides for contract negotiation between representatives of the two groups. The process "starts with a Federal outline in broad terms concluded at [the] national level between the federal organizations of practitioners and of the sickness funds; this is then expanded into a detailed contract between the individual fund and the local association of practitioners."[56]

A key issue of interest in past negotiations had been the method and level of remuneration for medical services. This too has been largely removed from the arena of conflict. For the most part, doctors are now paid on a fee-for-service basis. The amount of the fee is spelled out in an annually negotiated federal fee schedule, which includes approximately 2,000 procedures and their cost. In the event the two parties cannot agree on specific rates, the matter is submitted to the Federal Arbitration Committee, whose decision is binding. In effect, by agreeing to the procedure, the doctors have given up the right to strike.

Although sources of conflict still exist between the two groups (e.g., the sickness funds monitor medical and pharmaceutical costs, a procedure the doctors believe interferes with their professional freedom), the lack of direct contact between the two groups and the standardization of contract procedures have gone a long way toward eliminating conflict in the system.

The performance of the German health care system

In the final analysis the value of any public health care system lies in its ability to provide competent, affordable, and accessible health care. A problem in evaluating the performance of health care policy is to find acceptable standards for making what are essentially value judgments. For example, when one speaks of evaluating health care policy in terms of "accessibility," the first issue to resolve is: "Accessible to whom?" Some feel that publicly supported health care should be accessible to all; others feel that only those who cannot afford it should be provided with such care. Although personal value judgments legitimately have a place in policy analysis, we have chosen to avoid them wherever possible. We have minimized the likelihood of such value impositions in two ways: (1) we judge the performance of each health care system in terms of the goals it has set for itself, and (2) wherever possible we use generally accepted standards of health care achievement (e.g., increased life expectancy and decreased infant mortality rates). Some of the measures permit cross-national comparisons. Other measures evaluate problems that tend to be characteristic of a particular system and, therefore, less amenable to cross-national comparison.

In the case of Germany, our evaluation focuses on three performance areas: (1) the health status of the German people over time and compared with people of other nations, (2) the distribution of health care services, and (3) the problems of overtreatment by physicians and malingering by patients.

The state of health and health care

Almost one century has passed since the introduction of the pioneering German Sickness Insurance Law. During that time, the German people have enjoyed increasing physical well-being and access to health care facilities. The average German today lives about twice as long as his or her counterpart in 1883. The chances of a German infant surviving its first year are significantly greater now than in 1883: The infant morality rate has declined from 232 to 19.7 per 1,000 live births. These conditions are in part a function of the universal availability of medical care. Today there are 519 persons per physician compared with 3,000 per physician in 1883; and there are 88 persons per hospital bed compared with 545 in the year the insurance law was passed.

What is the contribution of German health care policy, and particularly of the insurance system, to these improved health conditions? In all nations mortality, morbidity, and life expectancy rates are related to a wide variety of factors. In part, the improved health status of the German people is a function of the progress in, and international diffusion of, medical knowledge. Since 1883 there have been extraordinary medical advances, many of which were initiated by German doctors and scientists. These advances have led to an improvement in the life chances of people throughout the world. Obviously, not all peoples have shared equally in the benefits of these medical advances. Those in advanced industrial nations have been more fortunate in this regard than those living in the less developed countries.

This latter point provides a second explanation for the improved health status of Germans. As noted in Chapter 4, health and health care indicators are closely related to the level of wealth and economic development of a nation. Such factors as diet, general sanitary conditions, education, workplace conditions, and personal health habits all affect the health of people. Generally speaking, the wealthier a nation, the healthier its people.[57] For most of the past century, Germans have enjoyed a relatively high standard of living. Clearly, this living standard and all it implies have contributed significantly to the improvements in health and the availability of health care facilities.

Table 5-5. *Health status in Germany, 1883-1975*

Indicator	1883	1900	1911	1933	1950	1960	1975
General mortality rate (per 1,000 population)	25.9	22.1	17.3	11.2	10.5	11.6	12.1
Infant mortality rate (per 1,000 live births)	232	229	162	77	55	34	19.7
Life expectancy (yr.)							
Male	35.6	40.6	44.8	56.0	64.6	66.7	68.3
Female	38.5	44.0	48.3	58.8	68.5	71.9	74.3
Population per physician	3,000	2,058	1,996	1,380	734	703	519
Population per hospital bed	545	N.A.	275[a]	111	94	105	88

N.A. = data not available.

[a]1906.

Sources: I. G. Gibbon, *Medical Benefit: A Study of the Experience of Germany and Denmark* (London: King, 1912), p. 232; W. H. Dawson, *Social Insurance in Germany 1883-1911* (London: Unwin, 1912), p. 207; *Statistiches Jahrbuch* (Wiesbaden: Statistisches Bundesamt), various years.

Has health care policy contributed anything to improved health and health care in Germany? There is no direct evidence on this issue. The general historical, social, and economic factors mentioned above confound any attempt to link directly, descriptively or statistically, the insurance system with health and health care indicators. A few speculative points, however, can be offered. First, as Table 5-5 indicates, improvements in life expectancy and mortality rates did not become significant until sickness insurance was extended to a substantial proportion of the population. Significant improvement did not appear until 1911 and became dramatic only in the 1930s. It is true that these figures may reflect a time lag between the introduction of an insurance system and, say, increased longevity. However, one might expect immediate improvement in infant mortality rates because many poor women who had previously gone without trained medical attention became eligible for such care. Between 1883 and 1900, the German infant mortality rate declined only slightly: from 232 to 229 per 1,000 live births. However, by 1911, when one-fifth of the population was insured, the decline was more pronounced: down to 162 per 1,000 live births. With the introduction of compulsory insurance for dependents in 1930, the infant mortality rates declined even more precipitously despite the poor economic conditions of the times. In 1933 the rate was 77 deaths per 1,000 live births. To repeat, these figures do not prove that the sickness insurance system contributed to the declining infant mortality rate. They are, however, suggestive.

A different kind of measure of the contribution sickness insurance has made involves the provision of medical care and medical facilities. It seems reasonable to argue that any public policy that discourages persons from entering the medical profession or inhibits the development of medical facilities is not performing well. Such is not the case in Germany. Despite predictions to the contrary, particularly from foreign opponents of national health insurance, medical facilities and personnel have grown steadily to meet the needs of the German people. In 1974 Germany ranked 7th among 138 countries in terms of population per hospital bed and 9th in terms of population per physician. In fact, throughout most of the century Germany has had more doctors than it has needed. It seems that, rather than discouraging or inhibiting adequate medical personnel and facilities, the insurance system has encouraged and facilitated their development.

When one moves from a cross-temporal comparison of health indicators within Germany to cross-national comparison, the record of German health achievements becomes somewhat more ambiguous. In 1974 Germany ranked 7th among 138 nations in terms of per capita gross national product. However, it ranked 22nd in terms of infant mortality and 18th in life expectancy. These gross indicators are somewhat surprising given Germany's rank in terms of population per physician and per hospital bed. No factors related particularly to health care policy appear to explain these figures.

The intervening impact of social, economic, and cultural factors on health conditions within a nation and on differences among nations limits the utility of aggregate statistics as a measure of the performance of the health care delivery system. It is necessary to find additional measures of the performance of the German sickness insurance system.

The distribution of health care

Over 90 percent of the German people receive medical attention under the national sickness insurance program. This includes persons who are most likely to need, but least able to afford, medical care: the poor, the unemployed, retired persons, the handicapped. Clearly, this by itself is an important achievement. Nevertheless, one must go beyond the general accomplishment and look at other measures. One of the most important of these is the distribution of, and access to, medical care among the population. Do all groups in German society enjoy equal access to the nation's health services? Is there reasonable uniformity in the quality and quantity of services available? In answering these questions one basic point must be understood. German health care policy, unlike current British and Soviet policy, has never sought complete universality or equality within the health care system. Its purpose has been to provide necessary health care, initially for the most vulnerable portion of society, and later for all but the most affluent. In doing so, German policy makers have established certain minimum benefit levels. Beyond these, each of the insurance carriers negotiates for greater benefits (and may require higher contributions) on behalf of its subscribers. Thus, the more affluent white-collar substitute fund members enjoy greater benefits than those belonging to other funds. The 1969 insurance law amendment, which provided blue-collar workers with full cash benefits, removed one of the most obvious and irritating class-based differences in the system. The differences that remain today involve discretionary rather than statutory benefits. Although not all persons receive the same benefits, all do enjoy a common minimum level of protection generally recognized as adequate to meet the health care needs of the people.

Although certain benefit differences related to income level exist, there does not appear to be any discrimination by the medical profession in terms of providing medical treatment. Unlike the case in the past, when many German physicians maintained two waiting rooms – one for private patients, the other for insurance patients – no such symbolic or real difference is reported to exist today. There are few complaints, similar to those heard in Great Britain, that private patients receive better, or at least speedier and more attentive, care. Nor are there any apparent differences in the quality of treatment according to the type of fund to which a person belongs. According to Fulcher, "fund doctors do not normally confine their practice to any particular fund or concern themselves with which fund their patient belongs to before treating him."[58]

One of the most commonly reported variations in access to medical care throughout the world relates to the geographical distribution of medical personnel and facilities. Typically, inequalities exist among regions and between urban and rural areas. In every country studied here, including Germany, urban residents have greater access (in terms of population per physician and per hospital bed) to medical care, and particularly specialist care, than their rural counterparts. The reasons for this are virtually identical in all four countries, as well as in the United States. Physicians prefer the social and cultural amenities and professional opportunities associated with urban living. In the case of Germany, this has resulted in 46 percent of all physicians practicing in the larger cities, which contain only 33 percent of the nation's population.[59]

In addition, and somewhat related, to the urban-rural variation are regional differences. In 1970, the national average of physicians per 100,000 people in Germany was 1,799. There was, however, considerable regional variation from the mean. At one extreme was the highly urbanized *Land* of Hamburg, which had 2,808 doctors per 100,000 population

(56 percent above the national average); Lower Saxony, on the other hand, had only 1,544 doctors per 100,000 persons (14 percent below the average).[60]

For the most part, geographical variations in access to medical care are a function of the social and professional factors mentioned above, rather than of a failure of health care policy. It should be noted, however, that the judicial decision in 1960, which prohibited the insurance companies from restricting physician access to health insurance practice, had an adverse effect on the geographical distribution of doctors. Up to that time, insurance companies could, and did, minimize maldistribution by refusing to accept doctors for insurance practice in heavily overdoctored (i.e., urban) areas. Similarly, they encouraged doctors to enter insurance practice in the underdoctored, typically rural areas. With the federal court's decision that any doctor who wishes to must be accepted for insurance practice, the companies lost most of their leverage in distributing medical personnel. The result, although it has not been fully documented, has been a trend toward greater maldistribution.[61]

The geographical maldistribution of medical personnel is one of the most intractable problems facing health care administrators. As we shall see with regard to the Soviet Union, even authoritarian regimes have been unable to deal effectively with this issue. It must be emphasized that of the four nations studied here, the problem is least severe in Germany and is generally recognized to be less significant than in many West European countries.[62]

Thus, although some social, as well as geographic, inequalities exist, the overall consensus is that the system is fair and accomplishes its goal. In this regard, perhaps the most important measure is consumer satisfaction, and "repeated surveys have shown that West German consumers are overwhelmingly satisfied with the national health insurance system."[63]

Consumer and producer abuses and their consequences for health care policy

Although generally the subject of praise, and a source of national pride, the German sickness insurance system is not without its problems. Two of these problems are closely related. They are the alleged (and sometimes documented) exploitation of the system in the form of malingering and excessive sick leave on the part of patients and overtreatment by physicians. These factors are related to, but by no means the sole cause of, a third, and more easily documented problem: rapidly rising health care costs.

The first two problems have plagued the system almost from its beginning and are viewed as a particularly, almost uniquely, German problem.

"Such complaints are heard far more in Germany than in any other country."[64] The charge against the patients is that cash benefits under sickness insurance are so attractive that they seduce Germans into taking "sick holidays" or malingering over inconsequential, if not nonexistent, illnesses. These claims have appeared throughout the history of the insurance program.[65] In the past, malingering took two forms. First, the statistics relating to the increased duration of illness since the beginning of the insurance system indicate that there was an increase from 14.1 days per illness in 1885 to 29.3 in 1932. Second, periodic control reexaminations of allegedly sick persons revealed that once the reexaminations were ordered, approximately 50 percent of those claiming to be ill, and collecting benefits, either reported back to work or, if examined, were found fit for work.[66] The practice of reexamination to catch malingerers and detect fraud was stopped only in 1970.

Although we are unaware of any recent studies on the subject, it is generally believed that consumer fraud is far less significant today than in the past.[67] Nevertheless, policy makers still treat it as a serious problem. In 1970 an amendment to the insurance law introduced a provision intended, in part, to discourage unnecessary use of medical services. Under the amendment, any insured person who did not use the system during a 3-month period would be reimbursed DM 10 per quarter, up to DM 30 in any given year. The rebate system had no appreciable impact on consumer demand and was dropped in 1973.

The issue of physician exploitation of the insurance system is closely related to that of consumer abuse. The major charge against the physicians is that the system of remuneration (i.e., fee for service) encourages the doctor to see as many patients as possible as frequently as possible and to administer as many treatments or procedures as possible. The income of the physician is a direct function of the quantity of services performed and persons treated. Because any insured person can go to any doctor, physicians, it is argued, are forced to compete with one another for patients. One way of attracting and keeping patients, so the argument runs, is to be generous in certifying eligibility for cash benefits.

Like consumer abuses, the charge that physicians engage in such practices has a long history in Germany. In the past, physicians who engaged in such procedures – and the evidence seems convincing that they did exist – were known as *Kassenlowen* ("Fund Lions"). These physicians saw between 20 and 30 patients an hour and were condemned by their colleagues for professional as well as pecuniary reasons. The charge of overtreatment by physicians is less frequently heard today than in the past. Without detracting from the professional integrity of the German physician, it should be noted that this decreased criticism may be a function of the rather elaborate monitoring and cost-control apparatus established jointly by the insurance funds and doctors' associations. Through a computer analysis of relevant medical practice data (e.g., location of practice, number of patients and contribution, type of treatment), norms for assessing the costs of a particular practice are determined. The claims of doctors on the insurance companies are then compared with the computed norm. If a physician appears to be overtreating (i.e., his claim for reimbursement for medicine, procedures, visits, etc. is above the norm) he or she is asked to justify the claim. Warnings may be issued and financial penalties may be assessed for abuses.[68]

As noted above, abuses by both patients and physicians are related to a third, and probably most serious, problem currently facing the German health care system: rapidly increasing health care costs. Rising health care costs are by no means unique to Germany. The issue, however, has become a preoccupation with German policy makers in recent years. The magnitude of the problem is revealed in a few cost figures. Between 1965 and 1970 average annual costs for health increased 8.5 percent. Between 1970 and 1975, however, they increased an average of 17.2 percent per year.[69] These increases have necessitated an increase in premiums. Between 1971 and 1977 the insurance premium was increased from 8.1 percent of the worker's salary or wages to 11.4 percent. The fact that similar increases have hit nations with very different types of health care systems, ranging from essentially private (the United States) to fully public (Great Britain) raises the question of the extent to which the health delivery system is itself responsible for health care costs. This issue is relevant if one accepts, as we do, that one characteristic of a "good" health care policy is that it be "affordable" to both the individual and the society in general.

A number of factors can explain the recent cost explosion in Germany and elsewhere. First, the worldwide inflation of the 1970s has affected the cost of most goods and services, but seems to have hit medical care with particular vengeance. Second, modern medicine, with its heavy reliance on sophisticated diagnostic and therapeutic paraphernalia, is very costly. German medicine, which has traditionally been in the forefront of modern techniques, relies particularly heavily on expensive technology. Third, as the insured population has become older, largely through the extension of coverage to retirees and pensioners, but also because of increasing longevity, the costs of medical care have risen commensurately. Older people simply make greater demands on health care services. Fourth, medical care has been redefined. Increasing reliance on preventive medicine, although intended ultimately to reduce costs by preventing long-term illness, has certainly added to the medical care bill, as has the inclusion of nonillness medical care such as abortions and sterilization.

Finally, it has been argued but not documented that people are simply more health conscious today and are therefore making greater use of the system.

We return then to the question of what role health care policy has played in Germany's cost explosion. It is doubtful that any single factor can adequately account for the rapidly rising costs. Even if it were possible to isolate the contribution of each of the factors mentioned above (which it probably is not), the analysis would take us too far afield. Although general economic inflation has undoubtedly played an important role, most of the other factors relate to health policy decisions. These decisions, particularly under the Social Democrats, have committed Germany to providing a comprehensive and modern health care system with a relatively broad definition of the concept of medical care. The unwillingness of the SPD and the inability of the CDU to impose cost sharing may or may not have contributed to the cost explosion. But this also reflects the values involved in directing the course of health policy in Germany. The satisfaction and sense of pride expressed by the public, the apparently acceptable level of inequalities, and the generally high level of health and health care indicate that the system is working well. The problem of health care costs must be evaluated in terms of the question: "How much is the society willing to pay for health care?" Thus far, Germans and German policy makers appear to be willing to bear rather high costs.

Accounting for German health care policy

This chapter deals with the evolution of German health care policy. Because the National Sickness Insurance Law has been the cornerstone of that policy for nearly one century, we focus attention on it. It is useful at this point to summarize the major findings concerning the factors that helped shape the structure and content of German health care policy in terms of the accounting scheme.

Situational factors

The evolution of German health care policy has been profoundly influenced by prominent personalities and extraordinary events. Although Bismarck's interest in and influence on sickness insurance was not as great as generally believed, or as great as in other areas of social reform, it was, nevertheless, considerable. Similarly, the rise of Adolf Hitler led almost immediately to changes in the content and delivery of health care policy.

The impact of events on policy was no less profound. The electoral successes of the Social Democrats in the latter part of the nineteenth century helped inspire Bismarck's social reforms, and the electoral successes of the Social Democrats in the 1960s and 1970s led to an expansion of the system. The overthrow of the monarchy after World War I and the democratic experiment that followed also led to changes in the insurance system. Two world wars, the inflation that followed each, and the Great Depression influenced both the content and structure of health care policy.

Environmental factors

Largely because of its innovative role in the development of national health insurance, Germany's health care policy has been less influenced by external factors than, for example, Great Britain's or Japan's. Rather than taking cues from the health policies of other countries, Germany has been a major source of policy inspiration.

The relative immunity from environmental influences in this area is illustrated by Germany's experience during the Allied occupation. It is, we feel, significant that although the American occupation strongly influenced Japanese health care policy, the Allied occupation of Germany had a minimal and transient impact. This is explained in part by the diversity resulting from the tripartite occupation of the western zone, but also by the resiliency of the prewar insurance system.

Structural factors

Though personalities and events loom large in the development of German health care policy, the impact of structural factors is unmistakable. The role of political regime type is particularly instructive. Under the authoritarian regimes of Imperial Germany and the totalitarian Third Reich, policy was almost exclusively the product of ministerial, rather than legislative or interest group, design. During the Weimar and the Federal republics, the formulation of policy was exposed to and influenced by a more diverse set of factors and interests.

Economic structure too has influenced health care policy. Despite early state involvement in the delivery of health care, from the very outset the provision of medical care has remained largely in the hands of private individuals and organizations (i.e., insurance carriers and physicians). Today, as in the past, physicians and insurance funds, not the government, negotiate over the condition of health care services. Only under the Third Reich was the basic economic and professional freedom of the physician compromised.

Of all the structural factors that have influenced the development of health care policy, one stands out most dramatically: the legacy of previous policy decisions and practices. As innovative as it was, the original

Sickness Insurance Law borrowed heavily from existing health care practices and institutions. Through its various political incarnations, ranging
from the most obnoxious form of totalitarian fascism to the pluralist
democracy of the Federal Republic, the basic structure of the German
system has remained intact. Each new regime and set of leaders have
accepted the basic structure as a given and carried on their own policies
within that framework. Bismarck would have little difficulty recognizing,
if not approving of, his creation.

Cultural factors

The Sickness Insurance Law of 1883 clearly was compatible with,
and in many respects made politically possible by, the prevailing paternal
ideology that had long characterized Prussian and, later, Imperial German
social policy. Bismarck, who was very much a product and proponent of
that system, undoubtedly was motivated in part by the values of the
regime he served so loyally.

The grotesque value system of Hitler's Germany also illustrates the
impact of political values on health care policy. The persecution of Jewish
patients and physicians, the prostitution of the medical profession in
implementing the policy of genocide, and the deterioration of medical
care for the ordinary citizen attest to the abhorrent ends to which Nazi
health care policy was applied.

6

Great Britain: health care in a modern welfare state

In July 1976 a British medical magazine, *World Medicine*, announced an informal contest to find the patient in Great Britain who had waited the longest for treatment by a specialist under the National Health Service (NHS). The winner of the competition would receive a Patient Patient's Award and a 1-year free subscription to one of Britain's private health insurance programs. The contest was started in response to a series of letters to the magazine from physicians complaining about the delays in getting specialist attention for their patients. Two of the more promising entries reported waiting 103 weeks to see an otolaryngologist and 138 weeks for an ophthalmologist. The winner, however, was a lady in Clitheroe, England, who as of August 1976 had been waiting for orthopedic surgery since September 1957!

The purpose of the contest was to dramatize the problem of inadequate hospital facilities in Great Britain. At the time of the study, the director of admissions at Saint Thomas's Hospital, a world-famous teaching hospital in London, reported that most of the 3,500 people waiting for admission to that institution probably would never be admitted because of its limited (850-bed) capacity.

This was not the first time in its history that the NHS had been the subject of critical attention. Since July 1948, when it was inaugurated, the state-run medical care system has been frequently criticized, and occasionally praised, by observers on both sides of the Atlantic. Not unexpectedly, the medical profession has been among the more vocal and persistent critics of the system. In 1975, for example, the NHS was threatened by the mass resignation of all its 23,000 general practitioners over complaints of poor pay and working conditions. But the notoriety surrounding the NHS should not obscure a basic fact: Public opinion polls indicate an overwhelming majority of British people support the state-run system. For example, the secretary of state for social services reported in July 1978 that 84 percent of those interviewed in a survey indicated that they were satisfied with the present health care system.[1] In fact, even its most vociferous critics have attacked provisions, not the principle, of the NHS. One doctor, who had been a member of Parliament, concluded an extraordinarily critical book on the NHS by commenting: "Whatever criticisms may have been made of the British National Health Service there can be no doubt in my mind, and in that of many fair-minded people, that the concept was right."[2] The doctor called for reform of the NHS, not its abolition. Despite its shortcomings and failures, the NHS has become a permanent, popular, although by no means flawless, part of the British welfare state. No government, Labour or Conservative, would or could abolish it.

At the end of this chapter, we examine some of the successes and failures of this ambitious and comprehensive medical system. First, however, we must turn our attention to the factors that led to its establishment, why it took the form it did, and what it was intended to accomplish. The analysis traces the evolution of state intervention in personal health care in Great Britain from its early twentieth-century beginnings, in the form of the National (Health) Insurance Act of 1911, to the National Health Service Act of 1946. These two pieces of legislation represent the most significant efforts in modern British politics in the area of medical care. In addition, they offer two distinct models or approaches to the provision of medical care: health insurance and health service. It is important that we understand why Britain chose first one then the other.[3]

National health insurance: 1912–48

The story of how and why Great Britain, the former bastion of laissez faire individualist thinking, adopted a state-sponsored medical insurance program in 1911 is the tale of a policy decision of considerable interest and importance to the student of comparative public policy. In the present context, the 1911 act takes on additional significance because it formed a vital part of the policy milieu in which the National Health Service developed. Furthermore, those interested in the possible and probable directions of an American health care system may find the earlier, more limited, British program of greater relevance than the more comprehensive National Health Service.

The National Health Insurance Act was one of a series of social reforms enacted by the Liberal government in Britain between 1906 and 1914. Many historians view these reforms, which included a school meal program, old-age pensions, unemployment insurance, minimum wage law, as well as health insurance, as the beginning of the British welfare state. The reasons behind these reforms are complex and have been the subject of careful scrutiny by historians and social scientists. Our task is to reanalyze the historical record in the area of health care policy using the accounting scheme presented in Chapter 3. The purpose of this section is to explain the adoption, content, and operation of the health insurance system that operated in Britain from 1913 to 1948.

The origins of health insurance

There is presumably a relationship between the objective needs or demands of a society and its public policies. It seems reasonable, therefore, to expect that the British health insurance program was in part a response to some felt need or articulated demand for an adequate health care system. The historical record suggests this was, in fact, the case.

The first decade of the twentieth century witnessed intense public and elite concern over the physical "condition of the British people."[4] This concern was expressed in government reports, medical journals, sociological investigations, socialist pamphlets, and the popular press. It was not the first time public attention had been drawn to the issue of the physical health and well-being of the population: Social investigators in the 1880s – for example, Charles Booth – documented the deleterious impact of industrialization on the personal circumstances of urban dwellers. The early exposés, however, did not attract significant political attention or support. To politicians, in and out of office, the "condition of the people" was not a salient political issue.

This attitude changed at the turn of the century largely as a result of the "inspection process" – to use Peacock and Wiseman's phrase – attending Britain's participation in the Boer War (1899–1902). The war had the effect of elevating an essentially esoteric issue to a full-fledged public policy problem.

The Boer War should have been won quickly and easily. It was not. It took 3 years and £250 million for the world's most powerful nation to defeat a ragtag army of Dutch farmers in what is now the Union of South Africa. Interestingly enough, a widely publicized and accepted explanation for this dismal military performance was the scandalously poor physical condition of working-class army recruits. Military leaders complained of difficulty in finding enough healthy recruits to fill their ranks and of the poor physical stamina and strength of many who were accepted for service. Published accounts suggested that 40 to 50 percent of the recruits were rejected as physically unfit; a 1904 government report noted that 8,000 of the 12,000 men examined at the Manchester recruiting depot in 1899 were rejected on this basis.

The implications of these findings went beyond the issue of military manpower needs. The condition of army recruits was seen as an indication of the general physical condition of the British working class who, after all, constituted over 80 percent of the population. Demographic data suggested that there was indeed cause for concern. Studies revealed that despite several decades of advancement in medical science and sanitary engineering, the infant mortality rate in 1901 was virtually unchanged from what it had been during the 1840s; roughly 150 per 1,000 live births. The dangers implicit in this situation were expressed in a *British Medical Journal (BMJ)* article in 1903 and reflected the attitudes of social reformers and military experts, as well as of the medical establishment. The *BMJ* warned that unless steps were taken to improve the living conditions of the working class, and particularly young children, "it is easily conceivable that the British race will deteriorate."[5]

The consequences of this "deterioration" were ominous. Physical deterioration was viewed as a manifestation of, as well as a contribution toward, the potential overall decline of the nation. Great Britain, it was argued, was in danger of losing its preeminence in the fields of education, industry, science, commerce, and international politics. The term that came to symbolize this concern was *national efficiency*. Were British educational, commercial, industrial, and scientific institutions as efficient and productive as they could be – or as they were in such countries as Germany and the United States? Was the working class as productive? Could Great Britain continue to compete with the other world powers? Some suggested that Britain's industrial productivity already lagged behind Germany's. But even here the issue returned to the question of the physical condition of the people. "At the center of the problem . . . lay the matter of physical efficiency. Great Britain was wasting her human resources. A great empire needed a martial and vigorous race. Instead there was a declining birthrate and a deteriorating incapacitated manhood."[6] Contemporary scholarly evidence supported such a contention. In 1901, B. S. Rowntree published a study of York, England, entitled *Poverty: A Study of Town Life,* in which he reported that "a low standard of health prevails among the working classes. It therefore becomes obvious that the widespread existence of poverty in an industrial country like our own must seriously retard its development."[7]

By 1903, the Conservative government could no longer ignore the issue of the "condition of the people." In that year, it appointed the Inter-Departmental Committee on Physical Deterioration. The following year, the committee issued a report that confirmed the essential conclusions of earlier social investigations: There were indeed widespread poverty, disease, and malnutrition among the British working class. The issue was kept before the public during the next several years by the Royal Commission on the Poor Laws, which held hearings, accumulated data, and issued reports between 1905 and 1909. The commission examined Britain's age-old public welfare system, including its provision for health care for the poor. Ultimately, both the conservative majority report and the more radical, and widely read, minority report called for some degree of state intervention in dealing with health care.

By the time the Liberal Party gained power in December 1905, there was general recognition that a problem existed and increasing political pressure and support for state action. The issue of personal health and health service had become part of the nation's policy agenda as a result of certain situational factors, foremost of which were the Boer War and the subsequent issue of national efficiency. Exactly how to deal with the matter was as yet undetermined. The Committee on Physical Deterioration recommended, and the Liberal Party adopted in 1906, a state-funded school meal and medical inspection program for children. But as yet no fundamental approach to the problem was contemplated. To understand why Britain chose national health insurance as the solution to its problem, we must examine certain additional factors.

Policy diffusion

Theoretically, the number and variety of policy solutions to every public problem are infinite. In practice, of course, the options available to policy makers are limited and guided by resource constraints, available technology, political culture, previous policy experience, and many of the other factors discussed in Chapter 3. Among the more influential of these factors is policy imitation. National policy makers frequently search for analogous policy problems and solutions in other countries and apply the experiences of others to their own situation.

During the late nineteenth and early twentieth centuries, Germany set the pace and standard for most of Europe in the area of social insurance legislation. "Bismarck's reforms of the 1880s – laws of 1882, 1884, and 1899 introducing compulsory insurance against sickness, accidents, old-age and invalidity – attracted immense interest in other European countries. Just as British factory legislation was copied overseas, so German social insurance stimulated foreign imitation."[8] By December 1911, when the British health insurance law was enacted, Austria (1888), Hungary (1891), Luxembourg (1901), Norway (1909), and Switzerland (1911) had all adopted health insurance programs modeled after the German system.

The impact of the German model on British policy makers was particularly strong. Most historians agree that it was as a result of a trip to Germany in 1908 that David Lloyd George, chancellor of the exchequer and major architect of the national insurance acts, was converted to the idea of a state-sponsored health program to deal with Britain's problem. Furthermore, it should be noted that this influence extended to the actual drafting of the British law. During the time the bill was being prepared, Lloyd George dispatched William Braithwaite, the civil servant assigned to drafting the proposed legislation, to Germany to study the content of the German health insurance law.

For Lloyd George and other Liberals, the importance and relevance of the German legislation involved more than simply emulating the substance and administrative structure of the law. Equally important were the political implications of Bismarck's social insurance programs. For Lloyd George and other European leaders, the major lesson to be learned from the German example was that social welfare reforms could be used by a conservative regime to undermine support for, and defuse the dangers from, the political Left. As noted in Chapter 5, this is precisely what Bismarck intended with his social insurance laws in the 1880s. "Bismarck was anxious to make German social democracy [i.e., socialism] less attractive to working-men. He feared 'class war' and wanted to postpone it as long as possible." With regard to the socialists' appeal, Bismark argued that "the thronging to them will cease as soon as working-men see that the government and legislative bodies are earnestly concerned for their welfare."[9]

In Britain, the threat from the political Left, as well as the increasing electoral strength of the working class, provided the Conservative and Liberal parties with the same dangers and opportunities Bismarck had confronted two decades earlier. In December 1905, the Liberal Party won a stunning victory over the Convervatives as a result of strong working-class support. The electoral message seemed clear: The working class wanted social reform. Thus the Liberal welfare reforms, including national health insurance, must be viewed in part as an attempt to preempt the political Left and to satisfy the increasingly powerful working-class voter.

The beauty and irony of a reform such as national health insurance were that it, like most of the Liberal program, was an essentially conservative measure – conservative not only in the sense of preempting the Left and thereby weakening its appeal, but conservative also in that it would strengthen and, thereby, help preserve the capitalist economic system in Britain. It was this latter point that made social reform so attractive to the Liberals. "The desire to retain as much as possible of the existing capitalist economic system, at a time when it was under increasing pressure from within and without, seems to have been the most important motive in the origins of the Liberal reforms."[10]

The link between national health insurance and strengthening the economic system was provided by the issue of national efficiency. The argument, simply stated, was that it was in the interest of national economic efficiency and productivity that workers stay healthy and, if taken ill, be returned to the job as quickly as possible. It is in this sense that reforms such as health insurance became, as Gaston Rimlinger so persuasively argues, "profitable, from the point of view of productivity . . . The workers' physical strength and good will had become important assets. Social insurance became one of the means of investing in human capital."[11]

That Lloyd George's primary concern was with the efficiency and productivity of the worker, rather than the state of health of the general population, is demonstrated by the fact that the health insurance bill limited coverage to workers, not their dependents and certainly not the nonworking population. The bill was not, nor was it ever intended to be, a primarily medical measure.

In sum, the origins of national health insurance lie in the concern of the British political and economic elite with improving national economic efficiency, defusing the dangers from the political Left, and, thereby, preserving the existing political and economic system. As one observer put it, Lloyd George's aim was "to spike the Socialist guns with essentially conservative measures derived from the Liberal arsenal."[12]

Pressure group politics

Lloyd George embraced national health insurance, in principle, as a result of his trip to Germany in 1908. In the following year, initial steps were taken in meetings with various private insurance agents to develop an acceptable bill based on the general principle of compulsory health insurance. Not until 1910, however, after having succeeded in pushing through budgetary reforms, was Lloyd George able to turn his full attention to wooing opponents and winning approval for his health insurance bill. The first phase of the process, beginning in the fall of 1908, essentially involved the two, often antagonistic, groups most likely to be affected by the proposed legislation: friendly societies and commercial insurance companies. The second phase began just prior to parliamentary consideration of the bill and extended beyond its actual enactment into law. During this phase, the major protagonist was the British medical profession.

Each of these actors had a great deal to lose or gain from a national health insurance program, and operating in a democratic political system, each exercised enormous influence over the ultimate substance and administrative operation of the reform. The compromises and bargains struck during these two phases affected not only national health insurance but ultimately, by negative example, its successor, the National Health Service. Scholarly analysis of the role played by these primary actors, and their impact on the law, has been critical and harsh. Harry Eckstein, for example, sees the seeds of the program's destruction in the role played by these groups.

The vested interests in opposition did not prevent passage of the measure, unlike their modern transatlantic counterparts. But they managed to make a shambles of it – and a considerable windfall to themselves – by imposing on it an incredibly

complicated administrative organization which doomed the system to ineffective-
ness, especially from a medical standpoint, from the outset.[13]

What were the interests and positions of the major actors and how did
these influence the policy outcome?

Let us begin with the friendly society movement. A *friendly society* was
a private organization catering to the needs of the British working class. It
combined the social functions and camaraderie of a fraternal lodge with
the economic protection of a commercial insurance company. From our
perspective, the insurance function was of primary importance. For a relatively small weekly premium, a friendly society member was guaranteed a
cash benefit to compensate for loss of wages during illness, free medical
care by a physician (usually) under contract by the society, and a death
benefit to cover funeral expenses. By virtue of their reliance on self-help,
the friendly societies were celebrated by nineteenth-century British Liberals
as an illustration of laissez-faire individualism at its best: industrious,
morally upright members of the British working class, protecting themselves without state intervention. Whatever the reason for their attractive-
ness, the friendly societies enjoyed enormous popularity and membership
during the nineteenth century. Bentley Gilbert estimates that around the
turn of the century nearly one-half of the adult males belonged to one of
the 24,000 registered societies and their branches.

By the latter part of the nineteenth century, however, the sense of
fraternalism, which played an important role in the development and
growth of the friendly societies, began to diminish as the organizations
became larger and less social in orientation. As a result, by the turn of the
century the insurance function of the societies became the primary induce-
ment for membership. In this context one begins to understand why the
societies became so concerned when Lloyd George announced his intention
of establishing a national health insurance program for the working class.
Such a program clearly would compete for the same clientele served by the
friendly societies.

Shortly after his intentions became known, leaders of the friendly
society movement met with Lloyd George to express their opposition to
the health insurance plan. The two sides held a series of meetings between
October and December 1908. The outcome of these meetings was a
compromise: In return for withdrawing their opposition, the friendly
societies were offered a key role – they believed, the exclusive role – as
administrative agents for the state-run insurance program. Many believed
the initial compromise was a victory for the friendly societies. This view
was based mainly on the fact that at the time many friendly societies were
in financial difficulty. The problem was that society members were living
longer and, therefore, more frequently drawing upon the sickness funds.

National health insurance would, it was hoped, relieve some of the financial burden of the friendly societies.

The first round, then, went to the friendly societies. And in at least two respects, this outcome was logical. First, it made sense to use a preexisting organizational structure and expertise to administer the program. This presumably would minimize costs and the size of the state bureaucracy. Second, the friendly societies still occupied a favored position in Liberal ideology. By incorporating them into the plan, Lloyd George hoped to legitimize national health insurance as an essentially self-reliant and democratic (each society elected its own leadership) program.

The friendly societies were not, however, the only groups involved in the insurance game. There was also the commercial insurance industry. The insurance industry in Britain was a formidable political and economic force. The industry's economic strength was based primarily on the sale of death benefits or burial policies. By 1910 there were over 30 million such policies in existence, with an additional 10 million added each year. To administer this mammoth enterprise, the industry employed about 100,000 full- and part-time employees. Financially, industrial insurance was a huge success. The largest single carrier, the Prudential, was wealthy enough to be one of the largest property and shareholders in the United Kingdom. The implications of all this were that industrial insurance in Britain

was an extremely large, profitable, and rather closely controlled business, that it engaged the talents and provided rewards for a great number of very able men, and finally, and most significant, that it had in the collecting agents an army of men in weekly contact with nearly every working-class home in the United Kingdom.[14]

It was, therefore, from a position of considerable strength that the insurance companies negotiated with Lloyd George, during 1910 and 1911, over the nature of the proposed state health insurance program. What did the insurance industry want? To begin with, it did *not* want funeral benefits included in any state insurance bill. There is some debate among historians whether Lloyd George ever intended to include death benefits. However, the insurance industry apparently thought he did and was vehemently opposed. Second, it did *not* want widows' or orphans' pensions included in the insurance plan as Lloyd George apparently did intend. Such a provision, the industry argued, would make death benefit policies, which were the lifeblood of the industry, virtually unnecessary. Third, it did *not* want the friendly societies to be the exclusive administrative agents or carriers of state health insurance. This, the industry claimed, would give the societies a strategic advantage in the death benefit market for which both the insurance companies and friendly societies competed.

The feeling was that health insurance agents would gain access to working-class homes and be in a position to sell private (death benefit) policies. Stated in the positive, the industrial insurance companies wanted to be part of the administrative structure of the national health insurance program.[15]

In November 1910, the Liberal Party was forced to call a general election. Not unmindful of the opportunity before them, the insurance industry – whose 100,000 or so collectors were generally considered to be Liberal Party supporters – marshaled its political forces and demanded from all candidates a pledge to oppose any provisions of a health insurance bill that would be prejudicial to the industry. The companies claimed to have received pledges from 460 of the 670 members of the House of Commons. They also received a letter from Lloyd George in which he promised a bill that would protect the interests of the insurance companies.

In the election of December 1910, the Liberals were returned to office. Shortly, thereafter, the efforts by the insurance companies apparently began to pay off: Widows' and orphans' benefits were dropped from the bill, the insurance companies were designated as "approved societies" (i.e., health insurance carriers), and there was no mention in the draft legislation of death benefits. Thus, another situational factor, an election, helped influence the content of health care policy. Round two went to the industrial insurance companies.

Of the three major interest groups involved, the medical profession, curiously enough, was the last to enter the debate over national health insurance. Lloyd George did not consult with the profession at all during the formative stages of the policy-making process: that is, late 1908 to mid-1910. In addition, discussions within the medical profession itself were rather limited, although articles on the subject in the *British Medical Journal* began to appear with greater frequency as 1910 wore on.

It was only *after* the insurance proposal was introduced in Parliament in May 1911 that the British Medical Association (BMA) began taking an active interest in the plan. In May the *BMJ* devoted a special issue to the subject. The BMA called a general meeting for the end of May to consider the position the profession should take on the bill. The result of that meeting was a list of six cardinal demands the doctors said had to be met before they would agree to support the bill. The demands were presented to Lloyd George when he met with BMA leaders on June 1, 1911. The demands were:

1. An income limit of £2 per week (about $5.60) on those eligible for national health insurance – to ensure that a significant proportion of the population would be available for private practice

2. Freedom of choice by both doctor and patient
3. Medical benefits to be administered by local health committees, rather than the friendly societies – with doctors represented on the health committees
4. Method of fee payment for health services to be determined by the doctors
5. Adequate compensation for medical services
6. Representation by the medical profession on all committees dealing with the medical dimensions of the law – the profession would police itself on such matters as malpractice and disagreements between doctors[16]

The doctors' demands reflected the unacceptable and often professionally degrading conditions under which many of them worked. Prior to national health insurance, most people in Britain (i.e., the working class) received ordinary medical care through some type of contractual system run by friendly societies, trade unions, and special medical "clubs." Under these arrangements, general practitioners were under contract to provide general medical care to members of the group or club. In return, the physician received a fixed per capita fee. Freedom of choice, a traditional concern among physicians, did not exist for either doctor or patient. Furthermore, doctors were often required by the club to accept non-working-class patients at contract rates. This deprived them of an important source of income: noncontractual (i.e., private) patients. Professional standards were further eroded by the fact that doctors were often required, either by contract or financial necessity, to solicit new members for the club. This, combined with fee schedules generally acknowledged to be inadequate, led to intense competition among doctors for club contracts and new patients. Lastly, the doctors did not have security of tenure; they could be dismissed by a club, society, or union at any time. In short, the majority of the doctors worked under demeaning professional conditions, enjoyed little freedom, inadequate compensation, and an uncertain practice. It was in this context that the BMA made its six demands.

Upon submitting these demands to Lloyd George, the doctors began an active campaign to win support in Parliament. Their tactics included a pledge signed by 27,000 of the 32,000 members of the BMA to refuse to serve under the National Health Insurance Act unless their demands were met. The campaign resulted in the adoption, in committee, of four of the six cardinal points – all but the income limit and the specified per capita fee. Despite continued medical opposition, the National Health Insurance Act was passed by Parliament and received royal assent on December 16, 1911.

The passage of the act did not end the matter as far as the medical profession was concerned. The law was not to go into effect until July 15, 1912, and no medical benefits would be disbursed until after a 6-month waiting period during which time weekly contributions would be made by the subscribers. The effective date of operation would be January 15, 1913. The medical profession, or elements within it, was not yet willing to concede the remaining demands: an income limit and "adequate" per capita fees. The debate and opposition were renewed. In February 1912, the BMA again called upon its membership to refuse to participate in the program until its demands were met. As the months passed, neither the government nor the BMA appeared willing to compromise. Finally, in October 1912, after the law went into effect but before patients could actually use the service, Lloyd George offered to raise the per capita fee beyond the level specified in the law. The new offer was considered inadequate by BMA leaders and rejected.

By the latter part of 1912, the bargaining power of the British Medical Association was considerably eroded. This erosion resulted from a loss of public support for the medical profession. The doctors appeared greedy – particularly after Lloyd George's latest offer – and insensitive to the needs of the working class, which eagerly awaited the start of the new insurance program. But perhaps more importantly, the BMA was becoming increasingly estranged from its own rank and file. The BMA leadership consisted mainly of specialists and consultants. These doctors were the most prestigious and affluent members of the profession – and the ones least likely to be affected by the insurance act. The vast majority of the doctors were underpaid general practitioners, who derived most of their income from contract practice. For these doctors, the National Health Insurance Act promised greater professional freedom, more security, *and* more money – in some cases as much as two or three times more each year. A study undertaken with the approval of both the government and the BMA in July 1912 reported that the average general practitioner in Britain earned about 4s 5d per year per patient (about 62 cents). Thus the last government offer of 9s (about $1.26) promised a considerable increase in income for the doctors.[17]

Defections from the ranks accelerated following publication of the income study. In the beginning of January 1913, Lloyd George announced that there were 10,000 doctors ready to provide medical care under the insurance law – a number sufficient to make the law work. With this announcement, the rush to sign up as a national health insurance doctor began. On January 17, 1913, in a face-saving move, the BMA released its members from their previous pledge of noncompliance. Two days earlier, January 15, 1913, working-class men and women throughout Britain had begun receiving medical care under the National Health Insurance Act.

Provisions of the National Health Insurance Act

At this point it is useful to summarize the provisions of the National Health Insurance Act.[18]

Eligibility

The act provided for compulsory participation by all wage earners, 16 to 65 years old, earning less than £60 ($448) per year. The income limit was periodically increased until the 1940s when the maximum was £420 ($1,176) per year. The law did *not* cover self-employed persons (including farmers), dependents, or the nonworking population.

Financing

The program was financed by contributions from workers, employers, and the state. Initially, the weekly contribution was about 3 or 4 cents for each worker, slightly less for the employer, with the state paying about one-sixth of the total. By the 1940s the worker's share was about 9 cents per week.

Benefits

The act provided for the following benefits:

1. A *medical benefit* that consisted of medical attention, treatment, and "proper and sufficient" medicine without charge. The medical care was limited to what ordinarily would be considered within the competence and practice of a general practitioner. It did not provide for hospitalization.
2. If unable to attend work owing to illness, each contributor was eligible for a weekly *sickness benefit* for up to 26 weeks. The amount of the benefit varied according to sex and marital status. Men received the maximum payment (which by the 1940s was $3.75 per week), married women the minimum ($2.50). In order to receive the sickness benefit, a worker had to be certified each week by a physician as incapable of working.
3. After 26 weeks of sickness benefits, the insured worker became eligible for a *disability benefit*. This benefit amounted to one-half of the sickness benefit and could be received indefinitely.
4. Insured workers were also eligible for a *maternity benefit*. This was a straight cash benefit of £2 ($5.60) either to a male worker whose wife gave birth or a female worker who gave birth.
5. Finally, any surplus or profits an approved society had accrued

could be used for *additional benefits* or to reduce the workers' weekly premiums. Such a surplus might result from a low incidence of sickness benefits paid to members of the society or from wise investments. Additional benefits had to be approved by the Ministry of Health and included money for such things as dental, ophthalmic, and convalescent care.

Administration

The administrative apparatus of National Health Insurance (NHI) reflected the compromises over the demands made by the medical profession and the insurance carriers. As the doctors had insisted, the medical benefits were administered, not by the approved societies but by local insurance committees. These committees were responsible for record keeping (e.g., which doctors served which workers) and resolving disputes between doctors and patients.

The sickness, disability, and maternity benefits were administered by the approved societies. An approved society was simply any organization that acted as an insurance carrier. As indicated earlier, the most common were friendly societies, industrial insurance companies, and trade unions, although any group of people could get government approval as a carrier. The requirements for approval included organizational control by the membership (a concession to the democratically run friendly societies), fiscal responsibility, and operation on a nonprofit basis. By the 1940s there were over 800 approved societies in Great Britain with memberships ranging from 100 to over 2 million. The approved societies received the weekly contributions (via the Post Office or Ministry of Health) of their members, invested them, and paid out nonmedical benefits.

It is important to emphasize that the only area of contact between the approved societies and the doctors occurred if a society questioned the certification of incapacity made by a doctor. Such disputes were resolved by regional medical officers, who were themselves doctors and appointed by the Ministry of Health. Thus, contact between the doctors and societies was kept, as the doctors had insisted, to a minimum.

Operation

In practice, the system operated in the following manner. A working young man or woman upon reaching the age of 16 years joined an approved society – typically a trade union, the friendly society to which his or her father belonged, or one of the aggressive insurance companies. Upon acceptance by the society – usually a physical examination was required – the young person chose any doctor he or she wished from a panel of doctors registered with the local insurance committee. Participation by qualified physicians in insurance practice was entirely voluntary, although ultimately two-thirds of the doctors participated. Those doctors who accepted NHI patients could still treat private patients, although most general practitioners earned the bulk of their incomes through insurance practice.

Once the young worker registered with a doctor, he or she became part of that doctor's "panel." The law allowed a doctor a panel of up to 2,500 patients, but the average physician's panel was between 1,000 and 1,500. A doctor received 9s (about $1.26) per patient each year, regardless of the number of times, if any, he saw each patient. A person could change doctors at any time, provided the doctor or the local insurance committee was informed.

This was the system that operated in Great Britain from July 1913 until July 1948. In the British context, it was a radical, even revolutionary, step. It involved the state for the first time in a direct way in providing curative and personal medical care to a substantial proportion of the population. NHI did not, nor was it ever supposed to, provide a comprehensive medical care system. It was a result of a series of compromises, concessions, and modifications involving competing interest groups, the prevailing ideology, and available resources. It was, in short, a workable program. The shortcomings and failures of NHI provide, in part, the background to the establishment of the more comprehensive and ambitious National Health Service. To this story we now turn.

The National Health Service

There are several important similarities in the circumstances surrounding the establishment of the National Health Insurance Act of 1911 and the National Health Service Act of 1946. First, in both 1911 and 1946 there was increasing popular and professional dissatisfaction with the existing medical delivery system. Second, awareness of the inadequacies of the existing system was stimulated and accelerated in both periods by an inspection process accompanying Britain's involvement in war – the Boer War and World War II. Third, the issue of medical care reform formally became part of the policy agenda with the publication of a widely read and much heralded government report – the Report of the Commission on the Poor Law (1909) and the Beveridge Report (1942). Fourth, adoption of the new health law was temporally proximate to a significant change in party control – the Liberals came to power in 1906 and the Labour Party in 1945. Fifth, leadership of the policy process fell in both instances to articulate, aggressive, and often abrasive Welshmen – Lloyd George and Aneurin Bevan. And, lastly, the content and implementation of both laws were affected by the eleventh-hour threat of nonparticipation by the medical profession. In both cases, situational factors played a key role in the policy process.

There were, however, significant differences in the factors influencing the adoption of these two monumental pieces of social legislation. First, policy imitation played an important role in 1911, but not in 1946. Whereas in 1911 Lloyd George was demonstrably infuenced by the German insurance scheme, in 1946 Great Britain set the pace and provided the model that a number of countries were to follow. Second, and perhaps most importantly, there was in 1946 overwhelming popular, professional, and political acceptance of, indeed insistence upon, the notion that health care was a *right* of all the people and an obligation of the state. The public was willing and eager for a comprehensive medical care system in 1946.

Let us now look more closely at the factors that led to the establishment and influenced the content of the National Health Service. Following this discussion, we examine the provisions of the law and evaluate the performance of the health care system that was described by the man who presided over its birth as "the most civilized achievement of modern government."[19]

Origins of the act

The National Health Insurance Act of 1911 represented an incomplete revolution in British health care policy. For the reasons discussed earlier, Lloyd George's scheme covered only a portion of the British people and provided only limited, general practitioner services. By the 1940s, about 40 percent of the population was covered by NHI. For the remaining 60 percent – the wives and children of workingmen, self-employed persons, and those with incomes over the specified limit – medical expenses still presented a danger to personal economic security. The middle class was particularly vulnerable and hard hit by medical expenses. Unlike the rich, who could handle ordinary and extraordinary medical expenses, and the lower class, who received medical attention through a variety of charitable and publicly supported programs, the middle class was left to rely on its own limited resources. "It was the middle-class which bore the principal burden of neglect. It received no concessions at all in the finance of its medical requirements and it was forced, by indirect means, to subsidize the medical coverage of the rest of the population."[20]

A second feature of the British medical delivery system that, although not created by NHI, was perpetuated by it, was the unequal distribution of medical personnel. Because doctors preferred to practice in areas where they could maximize the more lucrative private patient practice, they tended to gravitate toward affluent, typically urban or resort communities.

The result was an extreme maldistribution of medical personnel. Affluent sections of London and various resort areas were overdoctored; severe shortages of personnel existed in most working-class areas.

But perhaps the most obvious and important deficiency of NHI was its failure to cover specialized medical care or hospitalization. Aside from the obvious hardships this imposed on those who could not afford these services or who were not eligible for them under some sort of charitable system, the consequences of this omission were particularly profound for the British hospital system itself. The hospital system suffered from two major defects, neither of which was remedied by NHI: (1) a lack of administrative coordination among hospitals within the country and (2) financial uncertainty. Both defects ultimately affected the quality and quantity of medical care the hospitals could provide.

Much of the problem stemmed from the nature of the hospital system, if it could be called a system at all. There were essentially two types of hospitals in Great Britain prior to 1948. The first type was the municipal hospital run by county governments and, theoretically, available to all who resided in the county and needed hospital care. These hospitals were, in the main, former Poor Law institutions; that is, workhouses turned into hospitals to serve the indigent poor. In 1929, these institutions were taken over by the local governments. Although middle- and upper-class patients were eligible for treatment, the municipal hospitals continued to carry the stigma and appearance of their former status. As a result, they did not attract many non-working-class patients. One implication of the lower-class bias of the patients was that the municipal hospitals came to rely heavily on local taxes for their finances rather than on patients' fees, which were based on ability to pay. These taxes provided a level of funding that typically was inadequate to maintain, much less improve, the medical facilities. Finally, it should be noted that the municipal hospitals generally provided medical care geared either to routine problems (e.g., maternity services, tonsillectomies) or to chronic ailments (e.g., terminal cancer). The chronically ill patients, in particular, put increasing financial strain on the municipal hospital system. The fact that many municipal hospitals provided only routine care meant that those who required specialized hospital attention often had to travel some distance to receive it.

The second type of facility was the voluntary hospital. These were charitable institutions, founded during the eighteenth and nineteenth centuries, whose main purpose was to serve the sick, but "deserving," poor. Unlike the municipal hospitals, they tended to specialize in acute medical problems (e.g., crisis surgery, cardiology). A unique feature of the voluntary hospital system was that doctors provided their services free of charge. The motive behind this practice was not, however, entirely altruistic. Service in a voluntary hospital was the primary way for a specialist or surgeon to establish a reputation and thereby cultivate a wealthy private clientele. Doctors advertised their voluntary hospital affiliation, and patients who could afford to finance their own medical care sought such doctors out. In addition, most teaching hospitals were voluntary hospitals, and a specialist or surgeon could expect referrals from his former students.

Although the voluntary hospitals were originally established to serve the deserving poor, the fact that they were staffed by some of the best doctors in the country inevitably produced pressure to admit nonpoor patients – which they did. When this happened, a shift in the mode of financing occurred. Initially, the voluntary hospitals were completely dependent on charitable contributions from wealthy patrons. By the 1940s, however, about half of their income was derived from patients' fees. A substantial proportion of these fees were paid through private insurance schemes, which were becoming increasingly popular among the middle class. Despite this, however, the voluntary hospitals, like the municipal hospitals, faced severe financial difficulty; charitable contributions were dwindling as a result of the Depression, and patients' fees were inadequate to make up the deficits.

In sum, hospital care in Britain on the eve of World War II was characterized by critically inadequate financing, a lack of overall coordination to provide a rational geographical distribution of facilities, inadequate and deteriorating facilities, and costly conflict and competition between voluntary and municipal hospitals. Richard Titmuss estimated that on any given day in 1938–39, 100,000 people were waiting for admission to voluntary hospitals alone.[21]

The impact of war

It is almost certain that the British government would have responded to the organizational and financial problems of the health care system had World War II not occurred. What the war did was to hasten the process *and* help shape the nature of the solution. In the most literal sense, the war lead to an inspection of British medical facilities. In anticipation of war and the expectation that it would involve bombing of civilian as well as military areas, the Ministry of Health established in June 1938 the Emergency Medical Service (EMS). The initial mandate of the EMS was to inventory existing medical facilities and personnel, determine the steps necessary to prepare the nation's medical delivery system for war, and establish an organizational plan to coordinate the system to handle military and civilian casualties. Once the war began, the EMS (under the Ministry of Health) was responsible for the distribution and allocation of funds, hospital beds, and medical personnel throughout the country. Legally, the minister of health or the director general of the EMS could direct all hospitals to take the necessary steps (e.g., reserve a certain number of beds for war-related patients to handle war-related medical problems). In practice, the government had to act with political caution in dealing with the different interests and sensitivities of the *private* voluntary hospitals and the *public* municipal hospitals.[22]

The magnitude, varied problems, and considerable accomplishments of this undertaking are beyond the scope of this case study. From our perspective, the significance of the EMS and its activities is twofold. First, the EMS documented, in undeniable terms, the serious deficiencies in Britain's medical delivery system. On the subject of British hospitals, for example, the director general of the EMS wrote, in 1939, that prior to the survey of hospital facilities undertaken in preparation for the war "there was little appreciation of the low standard of hospital accommodation in the country as a whole. Even those institutions that are to be regarded as the centres of enlightened treatment and teaching in our large cities, are, with few exceptions, structurally either unsafe or woefully antiquated."[23] In virtually every area of medical care – nursing, utilization of hospital beds, quantity of doctors, medical equipment, and medical procedures – the surveys conducted by the EMS found gross deficiencies.

Second, the EMS imposed an unprecedented degree of order and coordination on the British medical system. The Ministry of Health, through the emergency doctor and hospital services, provided a centralized administrative apparatus for coordinating all aspects of war-related and many facets of non-war-related medical care. The government for the first time became directly involved in the direction, organization, delivery, and provision of health care. Although this involvement was supposed to be, and primarily was, limited to war-related (military and civilian) health care needs, the realities of modern warfare often made the distinction between ordinary (non-war-related) and emergency medical care unclear or irrelevant. Was it not as important to the war effort to get a sick airplane factory worker back on the job as to get a wounded soldier back to the front? The scope and experience of state activity in providing medical care for so large a number of people from 1939 to 1945 played an important part in the policy experience the postwar government drew upon in establishing the National Health Service.

The wartime experience – the bombings of the cities, the evacuation of children, the hardship, sacrifices, and suffering endured by virtually the entire population – led to an inspection process of another sort as well. This one was not limited to a specific social need, but concerned broader issues such as the quality of life, the equitable distribution of societal resources, social justice, and the proper role of the state in serving peoples' needs. In July 1940, shortly after the British navy evacuated trapped Allied troops from the European continent through Dunkirk, the *Times of*

London, hardly a radical newspaper, captured and articulated the change in philosophy that the war brought to Great Britain.

If we speak of democracy, we do not mean a democracy which maintains the right to vote but forgets the right to work and the right to live. If we speak of freedom, we do not mean a rugged individualism which excludes social organization and economic planning. If we speak of equality, we do not mean a political equality nullified by social and economic privilege. If we speak of economic reconstruction, we think less of maximum production . . . than of equitable distribution.[24]

The Beveridge Report

It now remained for the health care problems revealed by the surveys and experience of the EMS and the more informal inspection process accompanying the war formally to become part of the nation's policy agenda. This was accomplished by a report by the Inter-Departmental Committee on Social Insurance and Allied Services.

Despite its preoccupation with the war, the coalition government announced in June 1941 that it was appointing an interdepartmental committee to conduct "a survey of the existing national schemes of social insurance and allied services and make policy recommendations" to guide the government in the task of reconstruction following the war. The report, which was presented to the House of Commons in November 1942, carried the name of its author, Sir William Beveridge. The Beveridge Report became an instant best-seller; hundreds of thousands of copies were sold in Britain and abroad, and it was translated, in whole or in part, into seven languages. Excerpts from the report were read over the radio and discussed in newspapers and pubs. The importance of the report derived as much from the promise it offered of a postwar world free from the "Five Giants" – Want, Disease, Ignorance, Squalor, and Idleness – as for its specific recommendations. The *Times of London,* on December 2, 1942, called the report "a momentous document which should and must exercise a profound and immediate influence on the direction of social change in Britain."

In terms of our interests, we need be concerned only with the section of the report that dealt with health care. Beveridge linked freedom from want with the provision of a comprehensive medical care system. Although the section concerning health services was short on detail, its intention was unambiguous. The report called for "a comprehensive national health service [which] will ensure that for every citizen there is available whatever medical treatment he requires, in whatever form he requires it, domiciliary or institutional, general, specialist or consultant and will ensure also the provision of dental, ophthalmic and surgical appliances, nursing and midwifery and rehabilitation after accidents."

Furthermore this care should "be provided where needed without contribution conditions [i.e., the ability to pay] in any individual case."[25]

It is generally recognized that the Beveridge Report, at least with regard to its recommendation on medical care, was not particularly revolutionary or pathbreaking. Beveridge himself observed that "the Plan of my Report is a completion of what was begun a little more than thirty years ago when Mr. Lloyd George introduced National Health Insurance."[26] What the report provided, in addition to the significant boost to national morale, was a basis for the formal consideration of a universal, comprehensive medical care system. Political differences between the Conservatives and Labourites, plus Winston Churchill's unwillingness to support any controversial or innovative domestic policy as long as Britain was at war and ruled by a coalition government, prevented the immediate passage of legislation to set up a national health service. Instead, the report was sent to a committee for further study.

In February 1944, the committee, composed of members from both Labour and Conservative parties, issued a white paper on a national health service. The white paper echoed Beveridge's call for a comprehensive medical care system, available to every citizen, regardless of ability to pay. The service would include and coordinate general practitioner, specialist, surgical, ophthalmic, maternity, and dental care. These services would be free. Funding would come mainly from the national treasury, but be supplemented by insurance contributions and local taxes. Both municipal and voluntary hospitals would receive financial assistance from the central government, and there would be greater coordination and integration between the two hospital systems. The municipal hospitals would be taken over by the central government; the voluntary hospitals would maintain their private status. The principle of freedom of choice between doctor and patient, the panel system, and central administrative control by the Ministry of Health would continue. Neither doctor nor patient would be forced to participate in the scheme. In short, as many features of the old NHI system as possible would be maintained. One important issue left unresolved was remuneration. Suggestions included salary and/or capitation fees for various types of practice. The issue was left sufficiently ambiguous to allow for future negotiation – and conflict.

In March 1944, the House of Commons accepted, in principle, the white paper. Although work continued on the details of the new health service, formal legislative action had to await the end of the war with Germany and the much anticipated general election that would determine which party, Conservative or Labour, would usher in the era of freedom from the "Five Giants." Germany surrendered in May 1945, and on July 5, 1945, voters in Great Britain gave the Labour Party an overwhelming mandate to create a welfare state: Labour won 399 seats to the Conservatives' 213.

The task of translating the proposals of the white paper, which formed the basis for subsequent discussion, fell to the new minister of health, Aneurin Bevan – a Welshman of considerable political skill but abrasive personality. Bevan, like Lloyd George three decades earlier, was to find that his most formidable adversary was the British medical profession. Much of Bevan's time until July 1948, when the National Health Service Act went into effect, was devoted to winning support of the medical profession.

The doctors and the National Health Service Act

Contrary to apocalyptic predictions, the medical profession survived and indeed prospered under National Health Insurance. The doctors' worst fears of loss of clinical freedom and lay domination over professional matters were never realized. If doctors were not ecstatic about working under NHI, they were at the very least reconciled to it. A report by the profession in 1942 generously noted that NHI was "a greater success than was anticipated either by its supporters or by its opponents."[27] The degree to which the doctors had learned to live with state participation in the medical delivery system is reflected in the proposals for health reform initiated by the profession itself during World War II.

The activities of the EMS and the doctors' own experiences during the war led the profession to its own inspection of medical care in Britain. In August 1940, a medical planning commission was established by the BMA, the Royal Medical Colleges, and other professional groups. The resulting report, issued in 1942, has been described as "the most remarkable plan for self-reform in the history of the British profession."[28] We need not concern ourselves here with all its details. A brief review of its major recommendations is in order, however, for they reveal how far the medical profession had traveled since 1911. In addition, the report, like the Beveridge Report, which it preceded in time, provided much of the basis for subsequent discussions on the National Health Service. In fact, Beveridge himself quoted from the doctors' plan in his own report.

The commission recommended the following reforms. First, it acknowledged that the objective of medical service was "to render available to every individual all necessary medical services, both general and specialist, and both domiciliary and institutional." Thus, in addition to general practitioner services, the profession called for access to specialist, hospital, dental, and ophthalmic care. Second, to achieve this aim it would be necessary to have a centralized, *public* authority administer and coordinate these services throughout the country. Third, the commission called for organization of all hospitals on a regional basis. Fourth, it recommended that doctors establish group practices. This last recommendation was aimed at better utilization and coordination of medical personnel and equipment in treating patients. Aside from these generally innovative, almost radical, proposals, the commission's recommendations were moderate. It favored continued use of contributory health insurance to finance health care, but proposed extending NHI eligibility to cover dependents, self-employed persons, and many who were excluded by prevailing income restrictions. The eligibility extensions would result in coverage of approximately 90 percent of the population. Although this proposal appears revolutionary, it should be noted that the commission was aware that at the time only about 10 percent of the British people could afford private medical care. Finally, the commission repeated the traditional litany of freedom of choice and professional involvement in administration.

By 1944 it appeared that there was an emerging consensus, at least on fundamental principles, with regard to defining the major health care problems and specifying solutions to them. One can document the evolution of this consensus from the Interim Report of the Medical Planning Commission (June 1942) to the Beveridge Report (November 1942) to the parliamentary white paper (February 1944). Given the wide areas of agreement among the major parties, it is surprising that the first formal utterance of the profession's leadership on the white paper was negative. The *British Medical Journal* announced shortly after the white paper was issued: "It is difficult to see how, in the kind of evolutionary changes which are so persuasively outlined, private practice as we know it today can survive as much more than a shadow of itself."[29] As the *BMJ* saw it, the government was surreptitiously trying to exert bureaucratic control over the medical profession, limit the physician's freedom, and turn him into a civil servant.

One may well wonder at the apparent change in attitude on the part of the medical leadership. The most reasonable explanation has been offered by Eckstein:

What happened after 1942 is really very simple. Up to that time, planning for medical reform had been predominantly a professional enterprise and a paper enterprise. Now that the Government had shown its willingness to act on the paper schemes, the possibility of reform became concrete and imminent; moreover, the responsibility for reform was about to pass into the hands of laymen, and worse, into the hands of politicians and bureaucrats.[30]

For whatever reason, the official position of the profession's leadership changed dramatically. But what about the rank and file? What was the attitude of the general practitioner and the specialist? In an effort to determine this, the BMA sent out a questionnaire to its membership to gauge reaction to the white paper. About 48 percent of the doctors responded to the questionnaire, which solicited opinions on the white paper in general and on its specific provisions. Given the complexity of the issue, it is not surprising that the results were ambiguous. The overall reaction to the white paper, however, was negative: 39 percent favored it; 53 percent opposed it. On certain aspects of the proposed plan, the reaction tended to be more positive – and, therefore, more out of tune with the BMA leadership: 60 percent favored a free, comprehensive medical service for the entire population – a position opposed by the BMA leaders; 57 percent favored a central medical board to control doctors' entry into overdoctored areas – again, contrary to the leadership's view. On other issues, however, the profession seemed to speak with one voice. The doctors strongly opposed administrative control by local government authorities in any aspect of health care.

In sum, it appears that the doctors agreed with their leaders on opposing the administrative arrangements for the proposed health system, but disagreed over the principle of a free, comprehensive, and universally applicable medical care system. In addition, it should be noted that there were significant differences of opinion, even within the rank and file. General practitioners tended to take a more conservative (i.e., negative) position than the hospital-based specialists. Eckstein and Lindsey agree that this can be explained by the fact that specialists tended to practice under more structured and organized circumstances (i.e., a hospital environment) and, therefore, were less uncomfortable with the proposed administrative structure than the more independent general practitioners. Furthermore, it must be remembered that much of the specialists' work in voluntary hospitals was done gratuitously. Under the proposed health service they would be compensated for all services. Finally, to complicate matters even further, there was a generational split among the doctors: Younger doctors tended to be more favorably disposed toward the white paper than the older doctors.

In conclusion, as in 1911, the medical profession labored under two severe handicaps in its negotiations with the government over the proposed health service. The first was the division and ambiguity of opinion within the profession itself – a situation any astute Welsh politician could exploit. The second was the overwhelming popular demand for a national health service. Surely the doctors recognized by 1944–5 that the issue was not whether there should be a comprehensive national health service, but rather what the nature of that service was to be.

The legislative process

Aneurin Bevan, the major advocate and architect of the new health system, was well aware of the strength of his position. He was aware of the degree of popular support, manifested in the reaction to the Beveridge Report and Labour's mandate in the general election, for a new, comprehensive approach to medical care. And he was aware that, as in 1912, the medical profession did not speak with one voice; certainly the survey results on the white paper had shown that.

Given these conditions, it is not surprising that in the several meetings Bevan had with representatives of the profession, prior to submitting a formal bill to Parliament, the process was discussion, not negotiation. Bevan listened to the doctors and did, in fact, make some important concessions to them. After all, the service could not work without the support of the profession. The bill presented to the House of Commons in March 1946 included some of these concessions. Among them were a provision for "private" beds in nationalized hospitals; maintenance of the capitation fee as the basis of remuneration for general practitioners but, at Bevan's insistence, a small basic salary for younger doctors; and removal of local authority control over hospital and specialist services.

Despite these concessions, the bill clearly bore the ideological stamp of Bevan and the British political Left. For example, the sale of medical practices was to be abolished. It was common for a retiring physician to sell his practice or "good-will" to another, usually new, physician. The procedure was supported by the medical leadership, but opposed by the rank and file, and particularly by younger doctors. Bevan considered the practice tantamount to buying and selling patients and was adamantly opposed to it. The bill also provided for the nationalization of all hospitals, including the voluntary hospitals. Bevan felt that charity was an uncertain and essentially demeaning source of revenue. Finally, financing of the health scheme would come mainly from general taxation rather than insurance contributions. Weekly insurance contributions would continue, but would provide only a tiny fraction of the funding. General tax funding would mean that the rich would be paying more for the health service bill than the poor through higher taxation. Thus, the new law would be congruent with the redistributive inclination of the Labour Party.

It took 8 months of relatively uneventful deliberation for the National Health Service Bill to clear Parliament. On July 26, 1946, the bill passed the House of Commons by a vote of 261 to 113: Most of the opposition was to specific provisions rather than the general principle. Finally, on November 6, 1946, 4 years after the Beveridge Report, the National Health Service Act received royal assent. The service was not scheduled to begin operation until July 1948, to allow time to establish the necessary administrative apparatus *and* work out arrangements with the medical profession. As they had done three decades earlier, the doctors used the interim between passage of the law and its actual operation to confront the government on issues they had not been able to win in the legislative arena.

The extralegislative process

Following enactment of the National Health Service Act, the British Medical Association polled its membership on the question: Shall we or shall
we not enter into any discussion on the framework to be created within
the limitations of this act? And 90 percent responded no. As in the white
paper survey, the profession was divided: 55 percent of the specialists were
opposed to discussion; a majority of younger specialists and those physicians who were already salaried favored discussion. Nevertheless, the
overall tone and impression of the response did not bode well for the
future health system. Shortly thereafter, a special meeting of the BMA
leadership voted 252 to 17 to refuse negotiations with the Ministry of
Health over the doctors' role in the NHS.[31]

The remainder of the story reads like a replay of 1912–13. The doctors
threatened nonparticipation, and Bevan cajoled, charmed, and blustered.
Four main issues dominated the discussion during 1947 and on into 1948.
The first was the general practitioners' obsession with the prospect of a
full-time, salaried service that would turn them into "mere" civil
servants. The £300 basic salary for younger physicians ($750 in 1978
exchange rates, $840 in 1948) was just the beginning, a toe in the door,
which would eventually be extended to a complete, salaried service.
Second, the BMA opposed the abolition of the sale of practices. Although
the act did provide compensation, at the time of retirement or death, to
those initially entering the NHS, the BMA wanted the practice maintained indefinitely. Third, the doctors felt there were inadequate safe-
guards against capricious, unwarranted, and unjust dismissal from the
NHS. Clearly, in a medical system that the overwhelming majority of the
population was expected to use and wherein only a small proportion of
the doctors depended upon private practice, expulsion from the NHS
would be tantamount to ending a physician's career. Finally, the profession wanted greater assurance that the nationalization of the hospitals
would not extend to private nursing homes or eventual elimination of
reserved (i.e., private) beds in health service hospitals.

As the date of operation approached, Bevan conceded certain points.
While refusing to incorporate it in statute, he promised that private
hospital practice – either in nursing homes or reserved beds – would not
be abolished.[32] He was adamant about abolishing the sale of medical practices, but agreed to reexamine the level of compensation for those who
would be affected by retirement during the early stages of the new system.
Despite these and other conciliatory gestures, the profession was not
placated. A BMA poll of its membership in February 1948 found 90
percent of the doctors still opposed to the law and 88 percent saying they
would refuse to participate in the program.

In April 1948, just 3 months before the law was to go into effect, Bevan made further important concessions. He agreed to submit supplementary legislation prohibiting a full-time salaried service for general practitioners. In addition, the £300 base salary would be paid only to doctors just entering practice, rather than all young doctors. He also promised that the chairman of the Central Tribunal, the disciplinary body of the service, would be a lawyer of outstanding reputation, thus assuring the doctors of protection against capricious removal.

Given these further concessions, the BMA conducted still another poll of its membership, the results of which were published in May 1948. Once again the doctors indicated opposition to the NHS, but the margin had decreased to about 60 percent. More significantly, only a slight majority was now opposed to participating in the service. Not unmindful of the embarrassment and loss of prestige it suffered in 1913, when it had been left behind by its membership, BMA leaders decided in the latter part of May to recommend participation in the new National Health Service. By July 5, 1948, the appointed day, a majority of the doctors and about 75 percent of the people had registered with the service. Ultimately, over 98 percent of the people and medical personnel in Great Britain would participate.

The provisions of the National Health Service

We can now examine the actual provisions of the National Health Service. The description includes changes incorporated into the system since 1948 and thus represents the system as it operates today.

Coverage

Benefits under the NHS are available to all persons normally resident in Great Britain. There are no age, sex, contributory, occupational, social, racial, or any other exceptions to the basic assumption of universal applicability and availability. Over 98 percent of the people of Great Britain are currently registered with a health service physician.

Financing

The NHS is financed primarily from central and local government taxation: about 72 percent from central government revenue and 13 percent from local taxes. An additional 10 percent of the cost is covered by a fixed, weekly employee-employer contribution. This amounts to about 30 cents at the 1978 exchange rate per week for each male, 26 cents for a female, and 17 cents for the employer. Those who do not work, are unemployed, or are retired are exempt from this contribution. The remaining 5 percent of health service cost is provided through user fees or a cost-sharing provision. This involves relatively small fees for such items as dentures and eye-glasses, and a fixed 34-cent fee for each prescription. Most fees, however, are waived for expectant and nursing mothers, elderly and disabled persons, and the poor.

It is important to dwell for a moment on the significance of the shift in financing health care from the contributory insurance scheme under NHI to primary reliance on general taxation. The departure from a health insurance to a health service system represents an important administrative and ideological change. The change occurred in part because Bevan believed that contributory health insurance schemes were unwieldy to administer, too costly, and tended to exclude noncontributors. Beyond these administrative objections lay a more fundamental ideological point. This was the belief, shared by an increasing number of people in Britain and certainly by the Labour Party and its supporters, that everyone has a *right* to complete medical care services, regardless of ability to pay. And, as is true for other rights, such as justice or liberty or education, it is the responsibility of the state to provide that service. Beveridge had said in his report that "restoration of a sick person to health is a duty of the State," and so it was to be under the NHS. Ideology clearly influenced the financial provisions of the NHS.

Benefits

The National Health Service provides, with little or no cost to the user at the point of delivery, virtually the entire range of required medical services. For purposes of discussion (and until April 1974 as a matter of administrative organization), these services are divided into three areas: general practitioner, hospital and specialist, and local public health services. Sickness and maternity benefits (i.e., a cash allowance for working persons who must miss work because of illness or pregnancy) are financed and administered apart from the NHS and, therefore, are not described here.

Practitioner services

Practitioner services include out-patient care and dental, ophthalmic, and pharmaceutical services. The general practitioner or family doctor is the primary actor in the National Health Service. Except in emergency cases, the general practitioner has the first and most frequent contact with the average citizen. It is only by referral from a generalist that other (i.e., specialist) health services are made available to the public.

Every British citizen over 16 years of age who wishes to participate in the NHS is required to register with a physician of his or her choice. The doctor may refuse to accept a person for his list – although he may not refuse to give necessary treatment to a person not on his list or in case of an emergency. All medical treatment by a general practitioner, whether in his office or at the patient's home, is completely free.

A family doctor practicing on his own may have a list of up to 3,500 patients; the average is about 2,325. Doctors engaged in group practice may maintain a maximum list of 4,500 patients, provided the average for the group does not exceed 3,500 patients per physician. General practitioners are not permitted to treat patients in hospitals, nor are they equipped with x-ray or other diagnostic facilities. If medical tests or hospitalization are required, the general practitioner refers the patient to a specialist, who may then order hospitalization. In all other areas, the family physician enjoys complete clinical freedom.

Dental services

There is no list or registration system for dental care. Any person in need of care simply makes an appointment with a participating dentist (most do participate in the NHS). Examinations are free, but the patient must pay one-half of the treatment cost, up to a maximum of $17.40 per course of treatment. The remaining 50 percent of the cost is paid by the NHS. Children under 16 years (or under 21 if they are full-time students), expectant mothers, and women who have given birth within the last year are exempt from all charges. The clinical freedom of the dentist is somewhat limited by the fact that he must receive approval from the Dental Estimates Board before performing extraordinary procedures (e.g., oral surgery). This is primarily a cost-control procedure.

Ophthalmic services

General ophthalmic services are provided by a physician, optometrist, or optician. Eye examinations are free, but the patient must pay for eyeglasses; a $6.09 maximum is set by law. Children under 16 years and poor people are exempt from these fees. Any treatment beyond vision testing or prescribing eyeglasses is performed at special eye hospitals or hospital eye clinics.

Pharmaceutical services

There is a charge of 34 cents for each item prescribed by a health service doctor. Medicines are dispensed by pharmacists, who collect the prescription charge. The pharmacist submits monthly vouchers to the local

Family Practitioner Committee for reimbursement of costs beyond the fixed prescription fee. As in the case of other cost-sharing aspects of the service, the fee is waived for certain categories of people: children under 16 years old, retired persons, the poor, expectant mothers and those with children under 1 year of age, and persons suffering from certain, usually chronic, illnesses.

Hospital and specialist services

A National Health Service patient who requires medical attention that is beyond the competence of a general practitioner is referred to a specialist or consultant – the latter title indicating the highest ranking physician in a hospital. Most specialist care is performed in hospitals, either on an in-patient or an out-patient basis, and is free of charge. The service includes all surgical, diagnostic, pathology, x-ray, and rehabilitation procedures. Hospitalization in a public ward is completely free regardless of the length of stay or the procedures performed. NHS patients who wish to do so may pay about $1.70 to $3.40 per day for an "amenity bed" in a small (two- to four-person) ward or single room. In practice, until 1976, a certain number of "pay" beds – about 4,400 nationwide – were reserved in each hospital for private patients. The Health Service Act (1976) began phasing out private beds in NHS hospitals. Labour Party opposition to the private beds – which Bevan had promised 30 years earlier to retain – was based upon the fact that while NHS patients frequently had to wait long periods for noncritical, elective surgery, private patients who were willing and able to pay for health care could jump the queue and gain immediate or early admission to the reserved pay beds. Today, approximately 95 percent of all hospitals are nationalized. Under the amended law, private hospital care is possible only in the remaining 5 percent of the hospitals.

Local health service

Prior to the April 1974 administrative reorganization, local government authorities were responsible for providing certain public health and health education services. Under the reorganization plan, to be discussed shortly, these services have been transferred to 90 area health authorities. Among the nonadministrative functions performed by the area authorities are maternity and child care services, including pre- and post-natal care and family planning assistance; domiciliary services such as home nursing and health officer visitation; health and preventive education programs; vaccination and immunization services; ambulance services and services for the mentally ill and handicapped. These services, too, are free of charge.

Administrative organization

From July 1948 until April 1974 the National Health Service consisted of a tripartite structure under the administrative authority of the secretary of state for social services. The three branches were (1) hospital services, administered by 14 regional hospital boards, 330 hospital management committees and the boards of governors of 36 teaching hospitals; (2) practitioner services, administered by 134 local executive councils; and (3) local health services, administered by 175 local government units. Under this system there was little coordination or cooperation among the three branches of the health care delivery system. The 1972 government White Paper on National Health Service Reorganization in England found that

it has never been the responsibility – nor has it been within the power – of any single named authority to provide for the population of a given area of comprehensible size the best health service that the money and the skills available can provide. There has been no identified authority whose task it has been, in cooperation with those responsible for complementary services to balance needs and priorities rationally and to plan and provide the right combination of service for the benefit of the public.[33]

On April 1, 1974, in an attempt to rationalize the health care delivery system by unifying administration and integrating health services, the NHS was reorganized. Overall administrative authority remains with the secretary of state for social services under the Department of Health and Social Security (DHSS). (In 1968 the Department of Health and the Department of Social Security had been merged into a single agency.) The DHSS is responsible for budgeting, central personnel, and administrative guidance. The major organizational innovation is the establishment of a two-tiered administrative structure – regional and area health authorities – which administers, plans, and coordinates medical care across the entire spectrum of health services: hospital, practitioner, and public health care. Such coordinated administration is intended to reduce or eliminate inequities in the distribution of resources throughout the health care system. A major complaint about the old system was that disjointed administration had led to dominance by the more glamorous specialist services (particularly, care of acute illnesses) and neglect of the less glamorous, but no less important, care of chronic disorders, such as mental illness.

The highest administrative unit in the reorganized system is the Regional Health Authority (RHA), of which there are 14 in England and 1 in Wales. Each RHA is responsible for coordinating and planning hospital blood banks and computer facilities, allocating resources, and evaluating the performance of health care in its region. Below the regional health authorities are 90 area health authorities, which are responsible for coordinating health care at the local level.

The primary operational and health care delivery unit in the new system is the health district. There are approximately 205 of these (replacing about 580 units, authorities, and councils under the old system) with an average population of about 250,000 people. Each district, through district management teams and medical committees, coordinates and provides the full range of medical services to the community served.

It is too early to determine if the reorganization effort has been a success. There is general agreement that the effort was needed.

Reimbursement procedures

General practitioners are reimbursed in a variety of ways for the services they perform. The basic form of compensation is the capitation fee of $2.55 for each person under 65 years old on the physician's list and $3.57 for each person over 65. Beyond the basic capitation fee, there are several ways in which a doctor's income is augmented. To begin with, there are standard supplementary fees for (1) each patient on a general practitioner's list in excess of 1,000 persons, (2) night visits, (3) other duties performed outside office hours, (4) vaccinations, and (5) rural practice. Doctors are also reimbursed in whole or in part for office rental and ancillary personnel costs. Increased payments are provided for seniority and additional professional training. Finally, there are supplementary benefits for doctors who engage in group practices or who practice in areas where doctors are in short supply. Most of the supplementary fees were added in 1965 following a threatened mass resignation of general practitioners from the NHS. The main complaint of the physicians was the inadequacy of their incomes.

General practitioners may further augment their incomes by serving as physicians for insurance companies or hotels. It has been estimated that non-NHS income amounts to about 10 percent of a general doctor's NHS income. Using this as a guideline, it is estimated that the average general practitioner earned about $15,372 in 1974.[34]

Hospital physicians (i.e., specialists) are generally full- or part-time salaried employees of the nationalized hospitals. Their positions and salaries are based upon a rank or grade system ranging from house officer (the equivalent of an intern) to consultant. The salary scale ranges from approximately $4,860 (at 1978 exchange rates) for beginning full-time house officer to $18,171 for a senior full-time consultant. Consultants are eligible for merit awards in recognition of outstanding ability or professional work; these are awarded by an advisory committee of peers. About one-third of these awards are given each year and range from about

$3,400 to a few as high as $18,000. Consultants who accept only part-time hospital service may engage in private practice and earn from $5,000 to $20,000 per year in additional income.

Dentists are paid on a fee-for-service basis. There is a set schedule of fees for each procedure, and the patient pays up to one-half the fee and the NHS the other half. The average dentist earns approximately the same as a general practitioner.

Pharmacists are reimbursed for the prescriptions they dispense. The patient pays 34 cents for each item, and the NHS reimburses the pharmacist for the remainder of the cost. The reimbursement is based upon actual cost of the ingredients, plus a set percentage markup, cost of containers, and a professional fee.

This is how the National Health Service works. Now to evaluate how well it works.

The performance of the National Health Service

The British National Health Service has been in operation for nearly three decades. Thus, it hardly seems premature to ask: Has the NHS been a success? Despite the apparent simplicity of the question, there is no easy or simple answer. The most obvious difficulty lies in the definition and measurement of the term *success*. Before the reader grows impatient with what may appear to be an effort at semantic obfuscation, let me illustrate the difficulty.

It would seem that a reasonable measure of the relative achievements of the NHS would be to compare the intentions or purposes of the original act with its actual accomplishments. The purpose of the National Health Service Act was "the establishment in England and Wales of a comprehensive health service, designed to secure improvement in the physical and mental health of the people of England and Wales, and the prevention, diagnosis, and treatment of illness." Furthermore, it was the intention of the act "to divorce the care of health from questions of personal means or other factors irrelevant to it."

Medical care is available to every resident of Great Britain regardless of ability to pay. There is no evidence to suggest that anyone in Britain is ever denied necessary medical care because of financial circumstances. For most people, services are free or virtually free at point of delivery; for those in want, they are completely free. In this sense, "the objectives of the 1940's have been achieved. [The British] have created a system of health care in which, broadly, all types of medical skills are available to everyone, wherever they like, without financial barriers."[35]

Table 6–1. *Health status in Great Britain, 1948 and 1974*

Indicator	1948	1974
Life expectancy (yr)		
Male	66.3	69.3
Female	68.4	75.5
Infant mortality rate (per 1,000 live births)	31.4	16.0
Deaths per 100,000 population from:		
Tuberculosis	43.9	2.6
Influenza and pneumonia	79.0	68.0
Appendicitis	2.9	0.6
Whooping cough	17.0	0.0
Heart disease	311.0	368.5
Cancer	145.4	247.5

Sources: Demographic Yearbook (New York: United Nations, 1953 and 1977).

But what about health? Are the people in Britain healthier, mentally and physically, under the NHS than before? Are they receiving better medical treatment? And can their current health status and treatment be attributed to the health care delivery system? Table 6–1 presents for selected years health data that are relevant to these questions. Except in the areas of mortality rates from heart disease and cancer, there has in fact been significant improvement in the health status of the British people. Compared with the period at the start of the NHS, people today are living longer, are much less likely to die in infancy, and are less likely to die from such diseases as tuberculosis, influenza and pneumonia, appendicitis, or whooping cough. On the other hand, they are more likely to die from heart disease and cancer. Before we reach any conclusions on the basis of these data, several points must be stressed. First, the general trends that appear in Great Britain are similar to those appearing in economically developed countries such as the United States, France, West Germany, the Soviet Union, and Japan over roughly the same period of time. In some instances, the rate of improvement has been slower in Great Britain than in Japan, Belgium, or Italy, but this can be accounted for, in part, by the fact that the last three countries started from less favorable health positions. The explanation for these trends lies less in the nature of the health care delivery systems, which vary considerably, than in the general socioeconomic conditions in these countries. "In general, it would seem to be a reasonable assumption that health services as such have less influence on mortality rates than general social conditions in economically developed countries."[36] Higher and improved living standards – including better nutrition, housing, sanitation, health education – are just some of the factors that contribute to decreased mortality rates in most health areas. Second, improved mortality and morbidity rates can be attributed, in part, to the worldwide diffusion of medical progress. The development or availability of antibiotics, screening and treatment procedures for tuberculosis, and thousands of other advances in medical science in the past three decades have produced improvements in health and health care for people throughout the world.

On the other hand, progress has also contributed to certain health problems. Greater affluence, particularly in the West, has often meant less physical exercise (more people drive to work than walk or ride bicycles), consumption of foods high in cholesterol, and greater mental stress. Each of these, along with greater longevity, contributes to higher incidences of heart disease and stroke. Longer life expectancies, increasing air and water pollution, plus better diagnostic procedures have contributed to the detection of, and increase in mortality from, cancer.

Thus, although the overall health status of the British people is better today under the NHS than it was before the service was introduced, it would be difficult, and in most instances erroneous, to attribute these medical improvements to the British health care delivery system. As two experts, one a former surgeon general of the United States, have written: "There is no clear evidence that the increase in physician utilization apparently resulting from the NHS improved the health of the adult population."[37]

The ambiguity of aggregate health status indicators as a measure of the performance of a health care delivery system suggests additional standards are necessary. To begin with, improved mortality and life expectancy rates and what they represent in human terms are not the only results expected of a health care delivery system.

The yardstick of achievement . . . cannot be the mortality rate alone; other indices need to be brought in. One of them is the alleviation of anxiety by the very presence of personal health services. Another is how far the ideal of access to health services as a civil right has been realized.[38]

On these measures, the British National Health Service receives high performance grades.

The introduction of the National Health Service, making treatment available free or at nominal charge to the whole population, instead of only a limited service to a restricted number of employed persons before 1948, has undoubtedly greatly reduced the adverse effects of ill-health on opportunity. It has also removed a burden of anxiety about ability to meet doctors' bills or hospital charges, which in the past preyed heavily on many people of low or modest means.[39]

It is impossible to put a price tag on an achievement such as this. It is irrelevant to compare how much "peace of mind" is worth to a nation's people with how much the health system costs. No one, not even its most vociferous critics, have denied the NHS its due in this regard.

Beyond this basic achievement lie other aspects of the health care delivery system upon which an evaluation can be made. One of these is the question of distribution and access. Is there equal access, by all people, to the nation's health services? Is there reasonable uniformity in the quality and quantity of services available to all people? Both its critics and defenders acknowledge that the health system suffers from problems of inequality in at least three ways: (1) a geographical maldistribution of medical resources, (2) a related social class maldistribution of resources, and (3) irrational priorities within the medical community. In all instances, the results have been that, contrary to its original mandate, the NHS does not provide all sectors of the British population with equal health services.

The most serious and well-publicized problem is the regional variation in the availability of medical personnel and facilities. Although there are exceptions, in general the industrial areas of northern England and Wales have fewer and older hospitals, fewer hospital beds per population, higher patient/doctor ratios, and inadequate or in some instances no specialized medical personnel or facilities. Many examples can be given, but one seems to typify the situation. Cooper and Culyer, in a study of regional inequality, found that the Oxford region (in southern England) was better endowed on every single one of 31 measures of medical resources than the Sheffield region in the Midlands. One result of these regional differences is that there tend to be higher mortality rates in the northern regions of the country than in the southern. For example, the infant mortality rates in England range from 17 to 18 per 1,000 live births in the south or southeast part of the country to between 30 and 33 per 1,000 in northern countries. Similar trends exist for other mortality and morbidity measures. A government survey found that, based on a standardized mortality ratio, deaths in 1975 for adult males and females were higher in the north and northwest counties (111 for males, 108 for females) than in the southeast area, including London (94 for males, 95 for females).[40]

The second and related distributive problem involves the differences in the health status of people from different social classes. The convention in British social science is to rank people in a five-class scheme: class I, professional; class II, managerial; class III, skilled manual and nonmanual; class IV, partly skilled; class V, unskilled. Studies over the years have found that in general social classes IV and V have higher morbidity rates and lower life expectancies than classes I and II. A study of death rates for England and Wales between 1970 and 1972 found that the incidence of death for males and married females from cancer, heart disease, cerebrovascular disease, pneumonia, and other respiratory diseases was consistently higher the further down the social ladder one descended. To give one, but by no means exceptional, example, it was found that, based upon a standardized mortality ratio, deaths among men from pneumonia rose from 41 (professionals) to 53 (managers) to 78 (skilled nonmanual) to 92 (skilled manual) to 115 (partly skilled) to 195 (unskilled).[41]

Furthermore, the evidence seems to suggest that the differences among social classes have not, despite the introduction of the NHS, diminished in the years the system has been operating – and, in some instances, have actually increased. For example, between 1951 and 1961, while the mortality rate for men of all classes fell, the rate for class V men increased. What all this means in human terms has been graphically described by Peter Townsend. Townsend suggests that, with regard to all adults during the period 1959–63, "if the mortality experience of social class I had applied to social class V, only just over half of them would have died; 40,000 lives would have been spared."[42]

Again one must ask: To what extend has the NHS been responsible for this situation? It is clear that the regional and social class variations described were inherited by the service in 1948. At least since the nineteenth century physicians and hospitals tended to be located in certain areas of the country: wealthy residential and resort areas. In fact, one of the major criticisms of the pre-NHS medical situation was the serious inequalities of medical care throughout the country. Under the NHS, efforts in the form of negative and positive incentives have been used to redress some of the personnel problems. Since its inception, local medical committees have been directed to prohibit general practitioners from starting new practices or taking over existing practices in overdoctored districts. In addition, since 1965, annual allowances of significant proportions have been offered general practitioners who practice in "designated" or underdoctored areas. In most instances these are rural districts, particularly in the northern and midland regions, that are not considered attractive by the physicians. Despite these efforts, progress in the redistribution of medical resources has been slow and regional, and the closely related social class inequalities remain. Unfortunately, there has been a tendency for the NHS, through its system of funding health facilities, to perpetuate existing problems. "Those regions which had a great many hospital beds and doctors in 1948 have been given proportionately more money, while those with fewer resources have been given less. The result has been to perpetuate geographical inequalities which have little if any relationship to 'need' for medical care."[43]

Although the government has recently introduced a policy of reallocating resources to needy areas, it is too early to determine if these efforts will be any more successful than previous measures. If one accepts the self-proclaimed goal of the NHS to "secure improvement in the physical and mental health of the people of England and Wales," then the service cannot be considered a complete success. We hasten to add, however, that there are limitations to what a health system can accomplish. Clearly, the health problems of the British lower class are probably more a function of their overall standard of living than of the health system itself. One can assume that although a better distribution of health facilities and personnel would have some impact on the health status of the poor and neglected, an improvement in their standard of living would have a greater impact.

The third major distributive problem associated with the NHS has been the relative priorities, as measured by allocation of resources, assigned to different aspects of the health care delivery system. The greatest problem lies in the tendency for the less glamorous medical care problems to receive a disproportionately small share of the available resources. "Thus, although two-thirds of NHS activity is concerned with the care of the elderly, the mentally ill and the mentally retarded, these services get only one-third of the resources."[44] Financially more rewarding and medically more interesting acute health care problems attract more physicians and government resources than the areas of chronic illness. The unfortunate result is that those who are neither quick to die nor quick to recover tend to be short-changed under the NHS.

In conclusion, evaluated in terms of equal access to the best possible or available medical care, the NHS has yet to achieve its original goal.

Consumer and producer satisfaction

In addition to the problems discussed above, the consumers and producers of British health care have raised other issues concerning the NHS. From the consumer's point of view, the most irritating and frequently encountered fault is the long wait for admission to a hospital for elective (non-crisis) surgery. As noted earlier, it is not unusual for a person to wait 1 year or longer for a hospital bed. The situation at Saint Thomas's hospital described at the outset is reminiscent of the one referred to by Titmuss in his discussion of the situation between 1938 and 1939, when on any given day 100,000 people were waiting for admission to voluntary hospitals in Britain. This, from the patient's point of view, is the most serious failure of the NHS.

The greatest, or at least most vocal, criticism of the NHS comes, however, not from the consumers but from the producers of British medical care. The manifestations appear in critical writings and in continued avoidance of participation in the system. Avoidance comes mainly in the form of emigration. In the 1950s and 1960s approximately 300 to 400 doctors, or one-fifth of the annual medical school output, left Britain to practice in some other country – usually the United States, Canada,

Australia, or New Zealand. The problem *appears* to have accelerated in the 1970s. The *Economist* (London) on October 25, 1975, reported that 900 doctors emigrated from Great Britain in 1973–4, including 220 British and 680 foreign (mostly immigrant) physicians. The report went on to note, however, that 4,025 physicians immigrated during the same period. The immigrants came mainly from the Indian subcontinent and the Middle East. The net effect of all this has been a relatively stable supply of general practitioners and an actual increase in hospital doctors over the past decade.

More dramatic and highly publicized manifestations of professional discontent occurred in 1965 and again in 1975, when general practitioners threatened mass resignations from the NHS. In both instances, the major issues were money and working conditions. The basic source of doctor dissatisfaction with the service appears to be financial. For example, opposition to the abolition of private beds in nationalized hospitals was based upon the loss of income for the doctors from private patients. This is not to suggest that money is the only concern of the physicians. They have expressed concern over the adequacy of health facilities, clinical freedom, and the quality of doctor–patient relationships. The most persistent issue, however, has been the adequacy of income earned by the doctors.

It is interesting to note that the doctors' fear at the inception of the health service over arbitrary dismissal or discipline has proved unwarranted. For example, in 1972 in the inner London area, with 3 million patients and 2,000 doctors, there were only 50 complaints investigated by the local executive council. Of these, 37 were dismissed; in 12 the doctors were reprimanded for "failure or unreasonable delay in making house calls"; and in the other case the doctor was found to have falsified a certificate of illness. In addition, there appears to be a generally good doctor–patient relationship in Great Britain. One indicator of this, which may interest American physicians, is reflected in the premium doctors must pay for malpractice insurance. In 1972, a general practitioner received unlimited indemnity for about $52 a year.[45] In the United States the comparable figure in New York or Los Angeles was between $1,000 and $1,700. Both figures reflect, at least in part, the nature of the relationship between doctor and patient in these two countries.

Although the morale of the medical profession is important, from both the patient's and doctor's perspective, in the final analysis the perceptions and experiences of the nonprofessional under the NHS are of overriding importance. And from this perspective, the National Health Service can only be viewed as a great, although by no means flawless, success.

No doubt the accessibility of the general practitioner and the absence of worry about hospital costs account largely for the popularity of the NHS with the general public. Several surveys . . . have shown that the NHS is the most popular of the

Table 6–2. *Average income, taxes, and medical benefits for selected households in the United Kingdom, 1975* [a]

Total income per year (£) [b]	Total taxes paid per year (£) [c]	Value of medical benefits received under NHS (£)	NHS benefits as percent of taxes paid
1,032	204	200	98.0
1,276	327	205	62.7
1,540	360	228	63.3
1,766	463	210	45.4
2,023	629	195	31.0
2,546	889	228	25.6
3,376	1,234	234	19.0
4,706	1,758	217	12.3
6,636	2,529	230	9.1
10,694	4,355	246	5.6

[a] Data are for the United Kingdom (i.e., England, Wales, Scotland, and Northern Ireland) rather than simply England and Wales. They are certainly reflective of the two more populous areas we have been dealing with (i.e., England and Wales).

[b] Total income includes original income earned plus direct government benefits in cash (e.g., family allowances).

[c] Taxes include direct taxes such as employees' national insurance contributions, income tax, surtax, and indirect taxes such as user fees for goods and services.

Source: Based on data in *Social Trends: 1977* (London: Central Statistical Office, 1977), p. 108.

social services and that, in contrast with, say, housing and education, all groups in the community express themselves as surprisingly satisfied with the services they actually receive. It would be a political impossibility to change the basic features of the NHS from the consumer's point of view.[46]

The costs of medical care

One final aspect of the British health care system deserves our attention in this evaluation. At issue is the actual cost of medical care to the individual and the community. Although medical care in Britain is free, or virtually so, at the point of delivery, the taxpayer ultimately pays the bill. What is the financial burden on the average household for its medical care?

Table 6–2 presents data that address this issue. It seems to us that the data should be interpreted in the context of the welfare state commitment of British governments since 1945. In these terms, it appears that the NHS clearly reflects the redistributive inclinations of the welfare state. As Table 6–2 indicates, households in the first four (relatively low-income) groups

Table 6-3. *Public spending: annual average rates of increase in the United Kingdom, 1951-75*

| | Public expenditure (%) in | | | |
	1951–61	1961–71	1971–3	1973–5
Social services				
Social security	9.0	10.2	13.3	27.0
Health and personal social services	6.4	9.9	16.0	33.9
Education	9.8	11.6	16.2	29.4
Housing and environmental services				
Housing	3.2	8.4	38.9	33.9
Environmental services	7.3	11.7	20.1	18.9
Libraries, museums, the arts	10.1	13.2	20.9	30.0
Justice and law	9.6	12.0	15.3	31.3
Total	5.9	9.0	15.3	29.8

Source: Social Trends: 1976 (London: Central Statistical Office, 1976).

received in medical benefits alone between 45 and 98 percent of what they paid in taxes. In fact, if one totals the value of all benefits (medical and nonmedical) received by those with average incomes of £1,766 or less per year, they exceed the amount paid in taxes by between £769 and £1,156.

Higher income households received a proportionately lower return, in terms of value of medical benefits, for their taxes. Those earning £10,694 per year received medical benefits that accounted for only 5.6 percent of what they paid in taxes.

Another facet of financing involves the rapid rise in the costs of medical care – a problem that is not unique to Great Britain. Table 6–3 documents the problem with painful clarity. Between 1951 and 1961 health (and personal services) costs rose at an average annual rate of 6.4 percent. Between 1961 and 1971 they increased at an average annual rate of 9.9 percent. However, between 1973 and 1975 the average annual rate of increase was 33.9 percent. Critics claim that the rapid rise in costs threatens the ability of the government to continue to operate the NHS without either resorting to user fees or allowing medical services to deteriorate. We cannot possibly do justice to this very complicated issue, but two points should be stressed. First, as Table 6–3 indicates, the increase in medical costs is by no means unique – nor is it even the most precipitous. Second, as noted in the case of Germany, the rapid acceleration of these costs since 1971 is in part explained by the worldwide inflation. This, of course, does not make the problem any less severe, but it should put it in proper perspective. There does not appear to be any evidence that these cost increases are attributable to or inherent in the nature or operation of the NHS.

The British government is not unmindful of the problem. Faced with these and other extraordinary cost increases, the Labour government, in February 1976, issued a white paper setting out its expenditure plans through 1980. Included in its program is a commitment to limit increases in health care expenditures to 4.7 percent. The white paper argues that this can be accomplished by placing "greater emphasis on achieving the most effective use of available resources and obtaining savings by improvements in efficiency (including where necessary the closure of hospitals or units)."[47] In addition, the government indicated that additional savings can be achieved by encouraging cooperative and collegial health care delivery enterprises such as clinics, health care centers, and group practice. Whatever happens, it seems clear that neither political party will casually entertain the idea of imposing user fees unless it is absolutely necessary. Necessity, in this case, would be defined as the inability of the NHS to meet the nation's health care needs.

Accounting for British health care policy

This chapter deals with the evolution of British health care policy in the twentieth century, and focuses on two landmark legislative acts: the National Health Insurance Act of 1911 and the National Health Service Act of 1946. It is useful at this time to summarize the major findings concerning the factors that helped shape the structure and content of those policy decisions in terms of the accounting scheme.

Situational factors

Prominent personalities and extraordinary events helped shape British health care policy throughout the century. The inspection processes attending the Boer War and, especially, World War II helped place health care on the policy agenda by 1911 and 1946. Once on the agenda, the issues were in large measure guided and influenced by two of the most prominent personalities of their times: Lloyd George and Aneurin Bevan. Both NHI and NHS were timely and astutely managed issues, and their legitimacy was mandated by significant changes in government control: the Liberals' victories in 1905 and 1910, and Labour's victory in 1945.

Environmental factors

The most obvious external influences in twentieth-century health care policy were the lessons the British, and other status quo powers, had learned from Germany's social insurance program. This program served as a model for both sound social policy and practical political conservatism.

Structural factors

Despite the importance of personalities, inspection processes, and foreign models, British health care policy ultimately evolved in a structured political, economic, and demographic milieu. It was, after all, concern with maintaining the existing political and socioeconomic order that helped precipitate the concern for national efficiency at the turn of the century. British capitalism and democracy required a healthy and content working class. Industrialization required a healthy working class, and the government was called upon to ensure that industry received what it needed. Politically, between 1910 and 1913 and again from 1946 to 1948, the specific content and structure of public health policy were forged within the confines of British parliamentary democracy; an informed and articulate public opinion, aggressive interest group activity, political bargaining, and ultimately, legislative debate and enactment. Finally, in both 1911 and 1946, the legacy of the past, in the form of policies to be amended, expanded, or repudiated, provided the point of departure for future public policy.

Cultural factors

The passage of the 1911 National Health Insurance Act and the 1946 National Health Service Act coincided with basic redefinitions of the British political culture. By 1910, the notion that all men had certain political rights had become an integral part of British democracy: By 1945, the British political culture was expanded to include the notion of social rights, including the right to adequate health care regardless of ability to pay. The modern welfare state had come of age in Great Britain.

7

The Soviet Union: health care in a communist state

In November 1892 a political-literary magazine, the *Russian Idea,* published a short story by Anton Chekhov entitled "Ward Number Six." In the story Chekhov, who was a physician as well as a writer, described the medical care and medical facilities available in one rural hospital.

In wards, corridors and hospital courtyard you could barely draw breath for the stink. The ambulance men, the nurses and their children slept in the wards with the patients, complaining that the cockroaches, bed-bugs and mice made their lives a misery. There was endemic erysipelas [an infectious disease] in the surgical department, the entire hospital boasted only two scalpels and not a single thermometer, and potatoes were kept in the baths.

About 60 years later, another Russian writer, Aleksandr Solzhenitsyn, wrote about another hospital, perhaps the one in which he had been successfully treated for cancer. In his novel, *Cancer Ward,* Solzhenitsyn, a severe and persistent critic of the Communist regime, described a hospital and hospital life in a Central Asian city. Some patients still were kept in corridors because of overcrowded conditions, the surgical staff was overworked, and by American standards, there were few amenities. But there had been profound changes since Chekhov's time. The medical care was competent and the hospital staff generally concerned. Gone was the filth that characterized the hospital in Chekhov's story. In this hospital great pains were taken to keep surgical areas antiseptic and patient areas clean. The patients could enjoy fresh air and relaxation in an outdoor garden. In general, the patients, who included persons of varied ethnic and social backgrounds, were getting "good" medical attention. The hospitals described by Chekhov and Solzhenitsyn were probably typical of the hospital facilities available to the masses of people in their respective times. As the two literary descriptions suggest, the quality of medical care has improved substantially under communist rule.

This chapter examines the organization, content, and performance of the Soviet medical care system. The chapter begins with a historical overview of the system: the "sorry inheritance" from the Tsarist regime. It then examines the impact of ideology, historical conditions, and economic development on the nature of the Soviet medical system, and concludes with an evaluation of the performance of the Soviet health system: its accomplishments, its shortcomings, and its abuses.

A cautionary note must be interjected here. Soviet studies tend to be polemical: either excessively critical and abusive or uncritically appreciative. Rarely does one find a balanced, seemingly objective account of any aspect of Soviet society and polity. In most instances, the cold war has been and continues to be fought in scholarly books and articles. In this regard, Alex Inkeles once wrote: "Failure explicitly to condemn is viewed by some as tantamount to approval, and failure explicitly to praise is taken by others as the equivalent of criticism."[1]

Studies of the Soviet health care system have not been immune from the scourge of ideological wrangling. Depending on which account one accepts, the Soviet model is either an unparalleled achievement in health care delivery or a colossal failure. The problem for those less concerned with passing judgment on forms of governments and more concerned with understanding the development of public policy is to sift through the evidence and attempt to present a balanced account. This task is most difficult for the formative years of the Soviet regime: the 1920s and 1930s. For descriptions of this period, we have to rely heavily upon the accounts of Western observers, typically physicians rather than social scientists, who traveled through the Soviet Union at the time and who, one suspects, were generally sympathetic to socialism (if not Soviet socialism).[2] During this time many liberal intellectuals in the United States, England, and other Western nations became enamored of the promise of socialism and made the pilgrimage to the socialist Mecca. At best, the resulting accounts provide interesting, detailed, useful, but generally uncritical, descriptions of early Soviet medical care. At their worst, as in the case of Ravitch's *The Romance of Russian Medicine,* they are pure sycophancy. Nevertheless, these works, along with the writings of Soviet authors, provide the basis of our knowledge about this period. We have tried to separate fact from fancy and resist the role of advocate in describing the organization and operation of the Soviet health care system.

All this is not to suggest that opinions or values or, indeed, advocacy have no place in policy analysis. They do, provided they are labeled as such. We offer our own evaluation of the performance of the Soviet *health care* system at the end of the chapter, unclouded, it is hoped, by our bias against the Soviet *political* system.

One final prefatory remark is in order. This case study differs in some respects from those of Germany and Great Britain. Because the Soviet Union is a closed and controlled society, we find no published accounts or documentation of, for example, meetings among political decision makers, bargains and compromises forged, the activities of pressure groups, or the influence of public opinion on Soviet health care policy.

We simply do not have available the quality or quantity of information to describe in as intimate and personal detail the factors influencing the evolution of Soviet health care policy. For example, with but few exceptions, the following account does not detail the activities of specific individuals. In part this is because no one personality dominated the formation of Soviet health care as Lloyd George and Aneurin Bevan dominated British, and Bismarck dominated German, health care. But it is also true that even if specific persons had influenced Soviet health care, we would lack the detailed knowledge about them that we have about those who influenced health care policy in Britain and Germany.

Having said all this, we can now turn to a discussion of the Soviet health care system itself.

The Tsarist legacy

Despite the completely revolutionary and radical nature and intentions of the Communist leaders in 1917, they, like all policy makers, revolutionary or not, were constrained by the environment in which they operated and the decisions taken by their predecessors. Obviously, these constraints, particularly those involving Tsarist policy, were less limiting than they would have been in a nonrevolutionary situation. Nevertheless, the environmental and policy legacy inherited by the Communists did help determine and guide the course and content of both immediate and long-range Soviet medical care policy. In this regard, two major features of that inheritance stand out and require our attention. The first concerns the general state of health and medical care existing in Russia on the eve of the revolution. The second involves the nature and organization of the medical care delivery system in Tsarist Russia. Both factors influenced the course of Soviet health policy.

The sorry inheritance from the old regime

No matter what standard or index one uses, the medical care and health conditions in Tsarist Russia in the early twentieth century were appalling for the overwhelming majority of the people. Table 7–1 presents various quantitative measures of the state of health and medical care in Russia prior to 1917. These measures are compared with those in Germany, Great Britain, Japan, and the United States to give the reader a feeling for both the absolute and relative state of health and medical care of the Russian people at the time. As the table indicates, Russia lagged far behind each

Table 7-1. *Health status in Tsarist Russia, Germany, Great Britain, Japan, and the United States*

Indicator	Russia (1913)	Germany (1911)	Great Britain (1910)	Japan (1910)	United States (1910)
General mortality rate (per 1,000 population)	30.2	17.3	13.5	21.6	15.0
Infant mortality rate (per 1,000 live births)	269	162	105	161.2	99[a]
Average life expectancy (yr)	32	44.8[b]	48	44.2	50
Physicians per 10,000 population	1.5	5.0	N.A.	N.A.	15.7
Hospital beds per 1,000 population	1.3	3.6[c]	N.A.	N.A.	4.7[d]

N.A. = data not available.
[a]1915; [b]males only; [c]1906; [d]1909.
Sources: Mark G. Field, "Health as a 'Public Utility' or the 'Maintenance of Capacity' in Soviet Society," *Social Consequences of Modernization in Communist Societies,* ed. Mark G. Field (Baltimore: Johns Hopkins Press, 1976), pp. 244–61; Gordon Hyde, *The Soviet Health Service* (London: Lawrence & Wishart, 1974), p. 14; Y. Lisitsin, *Health Protection in the U.S.S.R.* (Moscow: Progress Publishers, 1972), p. 45; *Public Health in Japan* (Tokyo: Supreme Commander Allied Powers, 1949), 2, pp. A–1, A–12; *Journal of the American Medical Association,* February 16, 1929.

of these countries, and indeed most of the civilized world, on virtually every index of health and medical care.

In terms of medical personnel and medical facilities, the picture that emerges is of a medical system that was not only inadequate but also maldistributed.

For example, in 1913 only 25 percent of all the hospital beds and 22 percent (5,000 of 23,000) of the doctors in Russia practiced in the rural areas of the country, where 82 percent of the population lived. Thus, although the overall ratio of physicians per 10,000 population (1.5) was both absolutely and relatively low and inadequate, in certain outlying parts of the country the situation was even worse. In 1913 there was 0.2 doctor per 10,000 population in the region which is the Tadzhik SSR, 0.4 in the Kazakh SSR, and 0.7 in the Turkmen SSR.[3] Hospital facilities, too, were either inadequate or nonexistent in most areas. The national average of hospital beds was about 13 per 10,000 (or 1.3 per 1,000) population, but in those territories that now constitute the Republics of Turkmenistan, Uzbekistan, Kirghizstan, and Kazakhstan, there were only 1 to 3 beds per

10,000 people.[4] And according to one source, 35 percent of the towns had
no hospital at all.[5] Qualitatively, we can accept Chekhov's description as
not untypical of the standards of medical care practiced in those rural
areas fortunate enough to have some form of medical care. In fact, so
badly maintained were the public hospitals that their registries included
the category "patients who ran away."[6]

This is not to suggest that modern, first-rate medical care was unavailable in Tsarist Russia. In 1897 the International Medical Congress held its
annual meeting in Moscow. In anticipation of the occasion the British
medical publication, the *Lancet*, devoted a lengthy supplement to "Medicine, Past and Present, in Russia" (*Lancet*, August 7, 1897). The *Lancet*
correspondent described the modern and progressive medical facilities and
procedures found in hospitals in Moscow and Saint Petersburg. The report
noted: "It may be asserted without hesitation that some of those hospitals
will prove veritable revelations to many foreign visitors to the International
Medical Congress." Despite the undeniable achievements of Russian
medicine and medical personnel, modern medicine was limited geographically to major urban centers and available to only a minute portion of the
population.

The Tsarist government was not unaware of the state of medical care in
the empire and of its consequences. In 1912 an interdepartmental commission charged with examining existing medical and sanitary conditions
concluded that: "A vast part of Russia has as yet absolutely no provisions
for medical aid, the result of which is a distressing sickrate and mortality
from communicable diseases, as well as generally very low health standards."[7] And the morbidity and mortality rates were, indeed, distressing.
Tsarist Russia had the dubious distinction of leading most of the Western
world in the indexes of disease and mortality rates. In 1913, 269 out of
every 1,000 children died within their first year; about 430 of every 1,000
children died before the age of 5 years. It has been estimated that in 1914
one-quarter of the population of Russia suffered from infectious diseases
such as typhoid, typhus, and smallpox.[8]

In that same year, Russia reportedly had 19.7 cases of trachoma (a
chronic and contagious eye disease often leading to blindness) per 10,000
persons compared with 7.8 in England, 6.6 in Sweden, and 4.8 in
Belgium. It was as a result of the widespread incidence of trachoma that
Tsarist Russia ranked first in the world in number of blind persons.[9]
Plague and leprosy were endemic in parts of the country; diphtheria and
malaria as well as typhoid, typhus, and smallpox periodically reached
epidemic proportions.

The overall result of poor medical care and disease control was that the
Russian people had a high general mortality rate and a short life expec-

tancy (Table 7-1). The inadequate and depressing state of health and medical conditions in Russia prior to the revolution is forcefully brought home in a comparison with Great Britain at about the time the National Health Insurance Act began operation. In this regard Gordon Hyde, an ardent admirer of the Soviet system, makes the telling point that "to find comparisons with Russian conditions before the First World War it is necessary to go back 200 years in English history."[10] All this, of course, tells us nothing about the individual human suffering and misery that chronic disease and inadequate medical care meant to the overwhelming majority of the Russian people. It is unnecessary to detail the situation in order to reinforce the point that medical conditions in Russia on the eve of the Bolshevik Revolution were deplorable.

Thus, part of the policy environment in which the Communists had to operate was a legacy of inadequate health facilities and deplorable personal and public health conditions. Clearly, a regime committed to humanitarian goals and rapid economic development could not long tolerate such conditions. Whatever else they wished to do, the Communists had to turn their immediate attention to this much neglected policy area. In other words, the policy agenda for the new regime was in part inherited from the old regime.

The organization of medical care and the medical profession in Tsarist Russia

No matter what its ideology, no matter how radical its inclinations, every regime is to a certain degree constrained by its demographic environment. The Soviets could not wish away or outlaw epidemics or high infant mortality rates. They could, however, if they chose to do so, change the structure of the medical system. For this reason, an examination of the organization of medical care and the role of the medical profession in Tsarist Russia is relevant to our discussion. The purpose is to determine which features of that system were compatible and which features inconsistent with the policy plans and ideological predisposition of the Communist leadership.

From a comparative health policy perspective, perhaps the most important feature of the medical system was the direct and vital role played by the state. "The Russian medical profession developed within the rigid confines of the state's bureaucratic structure. The Tsarist government founded the first medical school in 1654 and during the following two centuries subsidized and supervised all medical education."[11] Having financed the doctors' education, the government then expected (and received) repayment in the form of obligatory government service. Despite the fact that the service was in no way attractive, financially or otherwise, about three-fourths of all Russian doctors worked for the government even after fulfilling their obligations. The reason for this was that few Russians could afford private medical care, and there were thus few employment opportunities for doctors in private practice.[12] Unlike their counterparts in Great Britain, government service rather than private practice was the primary employment for Russian doctors. Finally, most hospitals in pre-revolutionary Russia were state institutions. In general, these were operated either by municipal governments in the urban areas or, after 1864, by *zemstvos* (rural councils) in the towns. With the exception of a few prestigious institutions in major urban areas such as Moscow or Saint Petersburg (now Leningrad), these hospitals were generally poorly financed, badly equipped, and inadequate to the task of serving the health needs of the population. It should be noted that although hospitalization in public institutions was free or available at nominal charge, inadequate financing and facilities severely limited the services that could be performed.

The first point, then, to be emphasized is that the Russian medical system, including medical education, institutions, and employment of physicians, was in the main a public, state-run and state-controlled, operation.

The zemstvo

Among the features of the medical system of prerevolutionary Russia none is more typical and celebrated than the system of *zemstvo* medicine. Even the most severe critics of tsarism applaud the intentions and spirit, if not necessarily the accomplishments, of this system.

In 1861 Tsar Alexander II emancipated the Russian serfs. The abolition of feudalism produced the need for an alternative mechanism to provide some of the social services the feudal nobility had traditionally offered. Thus began a period of reform. Among these reforms was the establishment, in 1864, of local self-governing units in the rural areas, called *zemstvos*. Local residents elected a *zemstvo* assembly, which in turn elected an executive board whose responsibility was to administer and oversee the rules and regulations adopted by the assembly. Although all classes were supposed to be represented in the assemblies, indications are that they were dominated by the traditional elite. Among the responsibilities of the *zemstvo* was that of providing general welfare services, including education, medical care, and public health care.[13]

The health and medical responsibilities of the *zemstvos* included administration of hospitals, dispensaries, and public health facilities. In addition, they employed physicians to provide free medical care to all residents of the district. *Zemstvo* medicine thus provided organized modern medical and public health care to portions of the Russian population who had never been treated by trained doctors before.

As a result of the innovative nature of the system and the dedicated physicians it was able to attract, *zemstvo* medicine and the *zemstvo* physician, in particular, were much acclaimed both within and outside Russia. The reputation the system and the physicians enjoyed in Russia was reflected in a speech delivered in 1902 before a National Medical Association meeting.

The *Zemstvo* physician is a . . . new type of popular physician, able to speak with the common people, to understand their needs and interests . . . representing the ideal, the very best type of physician, who selflessly contributes to the welfare of his fellow man, sacrificing much, especially during epidemics – even his life (which happens often!) . . . The *Zemstvo* physician fulfills the highest Christian precepts and therefore deserves the title of "friend of humanity."[14]

Despite the accolades and the important contribution *zemstvo* medicine made to prerevolutionary rural Russia, its actual accomplishments were rather limited. The reasons for this are not hard to find. First, *zemstvo* assemblies and, therefore, *zemstvo* medical care, existed in only 54 of the 89 provinces of Imperial Russia.[15] Second, in 1913, fewer than 20 percent of the available doctors served in the rural areas of Russia, where 82 percent of the population lived. Third, the inadequate number of physicians was matched by the parsimonious funding for *zemstvo* medicine. Considering the task before them and the resources available, it is little wonder that the *zemstvo* physicians' accomplishments were limited.

More pertinent to our concern than its performance is the organizational and experiential legacy *zemstvo* medicine provided. "*Zemstvo* medicine paved the way for Soviet medicine in several respects. It created a medical organization, created a network of medical stations all over the country that could be improved and increased in number. Above all, it accustomed the people to the idea that medicine was not a trade but a public service."[16] A popular Soviet public health textbook similarly acknowledged that "*Zemstvo* medicine was a significant step forward . . . in that it set up a new network of *Zemstvo* hospitals, dispensaries, feldsher [paramedic] and midwife schools, and a sanitary organization."[17] The *zemstvo* system introduced the notion of a territorially based medical organization in which medical care could be provided, either free or for a nominal charge, in the form of a public service. This system proved quite compatible with subsequent Soviet plans.

One by-product of *zemstvo* medicine that proved incompatible with Soviet intentions was the increasing professionalization of the medical establishment in Russia. We have already seen that the Russian medical profession developed within the context of a public (i.e., state) practice. As a result, Russian physicians were a generally subordinate, nonassertive, and professionally unorganized group. Many were civil servants in a highly centralized and autocratic state. The development of the *zemstvo* system led to the decentralization of various governmental functions and controls, including, of course, medical service. Physicians saw *zemstvo* practice as an opportunity to assert their professional independence and exercise some influence over decisions affecting medical practice in the *zemstvo* assemblies. And indeed, as Frieden has noted, "by the end of the nineteenth century many *Zemstvos* did give considerable independence to the physicians in their employ." The *zemstvo* physicians were still government employees, but with the important difference that they were, through representation on local public health councils, able to exercise some influence over their professional lives.[18]

The medical developments within the *zemstvo* system were coincidental with two other factors that contributed to greater assertiveness and collegiality among physicians in the late nineteenth and early twentieth centuries. The first was an increase in the number of physicians from approximately 10,000 in 1864 to 23,000 in 1913. The second was the establishment in 1881 of a national medical society, the Pirogov Society, named after a famous Russian military physician. The society held annual medical congresses in either Moscow or Saint Petersburg.

Thus, by the eve of the revolution, the once small, docile, and unorganized medical profession had increased in size and achieved a degree of professional control and organization unknown just a few decades earlier. Under these circumstances, it is not difficult to anticipate that the profession would be reluctant to relinquish its newly acquired power, no matter how limited it might be.

Health insurance

One final feature of medical care under the old regime should be noted: passage of the Health and Accident Insurance Act of 1912. The model and motivation behind the law were similar to those behind the British National Health Insurance Act of 1911. The German law was the model, and the purpose was apparently to defuse workers' discontent. The act provided for hospital and out-patient care for workers and their families and was financed by joint employer-employee contributions. The law also required each factory owner to provide on-site first aid and dispensary facilities. Inadequate financing, lackadaisical administration, and the onset of World War I combined to make the health insurance law something less than the landmark it had been in Britain and Germany. We mention this here because the idea of social insurance was later adopted by the Soviet regime.

The evolution of Soviet medical care

The postrevolution medical environment

Among the most pressing concerns of the new Soviet regime in October 1917 was a critical public health problem. Tsarist Russia suffered from inadequate health facilities and personnel and high mortality and morbidity rates. Existing conditions were exacerbated by the socioeconomic and political dislocations caused by World War I and the Bolshevik Revolution. Shortages of food, fuel, soap, medicines, and medical personnel contributed to the rapid spread of various diseases. The most serious health problem was the prevalence of typhus. In 1913 there were 7.3 reported cases of typhus per 10,000 people. The rate in 1918 was 21.9; in 1919, 265.3; and in 1920, a record 393.9. Cognizant of the political, as well as the medical and humanitarian implications of the situation, Lenin noted shortly after the revolution: "Typhus among a population weakened by hunger without bread, soap, fuel, may become such a scourge as not to give us an opportunity to undertake socialist construction." Lenin reiterated his concern over the political consequences of the typhus epidemic at the Seventh All-Russian Congress of the Soviets in December 1919, when he said: "Comrades all attention to this problem! Either socialism conquers the lice [which transmit typhus fever], or the lice will conquer socialism."[19]

The public health problem facing the Soviets was not limited to typhus epidemics. Between roughly 1917 and 1921, Russia suffered epidemics of cholera, typhoid, dysentery, and recurrent fever as well as diseases associated with famine. The birth rate fell (from 45 per 1,000 in 1913 to 22 per 1,000 in 1919) and the general mortality rate increased (from 29.1 per 1,000 in 1913 for the overall population to as high as 90 per 1,000 in Leningrad in 1921). Such was the context within which the new Soviet regime formulated its health care policy.

Early health care policy

The formulation of Soviet health care policy and the development of a medical care delivery system began shortly after the revolution and reflected the influence of Marxist ideology, international imitation, the legacy of the past, and pragmatic adjustments to existing health conditions. The first formal action taken was the establishment of the Medical Sanitary Section attached to a local (Petrograd) Military Revolutionary Committee in late October 1917. The unit was responsible for organizing medical care for the "soldiers and workers."[20]

This institution set the pattern for similar medical organizations in other localities in the country. The decision initially to organize medical care along decentralized lines was taken by Lenin apparently in an effort to lay the foundation for a fully centralized system. Before a national health system could be created, Lenin felt, two tasks had to be accomplished. The first, according to Gordon Hyde, was to stimulate

activity from below, through the participation of workers and peasants in health activities. [Lenin] . . . therefore proposed the organization, locally, of sanitary sections attached to Soviets, with wide administrative participation by workers and peasants. The latter, together with Communist Party members could perform the necessary preparatory work, explaining the need for a central health organization.[21]

Beyond the apparently educative purpose of this initial action lay another, and perhaps more important, reason for delaying the establishment of a centralized health system. This was the practical political need for the Communists to identify and deal with "reactionary" physicians who opposed the new regime. One recent Soviet source explains the initial absence of a centralized medical system in the following manner:

The reason for this was that for some time after the revolution not all the doctors sided conclusively with Soviet power. Some of them failed to grasp the aims of the revolution, did not understand the essence of the democratic reorganisation carried out by the Government and the Communist Party and opposed the undertakings of the young Soviet state.[22]

We do not know the exact extent of the opposition or its manifestations within the medical community. One pro-Soviet source claims that "reactionary physicians were neglecting their duty, sabotaging the orders of the new government."[23] Others have been skeptical of these allegations. We do know that the number of "reactionary" physicians was considerable. Some opposed the new regime on ideological grounds, some on humanitarian grounds. Still others were unwilling to relinquish their recently acquired professional identity, status, and autonomy to the Soviet notion of complete state control. Much of the opposition was centered in the Pirogov Society mentioned earlier and in its newly (March 1918) formed political arm, the All-Russian Union of Professional Associations of Physicians. Unable to convert the medical opposition to its cause, in early 1918 the Soviets abolished the Pirogov Society.

The elimination of the major organized vehicle for professional opposition and the emigration of many physicians who opposed the regime cleared the way for neutralization of the medical profession. It took some time before this was ultimately accomplished. According to one Communist apologist: "It took considerable time for medical men, who clung to the idea of the old order, to realize the advantages of Soviet socialist medicine, but later they enthusiastically joined the ranks of the Soviet system."[24] As late as December 1919, at the Seventh Congress of the Soviets, Lenin acknowledged: "There are still doctors who regard the working-class Government with prejudice and distrust, however, they are a minority; their number is growing less and less."[25] And it was not until 1920 that the by then impotent All-Russian Union of Professional Associations of Physicians was dissolved.

Although the final neutralization of the medical profession did not occur until about 1920, by July 1918, the Soviet regime felt secure enough to establish the People's Commissariat (Ministry) of Health, whose purpose it was to unify medical and public health work in the Russian Soviet Federated Socialist Republic. Sigerist notes, with some exaggeration, that "for the first time in the history of medicine a central body was directing the entire health work of a nation."[26]

Actually it was not until the end of the civil war in 1920 and the establishment of the USSR in 1924 that the Commissariat of Health was able effectively to direct the health system of the *entire* nation. Nevertheless, it is accurate to portray the establishment of this ministry as a landmark in the centralization and state control and operation of a nation's health care system.

Basic principles of Soviet health care

Before we turn to a complete description of the Soviet health care system, it is necessary to examine the origin and application of some of its underlying principles. Although there have been substantive changes over the years in Soviet health policy, there has been a remarkable degree of continuity and consistency with the principles and practices begun with the establishment of the Commissariat of Health in 1918.

There appear to be six major principles of Soviet health care policy, some of which were set forth as early as the Fifth All-Russian Congress of Soviets in June–July 1918.[27]

1. Health care is a responsibility of the state.
2. Health care should be available to all citizens at no direct cost to the user.
3. The proletariat occupies a preferential position in Soviet society, including its health care delivery system.
4. There should be centralized and unified administration of health care policy.
5. "Public" health depends upon active citizen involvement.
6. The primary substantive emphasis in Soviet health care is on prophylactic or preventive medicine.

A responsibility of the state

The fundamental operating assumption of Soviet health care policy is that medical care, in all its dimensions, is properly the responsibility of the state and a function of government. The implicit corollary of this principle is that private medical practice is inappropriate in a socialist society, although some private practice still exists in the Soviet Union today. The origins of this basic principle are not difficult to find. Historically, the medical profession in Tsarist Russia developed under state control, and medical care was largely provided by either the national government or, later on, local (*zemstvo*) governments.

More important than the historical precedent, which in most instances would have been sufficient grounds for automatic rejection by the Soviet regime, was the impact of ideology. According to Marxists, the socialist state is dedicated to the elimination of suffering and the improvement of life for the exploited (working) class. The difference between socialist and capitalist systems is that under capitalism the medical system – like all social, political, and economic institutions – is an instrument of the ruling class, used to pursue its own interests by exploiting the working class. In a socialist state, classes are all but eliminated through the abolition of private property. The state is taken over by the proletariat and, therefore, serves the interests of the entire population and not just the ruling elite. Among the services performed by the state is the provision of medical care. Thus, in the Soviet Union, as in other socialist societies, the interests of the state (the collectivity) and the individual (the worker) are identical. One of these interests, based upon humanitarian and practical reasons, is the maintenance of public and personal health.

In addition to the historical and ideological bases for the principle of health care as a public responsibility was a practical reason: The rapid and continuing development of the nation required a healthy population. And the best way to ensure this was through state control and direction of the public health and medical care delivery system. We have already seen, of course, that the intervention of the state in Great Britain in the form of the National Health Insurance system was justified on the basis of national efficiency. And we have noted Rimlinger's more general argument that at some point in the industrialization process (i.e., when labor becomes scarce) it becomes profitable for the state to maintain a healthy and willing work force: hence, the introduction of social security systems.

In the case of the Soviet Union, the relationship between the health of the people and economic productivity is officially and explicitly recognized and emphasized, certainly more so than it was in Great Britain in either 1911 or 1946. The relationship is discussed in an official Soviet public health text.

The level of public health and the state and quality of medical care for working people have a great influence on the economy; they are important to raise the productivity of labor and to increase the nation's labor resources . . . The development of public health aids in improving the effectiveness of national production and in fulfilling the main economic task during the period of the full-fledged building of a communist society, and the creation of the material and technical base of communism.[28]

Furthermore, as Mark Field notes:

Although the establishment of a national health service cannot be said to be a sine qua non for the process of modernization and industrialization, it is difficult to conceive that the Soviet drive would have proceeded at the rate it did with a population afflicted by epidemic and other diseases, untreated trauma, a high level of mortality, and consequently a low life expectancy.[29]

A "free," universally available and accessible health service

The Constitution of the USSR guarantees the right to "free medical service for the working people." The major basis for the principle that health care should be available and accessible to all working people lies again in socialist ideology. In a socialist state there are theoretically no class distinctions; all citizens are treated equally. This means that competent medical care should be available and accessible to every citizen regardless of sex, age, nationality, occupation, and so on. Furthermore, such care should be given independent of any consideration of ability to pay; it should be free to all. The concept of free medical care was, of course, part of the zemstvo legacy and, therefore, part of the Russian tradition.

In 1917, however, the Soviet regime did not have the resources to implement, and indeed may not even have envisioned, such a comprehensive national health service. In actuality, the medical system initially developed along lines not dissimilar from those in Germany and Great Britain, although with important motivational and substantive differences. Within a week of the revolution, the Soviet government adopted a system of social insurance based on the German model and inherited in part from the Tsarist regime. The scheme, including the health provisions, covered all "wage earners" and their dependents (e.g., industrial workers, agricultural workers on state farms) and the "city and village poor."[30] The system, omitting as it did peasants and self-employed persons, had a clear working-class bias, reminiscent of the German and British schemes. The system provided free health care by government-employed medical personnel and was financed through contributions from factory, state, farm, and other employing organizations. Given the enormous disruptions during the civil war (1917–21), even this somewhat limited system could not be consistently and widely applied until about 1921 when the civil war (or war communism) ended and the period of new economic policy began. As noted above, the Soviet health insurance program introduced in November 1917, and reiterated in the Labor Code of November 1922, did not cover the peasant population, which constituted the single largest segment of the population. Two explanations have been offered to explain the omission. Rimlinger argues that "the exclusion of the peasants may have violated the spirit of the revolution, but the peasants' attitude, especially toward the end of War Communism, had made amply clear that they could not be relied on for the building of a socialist state."[31] Hyde, on the other hand, suggests that the decision involved a conscious allocation of scarce resources. "Health insurance, on class lines, played a significant role in establishing priorities in the provision of scarce medical resources."[32] It follows from these two arguments that once the reliability of the peasantry could be assured, and the scarcity of resources diminished, the regime could pursue a policy more compatible with its egalitarian ideology.

Both these conditions appear to have been met by 1937. The forced collectivization of agriculture begun in 1928 had the effect of subduing, if not eliminating, the peasants' opposition as well as reducing their numbers through emigration to the cities. In addition, the period of rapid industrialization initiated by Stalin in 1928 had begun to produce substantial economic growth. In 1937 the government abandoned the principle of financing health care through insurance contributions and made medical care free and available to all citizens. This was in fulfillment of a pledge of free medical service for all working people made in the 1936 constitution.

Preferential treatment for the proletariat

As the above discussion suggests, the Soviet regime has reserved a privileged position in the area of health care for the working class or proletariat. The basis for this preferential treatment is traceable to the combined dictates of ideology and economic necessity.

The Soviet Revolution was led by the Communist Party on behalf of the working class of Tzarist Russia and it is understandable that the top priority in health services should be accorded to the industrial proletariat . . . Moreover, the vast industrialization plans of the Soviet economy demanded a robust urban population, whose health would be constantly protected.[33]

In recent years, the preferential treatment accorded the working class, and particularly industrial workers, has been justified less in terms of their superior ideological purity – compared, say, with the less trustworthy peasantry – than on the economic grounds that progress and productivity require a healthy working class.

The preferential treatment accorded the proletariat was and is manifested in several ways. As already noted, during the first two decades of the new regime, the principle of free medical care through social insurance was largely restricted to the wage-earning class. During this period, the relative inequality in health care and services between the urban and rural population, which existed during Tsarist times, actually increased. The preferred position of the urban proletariat during this time, however, extended beyond the availability and accessibility of health care to another important health policy area: medical training. From the time of the revolution until the 1930s members of the working class and their children were given preference in admissions to medical schools and other institutions of higher education. In fact, it was virtually impossible for a student from a bourgeois family to be admitted to a medical school. This policy was presumably aimed at creating a loyal and Marxist-oriented medical profession. The practice was abandoned in the 1930s, but not before it had produced some unintended consequences. The members of the proletariat may have been ideologically acceptable, but they were often academically unprepared. Some were adults who had little formal education but had been selected by a committee of their fellow workers to go on to medical school.[34] Even the most sympathetic observers have acknowledged that the quality of medical training, and the resulting qualifications of many Soviet physicians, were inferior to those of prerevolutionary Russia.[35] Realization of this undoubtedly played an important role in the regime's decision to abandon a preferential admissions policy.

The current manifestations of the priority accorded the working class, and industrial and scientific workers in particular, are not as dramatic or discriminatory as they were in earlier years. We examine some of these later on and note just a few examples here. The most obvious manifestation of this preference is that a basic organizational feature of the health care system is separate health care facilities for factory workers. The care offered in these facilities can be quite extensive, and the staff, in the larger factories, may include several doctors, nurses, and paramedics. In addition, considerable emphasis on the job and in medical training is placed upon such things as industrial hygiene and safety. Finally, "within hospitals and polyclinics also, the worker is accorded priority. Polyclinic hours are scheduled to his convenience. He is put to the head of the line – ahead of housewives and oldsters."[36]

Centralized and unified administration

The most outstanding organizational and administrative features of the Soviet health care system are its centralized and unified administration. Centralization means that policy planning, supervision, and direction are the responsibility of a single administrative agency, the Ministry of Health of the USSR. Although some health services are provided by other agencies or institutions (e.g., the armed forces and the Ministries of Internal Affairs, Communications, and Transportation), these generally follow the standards established by the Ministry of Health. In addition, although each of the 15 republics of the USSR has its own Ministry of

Health, these are subordinate to the central ministry and responsible for the execution, not formulation, of health policy.

Unification of health services means that all aspects of the health care delivery system are brought into a single health service under the central control of the Ministry of Health. Included among these services and institutions are medical institutions (hospitals, polyclinics, health resorts, sanatoriums, and nurseries), medical personnel (doctors, nurses, paramedics, pharmacists), public health departments and activities, medical education, and medical research.

The principle of a unified and centralized health service is justified in terms of fulfilling the state's responsibility in providing health care in a socialist society. The concentration of authority within a single, unified system facilitates effective planning, coordination, and delivery of health services, and the integration of these services within the overall socioeconomic plan of the party and state.

The protection of the health of the workers is the task of the workers themselves

In the Soviet Union each citizen is expected to participate actively in the campaign for a healthy society. In this sense, both the state and the individual share this responsibility. The principle of public participation and *responsibility* in the health care system finds expression in a variety of formal and informal demands made upon the public. For example, nearly one-half of the adult population has taken first aid and hygiene courses. In addition, there is a nationwide system of health volunteers, organized through Councils of Voluntary Public Service, who freely give their services to hospitals, clinics, blood banks, and other health activities and agencies. The volunteers hold public health seminars, visit the homes of sick persons, and encourage people who have been treated at clinics to make follow-up appointments.[37] Membership on the councils includes those from the Communist Party and the youth groups of the party (Komsomol and Young Pioneers), trade unionists, collective farmers, housewives, and so on.

In addition to the collective mechanisms used to involve the public in the Soviet health system, emphasis is also placed upon the individual's duty to participate in maintaining his or her own health. Each person is *expected* to exercise regularly, participate in sports, have regular medical checkups, keep informed on health issues by attending seminars and discussions and, in general, maintain a high level of health consciousness.

The principle of active citizen participation in the health system derives from various ideological and practical impulses. One of these, discussed earlier, is the heavy emphasis placed upon the relationship among economic productivity, wealth, and the health of the worker. In this regard, the Public Health Act of 1969 explains the duty of citizen participation in health care as a derivative of the axiom that "the citizen's health is public wealth." There is clearly a pragmatic, utilitarian basis for the principle.

A second explanation for the emphasis on citizen participation relates to the politicization of all aspects of Soviet society. Each citizen is enlisted or mobilized in the struggle for the building of a Communist society. One way in which every citizen can participate is by being healthy and productive.

Emphasis on preventive medicine

Perhaps the most widely heralded feature of the Soviet health system, and the one that has been called "the basic principle of Soviet medicine," is the emphasis on preventive medicine. This principle received official party endorsement and encouragement as early as 1919 in the program of the Communist Party of the Soviet Union: "The C.P.S.U. will base its public health policy on a comprehensive series of health and sanitary measures aiming to prevent the development of disease." The principle has been reiterated ever since in pronouncements by party and state officials and underscored repeatedly in official statements, documents, and textbooks dealing with the nation's health care system.

The principle of preventive medicine is operationalized in a variety of ways. One technique has already been discussed: dissemination of health education and knowledge, encouraging a high level of health consciousness, and active citizen participation in the health care system. In addition, great emphasis is placed upon standard prophylactic procedures such as immunization, medical screening of vulnerable groups (e.g., miners), and routine medical examination for "special" groups such as industrial workers, pregnant women, and children. These prophylactic efforts are part of the so-called dispensarization scheme (because they are administered through medical dispensaries) and a vital link in the preventive program.

Two other types of medical facilities contribute to and illustrate the preventive emphasis in Soviet medicine: the prophylactoriums and the sanepids. *Prophylactoriums* are rest or convalescent facilities for Soviet workers suffering from such disorders as heart disease, hypertension, ulcers, or tuberculosis. Admission to a prophylactorium requires recommendation by a physician. Workers can be admitted for extended periods or simply on an overnight basis, during which time they are given proper diets, rest, and health surveillance. The purpose of the prophylactoriums is to provide preventive and curative medical care, preferably while allowing the worker to continue on the job.

Sanepids, or sanitary and epidemiological stations, are responsible for the administration of public health measures, including implementation of steps necessary for improving environmental and occupational hygiene and the prevention of communicable diseases. There are several thousand of these apparently well-equipped and well-staffed stations located throughout the country.

The bases for the preventive tendency of Soviet health care are similar to those discussed in the context of other health care principles. First, the epidemiological problems that plagued both Tsarist Russia and, later, the Soviet regime significantly contributed to the decision to emphasize preventive public health measures and personal medical care. Second, preventive medicine is compatible with the goal of achieving a high degree of worker, and hence economic, productivity, in this case by minimizing work hours lost because of avoidable illness. Finally, the Soviets have argued that preventive medical care is a product of the Soviet Socialist state in which power is in the hands of the workers (not an exploitive and unconcerned capitalist class) and in which there is unity of purpose and organization throughout the society, economy, and polity.

These, then, are the major principles of the Soviet health care system: state provision of a unified, centralized, free, universally available and accessible health service in which the citizen is expected to play an active role and in which the primary emphasis is on preventive medical care. Among the most prominent factors that account for the direction and content of the Soviet health care system are the impact of ideology, the concern for industrial productivity, and the legacy of the past. The remainder of this chapter examines the actual provisions and organization of the service and evaluates how well the system works.

Provisions of the Soviet health service

The following description of the Soviet health service represents the current (1978) status of the system.

Coverage

All residents of the Soviet Union are provided with complete medical care.

Benefits

Medical care is free (with some minor exceptions) and covers virtually every conceivable form of health service. The exceptions to free care are drugs taken at home and various appliances (e.g., eyeglasses, dentures). However, approximately one-half of the population is exempt from these charges (e.g., the chronically ill, veterans, pregnant women, children), and those who must purchase these items can do so at a government-owned store at nominal cost. Another exception to free care is termination of pregnancy by abortion, unless for therapeutic purposes. This must be paid for by the mother. The Soviet government has reversed itself serveral times on the issue of abortion. From 1920 to 1936 abortions, while not encouraged, were permitted and without cost. In 1936 they were out-lawed, except for therapeutic purposes. That law remained in effect until 1969, when the choice of termination was again left to the mother, but with the cost paid by the patient.

Among the health benefits provided are (1) routine and extraordinary primary health care by a physician, (2) hospital services, (3) pre- and post-maternity care, (4) dental and ophthalmic services, (5) physical rehabilita-tion and physiotherapy services, (6) ambulatory and institutional psychi-atric care, and (7) all prophylactic procedures such as immunizations, diagnostic tests, and x-rays. Also included as part of the health service are maternity, sickness, and disability benefits. In short, the Soviet health service provides all forms of medical service with no limitations placed on eligibility or on frequency and duration of use.

Financing

The Soviet health service is financed entirely by the state from government revenues. These revenues are derived from (1) profits from government-owned and -operated enterprises; (2) an income tax, which is not a signifi-cant source of revenue; and (3) a turnover or sales tax on consumer goods.

Organization of health services

Medical care in the Soviet Union is provided in a highly organized and institutionalized setting. The basic building block of the system is a neighborhood territorial unit called the "microdistrict" (uchastok). Each uchastok contains about 4,000 persons – roughly 3,000 adults and 1,000 children – a doctor/patient ratio similar to that of Great Britain. Every child and adult living in the neighborhood is automatically assigned to the general physician (usually an internist) or pediatrician serving that neighborhood.

The uchastok physicians and staff practice in health centers or poly-clinics. The polyclinic facilities (offices, examining rooms, diagnostic and medical equipment, etc.) are used by the physicians of several, usually 10, microdistricts. Thus, a typical urban polyclinic serves approximately 40,000 persons. In the larger cities, such as Moscow, Leningrad, or Kiev, there are separate polyclinics for children and adults; in the smaller cities and towns, each polyclinic serves both. In addition to general and pediatric medical care, polyclinics also offer specialist care for ambulatory patients. This includes dental, ophthalmic, psychiatric, and minor surgical care. Here, too, the organization is different for large and small cities. In the large cities specialist care is offered in separate polyclinics for, say, obstetrics and gynecology, cancer, psychiatric care, venereal and skin diseases. In the smaller towns and cities, both generalists and specialists work within the same polyclinic.

In addition to the residential polyclinics serving a specified territorial unit, there is a separate system of occupational medical facilities for industrial workers. The larger industrial factories have complete polyclinics providing the full range of preventive, curative, and sanitary hygiene services. In smaller plants there may be a single physician or paramedic, and the worker receives general medical care at a regular polyclinic, but on a priority basis. The special system of medical services for industrial workers and the priority assigned the worker in the regular system are, of course, manifestations of the preferential position of the worker in Soviet society. Medical care within this industrial unit is more convenient for the worker, reduces the amount of time spent off the job, and allows closer surveillance over the worker's health – all of which presumably contribute to labor productivity.

One final comment about the polyclinic system. Although the practice of providing medical care in an organized setting is neither original nor unique to the Soviet Union, it should be emphasized that the polyclinic has been a major factor in improving health conditions in the USSR and has provided a model for other, less affluent countries. In a society in which medical resources are limited, the pooling of such resources in a common institutional setting makes a great deal of sense.

In-patient health care in the Soviet Union is provided mainly in hospitals, sanatoriums, and prophylactoriums, although some in-patient care is available in clinics and facilities attached to medical and health departments. All hospitals are state-owned, state-operated, and affiliated with the polyclinics. The hospital is considered the administrative parent organization of the polyclinic. Persons requiring hospitalization can be admitted only upon referral from a polyclinic physician. An interesting feature of the Soviet system is the effort to integrate in-patient and out-patient care by requiring physicians to practice in both polyclinics and hospitals. A polyclinic physician may spend up to 4 months each year in a hospital, and a hospital specialist may be assigned periodically to a polyclinic. The program has helped to upgrade the skills of the polyclinic physicians, as most of the more advanced medical techniques are used in the hospitals, and has helped achieve greater integration of medical services. As we have seen, the lack of integration between first contact and specialist care has been a problem and a concern in Great Britain, where there is a strict differentiation between in-patient and out-patient medical care and personnel.

The Soviet hospital system is hierarchically and territorially arranged according to the type of care provided. At the first level is the large (300 to 1,250 beds) "district" (rayon) hospital, which deals with a wide range of medical problems. Patients requiring highly specialized treatment or having extraordinary medical problems may be referred to specialized "regional" (oblast) hospitals. These hospitals specialize in thoracic surgery, neurosurgery, and so forth. Finally, there are the republic-level hospitals, which are teaching hospitals and medical schools located in each of the 15 Soviet Republics.[38]

As in the case of primary medical care, workers are treated in specialized hospitals or given priority attention within territorial hospitals. A very large plant may have its own hospital. One automobile factory in Moscow built its own 1,000-bed hospital from profits made by the factory. The hospital provides complete medical and rehabilitation facilities for 60,000 employees. Workers in small industries use the regular, district, regional, or republic hospitals, but on a priority basis.[39]

We have already discussed the prophylactoriums in the context of the emphasis on preventive medicine. Little more need be said of this aspect of Soviet health care except to point out that these facilities are usually provided by trade unions and are located near where the worker is employed. In general, they specialize in treating occupation-related ailments (e.g., tuberculosis) or those that, when kept under control, do not result in undue interruption of work. The night prophylactoriums deal with persons suffering from ulcers, rheumatism, high blood pressure, and some forms of mental illness.[40]

Related to the use of, and theory behind, prophylactoriums is a heavy emphasis on the therapeutic value of health resorts, sanatoriums, and rest homes. These institutions, too, are preventive. Health spas offer a regimen of rest, relaxation, exercise, fresh air, proper diet and, in some instances, restorative therapy treatments (e.g., mud therapy, mineral springs). "Taking the cure" at a health spa has a long history in Russia and was popular among the Russian nobility and wealthy citizenry. Indeed, many of the current health resorts and rest homes are former Tsarist palaces in resort areas. Rest homes, resorts, and sanatoriums, like other aspects of the Soviet health care delivery system, give priority to industrial workers and are managed by trade union councils. Access to resorts and rest homes is obtained through free or subsidized passes allocated by the trade unions.

Public health services in the Soviet Union are performed by the previously discussed sanepid stations. We need only add here that there are functionally equivalent industrial and occupational medical-sanitation units that perform the same type of educative and preventive services as the sanepids.

The system of polyclinics, hospitals, public health services, and health resorts described above applies, in the main, to towns and urban areas in the Soviet Union. Health services in the rural areas do not differ substantially or organizationally from those described here. As in many countries, the size of the rural areas, their widely dispersed populations, and the reluctance of health personnel to serve in these areas have created various problems and unique situations. For example, there is considerable reliance on paramedical personnel (*feldshers*), midwives, and small (10 to 100 beds) and generally inefficient hospitals. By and large, however, the same organizational principles apply to both urban and rural areas.

Administration of health services

We turn now from the organization of the Soviet health service to its administration. As indicated earlier, one of the fundamental principles of the Soviet system is the centralization and unification of medical administration. The operation of this principle can be quickly discussed and described. Overall medical policy making and planning in the Soviet Union is the responsibility of the Ministry of Health. The principle of centralized administration is manifested by the presence of the minister of health in the Council of Ministers of the USSR. The council is the highest executive authority in the Soviet government, corresponding to the cabinet in parliamentary democracies. Traditionally, the minister of health has been an eminent practicing physician. The minister is assisted by four to six deputy ministers, who are also physicians, as are two-thirds of the 900 or so staff members of the Ministry of Health. The presence of so many physician-administrators, particularly at the highest administrative level, is in contrast to the pattern of lay control in Britain.

The specific functions of the Ministry of Health include (1) planning, coordination, and control of medical care and research within the country; (2) establishing qualitative standards for medical care (e.g., doctor/patient ratios); (3) producing and allocating medical resources such as drugs and medical equipment; (4) formulating the nation's health budget and thereby setting public health priorities; and (5) responsibility for 10 of the nation's 85 medical schools and 13 postgraduate institutes.

The Union of Soviet Socialist Republics is a federation of 15 union republics and several autonomous national republics. Each of these republics has its own Ministry of Health, headed by a minister who is appointed by the elected Central Soviet of the Republic, and subject to approval by the minister of health of the USSR. Republic health ministries implement national health policies and prepare and administer the budgets of their respective republics. They are more directly responsible for the actual administration of health care than the Ministry of Health of the USSR, which is involved more in policy planning. The revenues upon which the republic budgets are based come from the national government, as there is no local taxation. The union republic ministries are also responsible for the medical schools located within their jurisdictions.

Each of the republics is divided into administrative regions called *oblasti*. These regions vary in size from 1 million to 5 million persons, and such large cities as Moscow and Leningrad constitute a single region. Regions are governed by elected executive councils. The chief medical officer of the region is a member of the Executive Council. The medical officer in a town heads the Medical Council, which is responsible for the medical services provided by the polyclinics, hospitals, and public health agencies in the region. Responsibility for the clinical performance of the physicians and quality of medical care in the region is entrusted to the chief physician of the main regional hospital. Each specialty (e.g., cardiology, gynecology, surgery) has its own chief supervisory physician. Thus, it is at the regional level that the practical or clinical, as opposed to administrative, supervision and control are introduced in the Soviet health system.

The next administrative tier in the system is the city or rural district (*rayon*) level. Each region is divided into a certain number of districts serving populations of 40,000 to 150,000 people. There are one or more district hospitals, and the head medical officer of the district is usually the most senior physician of the central district hospital. The chief physician is appointed by the District Soviet and is responsible for the day-to-day supervision of health care in the polyclinics, hospital(s), and public health services in his or her area.

Finally, at the base of the entire structure is the microdistrict (*uchastok*), a subdivision of the district containing about 4,000 persons served by a general physician, pediatrician, and medical staff.

It is important to reemphasize that the guiding principle behind the entire administrative structure of the Soviet health system is centralized and unified control. This principle requires the subordination of lower administrative authorities to higher authorities. Thus, microdistrict personnel are subordinate to, responsible to, and take direction from the district; the district, in turn, is responsible to the region; the region to the republic; and the republic to the central Ministry of Health. This administrative organization ensures the implementation of nationally agreed upon health policies.

Soviet health personnel

We conclude this discussion of the Soviet health service by examining the most important, unusual, or characteristic features of the medical personnel system and conditions of medical practice.

We begin with the background, training, and conditions of practice of Soviet physicians. All physicians in the Soviet Union are salaried government employees. Some private practice legally exists, provided typically by an eminent physician in an urban area. Many physicians – no one knows quite how many – illegally accept fees from patients who expect better, or at least faster, medical attention. Salary scales are determined by the Ministry of Health and the Medical Workers' Union. A physician's salary is based on position, experience, postgraduate training, seniority, merit, and place of practice; salary incentives are given to physicians who practice in rural areas. Because the working day of a Soviet physician is relatively short (between 6 and 6.5 hours) and salaries are relatively low (between $140 and $187 per month, which is less than three-quarters of the average industrial wage), many physicians hold multiple jobs, although this too is officially discouraged. Physicians may also supplement their incomes by giving public health lectures after their regular working hours. This, of course, helps reinforce the emphasis placed on preventive medicine and health consciousness.

The relatively low rate of compensation for physicians may contribute to one of the outstanding features of the medical profession in the Soviet Union: Approximately 70 percent of Soviet physicians are women. In fact, "there are more women physicians in the U.S.S.R. than *in the rest of the world combined*, even including the other communist countries."[41] The relationship between salary scale and the feminization of Soviet medicine was recently explained by a Soviet scientist: "Men don't want it [work in the medical profession] because the pay is low."[42] Another explanation for the heavy concentration of women in Soviet medicine relates to the historical experience and resulting demographic composition of the country. "Because of the killing and wounding of men in wars and purges, women at times have constituted three-fifths of certain age cohorts in the population and a majority of the labor force from these generations."[43] Although the level of compensation and Soviet demographic structure have obviously contributed to the feminization of the medical profession, the *origins* of the situation lie less in personal economic motivation or demographics than in national economic necessity and regime priority. After the revolution, and particularly during the period of rapid industrialization, men were diverted to other, more industrially oriented, technical professions, such as engineering and scientific research.

The rapid feminization of Soviet medicine can be seen in the following figures. In 1913, 10 percent of all Russian physicians were women; this rose to 45 percent in 1928, and to 62 percent in 1940. The high point occurred in 1950, when 77 percent of all Soviet physicians were women. Since the 1950s, the regime has sought to encourage more men to enter medicine. In 1970, the proportion of women had declined to 72 percent of all physicians. It is interesting to note that in the same year, 1970, only 7 percent of all American physicians were women. Lest American feminists rally too quickly to the Soviet model, it should be pointed out that only a small proportion, 10 to 20 percent, of Soviet surgeons are women, and very few senior administrative posts in the health profession are held by women.

One final feature of the Soviet health personnel system requires comment: the position of *feldsher* or semiprofessional health worker or medical assistant. The *feldsher* is unique to the Soviet Union and occupies a position somewhere between a nurse and a physician. Originally introduced by Peter the Great in the seventeenth century, *feldshers* assisted military doctors in the field. In the late nineteenth century, the *feldsher* system was introduced into civilian medical practice in rural areas to compensate for shortages in trained personnel there. As the system developed, the *feldsher* came to be identified as the poor person's or peasant's doctor, while trained physicians served the upper class. Because of this class-based distinction, the Soviet regime originally intended to abolish the *feldsher* system. However, the same shortage of rural physicians that plagued Tsarist Russia continued after the revolution, and so did *feldsher*ism.

Today, *feldshers* receive formal training in special schools and are qualified and authorized to prescribe drugs for minor ailments, give innoculations, administer first aid to injured persons, and make sanitary inspections of industrial sites. They practice in both urban and rural areas and are responsible to physicians. However, because of the continued shortage of trained physicians in rural areas, the *feldsher* often performs independent of any supervision. Furthermore, in some rural areas, *feldshers* actually perform minor surgery.

We conclude this section with a brief comment about medical education in the Soviet Union. As one might expect, medical schools are state institutions, and medical education – including tuition, books, and living expenses – is state-financed. The one noteworthy political and policy-relevant feature of Soviet medical education is the heavy emphasis on political studies, including courses on Marxism, dialectic materialism, and the history of the Communist Party. In 1964, for example, the medical school curriculum for students in general medicine included 390 hours for social and political sciences compared with 190 hours for biology, 247 hours for physiology, and 189 hours for general surgery.[44]

This overt emphasis on political socialization clearly distinguishes the Soviet from the German, American, British, and Japanese systems of medical education. There is no indication that this emphasis detracts from the competence of Soviet physicians, but it does represent the impact of ideology on policy. In the Soviet Union physicians must be politically, as well as professionally, competent and acceptable.

The performance of the Soviet health system

As stated at the outset of this chapter, a major problem in Soviet studies, from which research on health care is not immune, is the intrusion of ideological bias into scholarly analysis. This danger is particularly acute in evaluating the performance of the Soviet system. An effort is made in the following account to avoid such bias. Nevertheless, this evaluation is judgmental, reflecting certain values of the author. The basic conclusions about the performance of the Soviet health care system are: (1) health care policy has been enormously successful in providing all Soviet citizens with professionally competent, comprehensive, free medical care; (2) the system has contributed to the improvement of the nation's health condition; (3) certain distributive problems, by no means unique to the Soviet Union, persist despite the regime's commitment to equal health care for all; and (4) in some important cases, medical care and medical practice are influenced by ideology and political considerations.

We offer no evaluation of the organizational assumptions of Soviet health care – that is, centralization and state administration. Nor do we comment upon the role and status of Soviet physicians. These are obviously important and controversial issues, but they are not, it seems to us, the basis for a systematic comparison of health system achievements. This evaluation is based upon certain assumptions that appear to be part of an emerging consensus about health care. Among these assumptions are: (1) competent medical care is a civil and human right and should be made equally available and accessible to *all* citizens of a nation independent of political, financial, or social considerations; (2) medical care should not be used as a political weapon, to punish opponents or reward supporters; and (3) appropriate medical procedures should not be determined by political ideology. These are the values on which the following evaluation is made.

The state of health and health care

Earlier in this chapter we examined the state of health and health care in Tsarist Russia on the eve of the revolution. We concluded that the situation was indeed a sorry inheritance from the old regime. An examination of Table 7–2 reveals the enormous progress the Soviet Union has made in reducing general and infant mortality, increasing life expectancy, and providing medical personnel and facilities for its people. Since 1913, life expectancy has more than doubled; general mortality has declined by 71 percent and infant mortality by 90 percent. In 1913, there were 1.5 physicians per 10,000 people in the Soviet Union; in 1970, there were 23.8 doctors per 10,000 people. In 1913, there were 1.3 hospital beds per

Table 7–2. *Health status in Russia (1913 and 1973) and in Germany, Great Britain, Japan, and the United States (1973)*

Indicator	Russia (1913)	USSR (1973)	Germany (1973)	Great Britain (1973)	Japan (1973)	United States (1973)
General mortality rate (per 1,000 population)	30.2	8.7	11.8	11.9	6.5	9.4
Infant mortality rate (per 1,000 live births)	269.0	26.0	20.0	17.0	12.0	18.0
Average life expectancy (yr)	32.0	70.0	71.0	72.0	73.0	71.0
Population per physician	6,862.0	369.0	532.0	756.0	864.0	612.0
Population per hospital bed	767.0	86.0	87.0	106.0	97.0	135.0

Sources: Mark G. Field, "Health as a 'Public Utility' or the 'Maintenance of Capacity' in Soviet Society," *Social Consequences of Modernization in Communist Societies,* ed. Mark G. Field (Baltimore: Johns Hopkins Press, 1976), pp. 244–61; Gordon Hyde, *The Soviet Health Service* (London: Lawrence & Wishart, 1974), p. 14; Y. Lisitsin, *Health Protection in the U.S.S.R.* (Moscow: Progress Publishers, 1972), p. 45; *Public Health in Japan* (Tokyo: Supreme Commander Allied Powers, 1949), 2, pp. A–1, A–12; *Journal of the American Medical Association,* February 16, 1929; Ruth L. Sivard, *World Military and Social Expenditures: 1976* (Leesburg, Va.: WMSE Publications, 1976), pp. 24–9.

1,000 people; in 1971, 11.1 beds per 1,000 population. In 1913, there were 6 medical schools in all Tsarist Russia; today there are over 80. In addition, the incidence of specific diseases has shown a dramatic decline between 1913 and the present: Typhoid fever declined from 257 to 10 cases per 100,000 people; diphtheria declined from 314 to 0.9 cases per 100,000 population; and whooping cough dropped from 300 to 50 cases per 100,000. Epidemic typhus, which Lenin had warned threatened the very existence of the new Communist regime, was down to 1.3 cases per 100,000 in 1968 from its high of 4,000 per 100,000 population in 1920.

In part, the decreases in mortality and morbidity rates and the increase in life expectancy can be attributed to the international diffusion of medical knowledge and advancement. Although medical improvements are, for the most part, available for the entire world to enjoy, they are not automatically adopted or disseminated. In every society, government officials or private physicians must take the initiative and allocate the resources to make new procedures, drugs, and facilities available in a particular country. That the process is neither automatic nor uniform in impact is illustrated in the case of India. In the first two decades of the twentieth century, Russia and India had similar health profiles: The infant mortality rate in each country was about 250 per 1,000 live births; general mortality in India was 34 per 1,000 people and in Russia 30.2 per 1,000. By 1973 the comparable figures for the two nations were: an infant mortality rate of 139 in India compared with 26 in the USSR; a general mortality rate of 16.7 in India and 8.7 in Russia. Although there are important differences between these two countries now, they started with roughly the same demographic base. A good deal of the difference can be attributed to the policy commitment of the Soviet regime to improving health conditions in that country.

That commitment is reflected in the magnitude of the health care establishment of the Soviet Union. One-fourth of all the doctors in the world today are Soviet doctors. The USSR ranks second, behind Israel, in the number of physicians per population, and eighth in the number of hospital beds per population. On both these measures, the USSR ranks above the United States, Great Britain, Japan, and Germany (see Table 7–2). And the annual rate of increase of both doctors and hospital beds is higher in the USSR than in the other countries. Every year the USSR graduates almost 38,000 new doctors. In addition to the over 700,000 doctors in the country, there are approximately 2.5 million auxiliary health personnel: nurses, *feldshers,* pharmacists, and so on. In terms of nursing, the ratio of nurses to population is higher than in the United States, Great Britain, Germany, or Japan.

The Soviet state is committed to making competent medical care available to all its citizens. It has implemented that policy commitment by allocating sufficient resources to produce the world's largest medical establishment. The results of this effort have been spectacular. The health care profile of Tsarist Russia resembled that of a backward Asian or African country. Russia was ravaged by epidemics; it had high mortality and morbidity rates, a short life expectancy, and totally inadequate medical facilities. Health and health care statistics in the Soviet Union today portray a nation equal or superior to most modern Western nations. There is no denying the quantitative achievements of the Soviet health care effort.

The Soviet regime has apparently succeeded in providing virtually cost-free medical care to all its citizens. But what about the *quality* of the Soviet health care system? It is almost impossible to answer this question with any degree of certainty for several reasons. First, there has not been, to our knowledge, any systematic analysis of, say, survival rates after various surgical procedures. Nor has there been any systematic study of medical equipment in the more than 25,000 hospitals of the Soviet Union. Data on the quality of Soviet medical care tend to be anecdotal and, therefore, unrepresentative and unreliable. A case in point is David Shipler's fine article in the *New York Times,* entitled "Soviet Medicine

Mixes Inconsistency with Diversity" (June 26, 1977). In the article, Shipler describes a system of technical and administrative inconsistency. "Pioneering heart research is done, but a young man is transfused with incompatible blood until he nearly dies. Artificial plastic lenses are implanted into eyes, but a Muscovite who breaks his glasses cannot get new ones for months." Similarly, with regard to the doctor-patient relationship in the Soviet Union, one source notes: "One sometimes reads complaints of hurried work or brusque behavior." However, another commentator writes that there is general agreement by observers that "splendid human warmth and attention is shown to Soviet patients."[45] However revealing, these accounts are hardly the basis for scholarly evaluations of the performance of the Soviet health care system.

A second problem in evaluating the quality of Soviet medical care is determining the standard by which that quality should be measured. Milton Roemer, for example, notes that by American standards there are a number of qualitative deficiencies, including weakness in routine diagnostic procedure. Roemer goes on to suggest, however, that "it may not be fair to compare Soviet resources with those of the wealthy United States. The technical level of hospitals is certainly as good as much one sees in Western Europe, not only in France and Italy, but also in Great Britain."[46]

Given these limitations, is an overall assessment of the quality of Soviet health care possible? Despite the problems listed above, there are some areas of agreement among various observers of the Soviet health scene. The following is a composite of those views, recognizing that in the Soviet Union, as in all other countries, quality does vary. Medical facilities – polyclinics and hospitals – in the Soviet Union are clean, well kept, and by American standards, modestly furnished. "The beds are simple, flat cots, usually without the mechanical features – bedside lamps, call-buttons, and other gadgets – that add to patient comfort in the United States."[47] Medical equipment and medicines tend to be of poorer quality and not as widely available as in the United States.

In terms of medical personnel, supporters and detractors of the Soviet system seem to agree that medical training and the resulting level of personnel competence are generally lower in the USSR than in the United States. This is not to suggest that Soviet physicians and nurses are incompetent. It does appear, however, that greater attention has been paid to making medical care available to all by producing an enormous number of physicians, nurses, and allied personnel than to achieving the highest possible levels of competence among that personnel.

In the final analysis, however, as far as Soviet citizens are concerned, the availability and accessibility of medical care are of primary importance. After discussing some qualitative shortcomings of the Soviet health care system, Hedrick Smith, who covered the USSR for the *New York Times* for several years, observes: "Nonetheless, for most Russians, such problems are outweighed by the improvements over the past. They regard the system of free health care as one of the most positive features of Soviet socialism."[48]

The distribution of medical services

Despite the regime's genuine commitment to an equitable distribution of medical services throughout the country, substantial variation persists in the Soviet Union today. This problem is openly acknowledged by Soviet officials. A deputy minister of health recently observed: "In the health services system of the U.S.S.R. there are still some unresolved problems and difficulties. Particularly notable is the task of raising the level of medical care in rural areas to the standard in the cities."[49]

The quantitative inequalities between urban and rural areas are represented in the data on the distribution of physicians and medical facilities. Overall, it has been estimated that although 42 percent of the Soviet population lives in rural areas, only about 11 percent of the physicians practice in these areas. Unfortunately, it was not possible to find recent figures on the disparity of physician/population ratios for the rural versus urban areas of each Soviet republic. Although the following figures are obviously dated, they do illustrate the nature of the problem. As Table 7-3 clearly demonstrates, there were, in 1961, enormous differences in the ratio of physicians to population in each of the 15 republics. Indications are that, although the inequalities are not as great today as they were in 1961, they remain substantial. Somewhat more recent data (1964) indicate that the discrepancy applies to availability of hospital beds as well, but not in as exaggerated a fashion. For example, in 1964 there were 8.8 hospital beds per 1,000 people in the urban areas of the Soviet Union and 7.3 per 1,000 people in the rural areas. This represents substantial improvement since 1950, when the corresponding figures were 7.6 (urban) and 3.1 (rural) beds per 1,000 people.

The explanation for these inequalities is not unique to a communist society. Soviet physicians, like their colleagues throughout the world, do not like practicing in the boondocks. Whether for professional reasons (e.g., isolation from major centers of medical research and advanced practice) or personal reasons (e.g., the desire for the creature comforts associated with urban living), Soviet physicians have been as reluctant to practice and as ingenious in avoiding service in rural areas as their Western counterparts.

To its credit, the Soviet regime has made great efforts to attract qualified medical personnel to all areas of the country. Theoretically, a new

Table 7–3. *Urban-rural differences in number of physicians per 10,000 population in the Soviet republics, 1961*

Republic	Total	Urban	Rural
Russian SFSR	19.4	27.3	9.4
Ukrainian SSR	18.9	27.6	10.5
Belorussian SSR	16.7	27.2	11.0
Uzbek SSR	15.4	28.8	8.2
Kazakh SSR	15.5	24.3	8.5
Georgian SSR	22.8	34.0	13.5
Azerbaijan SSR	19.9	31.4	8.6
Lithuanian SSR	19.4	30.1	12.0
Moldavian SSR	14.8	33.7	8.8
Latvian SSR	24.2	29.4	17.1
Kirghiz SSR	15.7	24.7	10.4
Tadzhik SSR	14.4	28.0	7.2
Armenian SSR	20.4	29.0	10.9
Turkmen SSR	18.6	29.6	8.5
Estonian SSR	24.4	30.9	15.1
Average USSR	18.8	27.6	9.8

Source: Mark G. Field, *Soviet Socialized Medicine* (New York: Free Press, 1967), p. 113.

physician must accept a compulsory 3- to 5-year assignment to an under-doctored area. The assignment is viewed as repayment for the free schooling the state has provided. However, there are various ways of avoiding this, including "self-assignment," which allows a new physician to find a job on his or her own instead of being placed by the medical institute.[50] Another factor that inhibits the assignment of physicians to rural areas is the high proportion of women doctors. In a situation where the doctor is a married woman, there is an apparent reluctance to force her to separate from her husband (and perhaps children). Although the husband can, of course, go with his physician-wife to her new assignment, it is often difficult, if not impossible, to find an appropriate job for him in the rural location. Thus, many women avoid rural assignments. Finally, most of those who do accept initial rural assignments, leave them upon completion of the specified tour of duty.

The Soviet regime has also offered various incentives to attract and retain greater numbers of physicians in the rural areas of the country. Characteristically, nonsocialist incentives include higher salaries, longer vacations, better opportunities for postgraduate medical training, and, in some instances, rent-free homes or apartments. Despite these inducements, the availability of physician care, and indeed the quality of medical care, are poorer in the rural areas of the country than in the cities.

The geographical maldistribution of health services is understandable and, given the apparently genuine regime commitment to its elimination, in a sense defensible. But there is another distributional issue that is less defensible – either ideologically or pragmatically. Despite its commitment to equal medical care for all, regardless of financial or political considerations, the quality and accessibility of health services in the Soviet Union *are*, in some instances, dependent on the ability to pay or on political (i.e., Communist Party) standing. It is not uncommon for some persons to get more attentive, responsive, and reputedly, competent care than is available to the general public. For high-ranking officials in the party and state bureaucracies, preferential treatment is routinely provided. For others it must be purchased. Shipler reports that payment may be in rubles or in scarce commodities. One physician told Shipler of an arrangement he had with a meat dealer: "There is no meat in the stores, so he comes to me for [preferential] treatment and my wife goes to him for [unavailable] meat." Whichever the case, political or economic influence, the practice of preferential treatment is hardly in keeping with the ideological precepts of the regime.

Politics, ideology, and medicine

Among the shortcomings of the Soviet health care system, none is more objectionable than the imposition of politics and ideology on the practice of medicine. Consider, for example, the following celebrated episode. On May 29, 1970, Zhores Medvedev, a prominent and internationally respected scientist, was forcibly removed from his apartment in Obinisk City, 80 miles southwest of Moscow, and taken to a psychiatric hospital, where he was kept, without legitimate medical justification, until June 17, 1970. His release was gained only after intense pressure from scientists and intellectuals both within and outside the Soviet Union. The "medical attention" given Medvedev apparently resulted from his outspoken and published criticisms of certain aspects of Soviet science and the scientific community. What happened to Zhores Medvedev was not an isolated incident. Rather, it was part, in Medvedev's words, of "the dangerous tendency of using psychiatry for political purposes, the exploitation of medicine in an alien role as a means of intimidation and punishment – a new and illegal way of isolating people for their views and convictions."[51] This tendency was attacked by another prominent Russian dissident, Andrei Sakharov who, in a letter to Leonid Brezhnev on Medvedev's behalf, argued: "Psychiatric hospitals must not be used as a means of repression against undesirable persons. They must be used for one purpose only – namely, to treat patients who are really ill, while at the same time, respecting all their human rights."[52] It is also apparently routine practice to admit all socially dangerous persons to psychiatric hospitals prior to major Soviet celebrations such as May Day or Lenin's Birthday or other occasions when foreign dignitaries may be in the country.

The case of Zhores Medvedev illustrates one of the paradoxes of the Soviet health care system. Medvedev himself pointed out this paradox in his book, *A Question of Madness:* "Totalitarian centralisation of the medical service, while introducing the progressive principle of free health care for all, has also made it possible to use medicine as a means of government control and political regulation."[53] In other words, the same system that is able to organize and deliver competent health care virtually cost-free to an entire nation can and has been used as a means of political repression. This, it seems to us, is an unacceptable, illegitimate use of medicine.

The area of psychiatry provides another quite different and less obnoxious illustration of the impact of politics on medical practice. We refer to the influence of Marxist ideology on the attitude toward and treatment of mental illness. There is, to begin with, the unsubstantiated claim that there is a lower incidence of mental illness in socialist than in capitalist societies owing to the social and cultural achievements of socialism. One Soviet source claims: "In the USSR the incidence of mental diseases among both urban and rural population is only one-third or even one-quarter of that registered in several economically developed capitalist countries."[54] The absence of class conflict and the collective orientation in socialist societies produces less stress, greater happiness, and lower rates of mental illness. In fact, however, the available data suggest there is little difference in the rates of mental illness among, for example, the USSR, the United States, and Great Britain.[55]

The importance attached to the contribution of a communist social environment to mental health has led to reliance on a particular approach to, and explanation of, mental illness. Specifically, Soviet psychiatry is based on Pavlovian rather than Freudian theory. Pavlov argued that people could be conditioned, given a properly controlled environment, "to achieve almost any kind of social adaption."[56] If you create the proper social environment, people can be conditioned to behave properly. Thus, Pavlovian psychology and communist ideology both emphasize the importance of social factors. The logical extension of the acceptance of Pavlovian theory is explained by Ari Kiev.

> The acceptance of Pavlovian theory is accompanied by a rejection of those theories which regard unconscious thoughts as motivating forces over which man has little control [e.g., Freudian psychology]. Such theories are obviously incompatible with a system which sets great store in rational planning for society and for the individual.[57]

Because the Soviet Union has created the proper environment for maintaining mental health, it follows that most mental illness must be caused, not by an improper environment but by organic problems. "The predominant view seems to be that mental illness is associated with organic changes in the brain." These changes "are believed due largely to chemical processes induced by metabolic disturbances, trauma, infection, or other physical causes."[58]

Finally, Marxist theory and Soviet psychiatry again dovetail in recommending the appropriate form of therapy for mental illness: Great reliance is placed on work therapy. "In Marxist theory work is viewed as man's most important activity. It is felt that man's consciousness grows and his relations with other men develop within the framework of economic activities. According to the Soviet Constitution, work is a duty and a matter of honor."[59] This attitude is shared by Soviet psychiatrists. "Russian psychiatrists feel very strongly that the continuation of work habits while under treatment keeps the patient from regressing into dependency and losing his self-esteem."[60] The result is that psychiatric treatment for working adults involves, along with necessary chemotherapy and physical therapy, an effort to get the individual into a work situation. The individual is assigned a job commensurate with his skills and receives just compensation.

One should not conclude from the above discussion that the Soviet approach to mental illness is necessarily wrong. Psychiatry is by no means a hard science in which "truth" can be definitely determined. There are many psychiatrists in the United States who reject, for example, Freudian analysis – although perhaps for different reasons than their Soviet colleagues do. Indeed, some aspects of Soviet psychiatric care – the emphasis on work therapy, attempts to maintain those with mental illness in their community rather than institutions, and the very high doctor/patient ratio in Soviet psychiatric hospitals – are widely acclaimed throughout the West. Our purpose is not to debunk these aspects of Soviet psychiatric care, but to explain their genesis in political ideas – that may or may not be valid.

Conclusion

In the final analysis, one seems always to come back to the same point when considering the Soviet health care system: The system has provided an extremely large, diverse, and previously deprived people with (at least) adequate, universally accessible and available, free health care. It has turned, through sheer quantity of effort and personnel, a country ravaged by epidemics and ill health into one that is on par with most advanced nations today. Problems of equitable distribution remain, but the regime does appear genuinely committed to minimize, if not eliminate, these. We can and should condemn the political abuse of medicine in controlling political dissidents. But, after all the qualifications, despite whatever reservations one may have about a state-run health system, as far as objective health standards are concerned and as far as the overwhelming majority of Soviet citizens is concerned, the Soviet health service is a success.

Accounting for Soviet health care policy

As one might expect in a communist society, ideology has had an enormous influence on the direction, content, and implementation of health care policy in the Soviet Union. Nevertheless, other factors have contributed to the nature of health care policy since the Bolshevik Revolution of October 1917. By way of summary, we can itemize some of the more important of these influences.

Situational factors

Epidemics rather than polemics determined early Soviet health care policy. As Lenin clearly recognized, Bolshevik survival depended in large measure on containing and reducing the ravaging effects of hunger and illness in the country. As a result, several policy concessions, including the initial decentralization of health administration, toleration of opposition from segments of the medical profession, and continuation of certain Tsarist practices (e.g., *feldsher*ism and health insurance), were made in response to the demands of the moment. Similarly, when the ideologically inspired policy of restricting medical school admissions to workers proved a failure, the regime responded to the situation by changing policy.

Environmental factors

Not unexpectedly, environmental factors have been less significant in determining health policy in the Soviet Union than in either Great Britain or Japan. The authoritarian nature of the Soviet regime, the fervent belief in the rectitude of socialism, and a strong xenophobic strain in Soviet history dating back to the civil war period have kept policy imitation and diffusion to a minimum. When the Soviet leadership has borrowed at all, it has tended to reach back to its own rejected (i.e., Tsarist) past rather than to the outside world.

Cultural factors

The most obvious and important impact on Soviet health care policy has been the regime's ideology. The basic organizational and substantive health policy principles discussed in this chapter – complete state responsibility for a highly centralized, free, comprehensive and universal medical care system, with priority given to the proletariat – are essentially efforts to spell out the humanitarian, egalitarian, and collective implications of socialist ideology. The impact of ideology is so complete that it has filtered down to the actual practice of medicine, particularly in the Soviet approach to psychiatry.

Structural factors

The primary impact of the humanitarian, egalitarian, and collective content of socialism on Soviet health policy has been rivaled by the authoritarian nature of the regime. This impulse has led to, among other things, the political neutralization of the medical profession and, more importantly, the abuse of medicine for political repression.

The structure of the Soviet economy, and particularly its emphasis on rapid and sustained industrialization, also has influenced the delivery and content of health care policy. Particularly relevant has been the emphasis on industrial health centers and concern with industrial safety, worker rehabilitation, and so on.

In addition, the demographic structure of the Soviet Union has tempered and qualified certain socialist tendencies in health care policy. One example of this has been the continued reliance on *feldshers* to carry the burden of health care in the remote rural areas of the nation. Although this system has clear class-based origins and is a departure from the principle of equally competent and qualified medical care for all, the physical size of the nation and the reluctance of physicians to serve in remote rural areas have led to the institutionalization of *feldsher*ism.

In conclusion, ideology has been predominant in influencing Soviet health care policy, but that ideology has been tempered by other policy-relevant considerations and in some instances abandoned.

8

Japan: health care
in an Asian nation

In 1968 Japan celebrated the one-hundredth anniversary of the Meiji restoration. The restoration of 1868 marked the beginning of Japan's radical transition from a predominantly agrarian and feudal society to a modern industrialized nation. In honor of the centennial, the International Medical Foundation of Japan published *One Hundred Years of Health Progress in Japan*, by Dr. F. Ohtani, of the Ministry of Health and Welfare. The book, published in March 1971, chronicled the impressive developments in Japanese health care since the restoration. About 4 months later, the Japan Medical Association offered its own commentary on the Japanese medical system when 67,000 of its 87,000 members resigned from the state-sponsored health insurance program.

This curious, and fortuitous, concatenation of celebration and condemnation nicely symbolizes the complicated, diverse, but always intriguing story of the development of health care policy in Japan. As does so much of Japanese politics over the past century, health care policy reflects a curious mixture of traditional Japanese concerns (e.g., reverence for the past) and modern Western institutions (e.g., use of organized interest groups). This chapter examines the evolution of Japan's health care delivery system, underscoring how public policy has attempted to incorporate and reconcile the health needs of the nation, the impact of external forces, and the preservation of cultural integrity.

Historical development

The Meiji restoration

The period of Japanese history that began in 1868 received its name from the nominal "restoration" of imperial rule and the removal from power of the feudal shoguns and barons. The new emperor, who had come to the throne in 1867, assumed the reign name of Meiji.

The restoration was led by a small group of disaffected *samurai* warriors, who were concerned about Japan's increasing concessions and vulnerability in the face of Western demands for opening the country to foreign trade. The problem had begun in 1853, when Commodore Matthew C. Perry forced trade concessions from the Japanese that were quickly followed by similar demands from, and resulting treaties with, several European nations. The concessions were viewed with increased hostility by the young *samurai,* who demanded expulsion of the "barbarians." In their view, Japan had to modernize in order to control the Western threat and be assured a place of equality among nations. As Edwin Reischauer describes it:

> The young "samurai" of western Japan embarked on a daring course of rapid modernization which amounted to a revolution in Japanese society and government. This revolution did not, like those in nineteenth-century Europe, boil up from below. It was carefully planned at the top and forced upon the people by a relatively small but extremely vigorous group in control of the government.[1]

The irony of the situation is that in the process of modernizing to protect themselves from the Western powers, the Japanese engaged in wholesale borrowing from the very same nations. Indeed, the process of cultural borrowing was elevated to a position of imperial policy in the famous Charter Oath of Five Articles issued in April 1868. Article five declared that "wisdom and knowledge shall be sought from all over the world and thereby the foundations of Imperial rule shall be strengthened." In an explicit and conscious effort to emulate their adversaries, Japan's new leaders studied Britain, France, Germany, and the United States. They hired advisors from these countries and modeled new Japanese institutions after those of the other nations. In each case, the Japanese selected the area in which a nation was reputed to excel – the British navy, the German army, the French legal system, and American business practices.

Among the various policy activities, of particular interest to us are the Japanese efforts to modernize their medical system. Although Western medicine had been introduced by the Portuguese as early as the sixteenth century and was firmly established by the nineteenth century, the majority of physicians in Japan practiced *kampo* (Chinese medicine). *Kampo* includes massage, acupuncture, moxibustion or moxicautery (a process in which cones from wormwood trees are burned at specific places on the body), and herb medicines. The restoration leaders decided that in medicine, as in other areas, modernization required Westernization. And in line with their policy of adopting the most advanced system in each field, they surveyed various medical systems in Europe and America. The choice, however, was a foregone conclusion. By the second half of the nineteenth century, there was general agreement that the German system of medicine was the most advanced in the world.

In 1870 the Japanese government contracted with two Prussian medical instructors to come to Japan and teach Japanese medical students German practices. At the same time, Japanese students were sent to Germany and Austria to study medicine. All aspects of Japanese medicine – hospital organization, medical education, scientific procedures – were Germanized. In fact, German became the language of medicine in Japan. The impact this had on Japan was so complete and persistent that as late as the 1960s German was still required in Japan's medical schools, and many practicing physicians, hospital staff doctors, and medical professors continued to use German for their medical records, professional papers, and so on. Not until the 1970s did English begin replacing German as the professional language of Japan's doctors. In sum, the influence of the German model (i.e., policy diffusion) was overwhelming. "It is unlikely that there is an instance in history of a country not under the political domination of another, adopting a pattern of medical education as completely as the Japanese adopted the German system."[2]

The government-sponsored modernization of the Japanese medical system proceeded along several fronts. In 1872 the Medical Section was established in the Ministry of Education; it was elevated to the status of Medical Bureau in 1874. The bureau's first director, Dr. Chian Sagara, had played a prominent role in introducing the German model into Japan. The bureau's main concern was with administering medical education and public health services. In 1875 the Medical Bureau was transferred to the Ministry of Home Affairs; it was eventually renamed the Sanitary Bureau and given exclusive public health responsibilities.

In 1874 the government issued the nation's first omnibus Medical Law. The law contained provisions dealing with public health organization and administration, medical education, dispensing of medicines, and licensing of hospitals and medical personnel. As a practical matter, many of the provisions of the law were either unenforceable or unattainable at the time. Therefore, the Medical Law of 1874 was largely a statement of intention rather than a description of reality.

One of the Medical Law provisions the government was anxious to enforce was the licensing of physicians. According to the law, licenses to practice medicine would be granted only to those who passed government-run, uniform medical examinations; those examinations were to be based on Western medicine. Provisional licenses would be granted to all practicing physicians, thereby recognizing, at least temporarily, practitioners of Chinese medicine. However, every physician was given 10 years to pass the examination and qualify for a license to practice. All new physicians would have to qualify under the Western examination system. Examinations began in 1876 and were regularly conducted throughout the country by

1878. The medical examination system had the effect of institutionalizing two fundamental principles of Japanese health care policy: (1) the primacy of Western medicine and (2) the right of the imperial government, not the medical profession itself or local governments, to license and regulate the medical profession.

As one might expect, the decision to license only physicians who could demonstrate competence in Western medical practices was a matter of considerable concern and professional disability to *kampo* physicians. The failure rate on the examination by these physicians was quite high; in the spring of 1887, only 259 of 1,125 taking the examination passed it.[3] As a result, *kampo* physicians began a campaign to revise the examination system. In 1890, when the first Imperial Diet (or parliament) met, they petitioned the legislature for a change in the system. Despite their efforts and numbers – in 1874 over 80 percent of Japan's 28,262 physicians practiced *kampo* – this and all subsequent appeals were rejected and eventually all recognition of *kampo* was withdrawn.[4] We should point out here, however, that the practice of *kampo* was not prohibited. Physicians licensed to practice Western medicine could use Chinese medical practices. Even today, there is widespread use of Chinese herb medicines and medical practices in Japan. In 1967, for example, there were 125,000 masseurs, acupuncturists, and moxicauterists in Japan compared with 110,000 physicians.[5] Even in their pursuit of modernization, the Japanese leaders were willing to make concessions to traditional practices.

By the turn of the century, the process of modernization had been virtually completed. Instruction at most medical schools was conducted by German-trained Japanese instructors. In addition, most of the paraphernalia of a modern, professional medical system were in use; medical research institutes, professional associations, and medical journals were all available in Japan. The last significant and culminating action of the Meiji period in this area was the Medical Practitioners Law of 1906. The law was promoted by the medical profession itself in order to protect its newly acquired and improved status. Whereas historically the social standing of the physician in Japan had fluctuated, the Japanese not only adopted the methods of Western medicine but also attributed to Japanese physicians a social status comparable to that of their Western counterparts. In essence, the law (1) prescribed who could be licensed – those graduating from accredited Japanese medical schools, those passing the medical practitioner's examination, those graduating from recognized foreign medical schools or holding recognized foreign medical licenses; (2) prescribed procedures for suspending or rescinding medical licenses; (3) prescribed penalties for practicing without a license; and (4) recognized and granted certain powers to medical associations. The intent clearly was to establish a professional medical community firmly in Japan.

Although the Meiji period formally ended in 1921 with the death of the emperor, in terms of medical policy the 1906 Medical Practitioners Law marked the end of the modernization period. The restoration leaders had set out to establish a modern system of medicine based on Western scientific principles and, within a remarkably short time, had done so. In the process they also had established the basis for private medical practice and government oversight of the medical system.

The establishment of national health insurance

By the beginning of the twentieth century, Japan had entered a stage of rapid industrial development in an essentially free market environment. Although the Meiji government had played an active role in the early stages of Japan's industrial development in the form of government ownership and management of key industries, in 1880 it divested itself of virtually all enterprises. From 1880 on, the Japanese economy was essentially capitalistic.

In Japan, as in the West, industrialization was accompanied by urbanization, rapid population growth, and considerable social dislocation. These, in turn, spawned two problems related to health policy: (1) a deteriorating public health situation, and (2) demands by the working class for security against the uncertainties of urban living and working conditions.

In terms of public health, the area of principal concern was the high incidence of tuberculosis. In 1902, the death rate from tuberculosis per 100,000 persons was 183.6; in 1910, 234.0; and in 1918, 257.1. The number of deaths from tuberculosis in these years rose from 82,559 (1902) to 133,202 (1910) to 140,747 (1918). Aside from the humanitarian interest, the prevalence of tuberculosis particularly concerned authorities because of the unusually high rate among Japanese textile workers. The textile industry was Japan's key industry; at the turn of the century between 60 and 70 percent of all factories and workers were involved in the manufacture of textiles. In response to the threat to human life and industrial productivity, the government undertook various public health measures. In 1904, the Ministry of Home Affairs issued an ordinance requiring spittoons and disinfection of sputa in public places; in 1914, the government passed a law providing for the establishment and public subsidization of tuberculosis sanatoriums. The law required any urban area of 300,000 or more persons to establish a sanatorium and provide treatment, free of charge, to anyone unable to afford it. These laws were updated and expanded in the Tuberculosis Prevention Law of 1919.

Although the government attempted, not too successfully, to deal with tuberculosis from a public health angle, the implications of the problem from a personal economic and social perspective were largely ignored. No public provisions were made for routine medical care for vulnerable segments of the population or for compensation for job-related illness or injury. Given the prevailing free market orientation in Japan and the sense of paternalism that came to characterize Japanese industrial relations, it is not surprising that the first efforts to provide social insurance came from private enterprise rather than the government. One of the first and most celebrated of these efforts was the introduction of a health insurance program at the turn of the century by the Kanegafuchi Spinning Company, one of Japan's leading textile firms. Its president, Sanji Muto, introduced the employer-sponsored program apparently in response to the high incidence of tuberculosis among his female spinners. Similar company-sponsored mutual benefit associations were introduced by other employers and became the primary form of social and health protection in the first two decades of the twentieth century. These organizations constituted, in part, the origin of social security in Japan. Although we have no record of the numbers or proportion of urban workers covered by these programs, all indications are that the programs were clearly inadequate to the task. The need to protect the urban working class remained.

The primary impetus for the development of a state-sponsored social insurance program, however, lay not in the public health problem but in the increasing unrest among the urban working class. Although industrial paternalism inhibited the growth of organized labor in Japan, by 1900 unions had become strong enough to force the government to pass the Peace Preservation Law, which declared unions subversive and, therefore, illegal organizations. Similarly, in 1910 an attempt to start a socialist party was halted by the government.[6]

Despite the absence of an organized labor movement and the practice of industrial paternalism, manifestations of labor dissatisfaction continued. Among the more dramatic episodes was an alleged assassination attempt against the emperor in 1910 by a group of anarchists. Although the alleged attempt is shrouded in mystery, along with the general level of labor unrest, it led to an imperial speech in 1911 in which the basis for a mixed public-private charity health service was established. In typically noblesse oblige fashion, the emperor declared:

We are most seriously concerned over the situation in which the poor people, who cannot afford a medicine, die before their time. So, desiring as We do to promote welfare by serving out medicine and giving medical treatment to the poor, We wish to apply the money from our private purse to this purpose.

The emperor's contribution of 1.5 million yen, besides various private contributions, was used to establish the *Saiseikai*, an imperial endowment providing free medical care to the needy. The system began in 1912 and ultimately included several hospitals, clinics, sanatoriums, and traveling health units, all offering free medical care.[7]

Obviously such a system was inadequate to the need and demand for medical care and other social security benefits. World War I brought both industrial progress and increased labor activity and unrest to Japan. Despite the existence of the Peace Preservation Law, labor began to organize, and in 1919 the government acknowledged reality by declaring it would not oppose "wholesome development of trade unions."[8] Clearly mindful of the German experience, the Japanese, faced with a militant and socialist-oriented labor movement, decided to buy industrial peace through enactment of a health insurance law. A bill was drafted by the Ministry of Agriculture and Commerce in 1920 and the Health Insurance Law was passed in 1922. Operation of the program was postponed, however, owing to a catastrophic earthquake (and subsequent fires) in September 1923, which destroyed almost half of Tokyo and nearly all of Yokohama. The law actually went into effect on January 1, 1927. Japan thus became the first Asian nation to adopt some form of social insurance.

The Health Insurance Law, sometimes referred to as the Employee's Health Insurance (EHI) Law, like the British law of 1911, was patterned after the German system. The Japanese law was limited to only a portion of the urban working class. Specifically, it called for compulsory participation of miners and workers in factories with 10 or more employees who earned less than 1,200 yen per year – about $600 at the prevailing 1927 exchange rate. As in the British and German cases, the law did not apply to self-employed persons, those engaged in agriculture, or the dependents of miners and factory workers. In 1927 the insurable population numbered about 2 million out of a gainfully occupied work force of over 16 million and a total population of about 62 million. The law did provide for voluntary participation by certain categories of workers. For example, an *employer* of a factory with fewer than 10 employees could petition the minister of home affairs for participation, provided a majority of employees consented.

The EHI Law provided sickness, m .ernity, and funeral benefits. The sickness benefits went beyond those provided by the British system by including provisions for surgical, dental, and home nursing care as well as routine out-patient care. Sickness benefits were limited, as they were in most other countries at the time, to 6 months. In addition to paying for medical treatment, EHI provided for a cash benefit equal to 60 percent of the worker's daily wage in the event the sickness or injury caused him to miss work.

The insurance scheme was financed through equal contributions by employer and employee. Unlike the British system, which required different contributory rates for men and women, the Japanese law provided that contributions would vary, not by sex but according to the wages of the employee. Sixteen wage categories were established and each worker contributed on the basis of ability to pay. Lastly, the government contributed up to 10 percent of the cost of the program, not to exceed 2 yen a year per insured person, to cover administrative costs.

Administration of the program was undertaken either by the government through health insurance offices located throughout the country and administered by the Ministry of Home Affairs or by health insurance societies. The latter could be formed voluntarily by an employer or groups of employers of at least 300 workers, provided more than one-half of the workers gave their consent. Ultimate approval for forming these societies had to come from the Ministry of Home Affairs. Once a factory or mine formed a society, all employees were required to use that society as their agent. Health insurance or mutual benefit societies were mandatory• in factories and mines that employed 500 or more workers. Thus, all workers covered by EHI were insured by either a company-based health society or a local health office. Ultimate administrative authority for the entire program was vested in the Ministry of Home Affairs.

Lastly, under the scheme the insurance offices and societies appointed doctors, dentists, and pharmacists who chose to affiliate with the program to provide insured persons with necessary medical care. Reimbursement for services rendered was administered by the Japanese medical, dental, and pharmacists' associations. Physicians, dentists, and pharmacists joined the insurance program through their respective professional associations, and the government paid a monthly lump sum to each of these associations based upon the number of patients treated or prescriptions filled. Each association then reimbursed its members for the services they had performed.

The EHI continues to constitute an important part of the compulsory health insurance program in Japan today. The original law has been amended 54 times since 1927, with the effect of expanding its scope and benefits. Among the more significant prewar changes was the extension of coverage in 1939 to the dependents of workers. Later in this chapter we examine the current provisions of the scheme. The important points to remember about the first effort to provide social insurance in Japan are that (1) it was limited in scope, (2) it was intended primarily as a mechanism for defusing labor conflict and ensuring industrial productivity, and (3) wherever possible it used existing private institutions for administrative purposes. In short, its origins, content, and organization were remarkably similar to those of the German model upon which it was implicitly based.

Economic depression, preparation for war, and health care

The next major step in the development of a national health care program came in response to the economic and military crises confronting Japan in the 1930s. The worldwide economic depression severely affected Japan's rural sector, which contained approximately 48 percent of its labor force.

Among the more serious problems attending the economic crisis was a deteriorating medical situation. One manifestation of this was the exodus of physicians from the rural areas. For example, in the period 1928 to 1936, while the number of physicians in urban areas increased from 16,440 to 30,878, the number practicing in rural areas declined from 26,833 to 22,498. In addition, the number of rural towns and villages *without* doctors increased from 1,960 in 1923 to 3,243 in 1936. The latter figure represented about one-third of all rural localities in 1936. Lastly, the ratio of physicians to population was 3.6 per 10,000 in rural areas compared with 13.6 per 10,000 in the cities.[9]

The maldistribution of medical personnel and facilities in rural Japan was attributable, in part, to those factors that produced similar problems in Germany, Great Britain, and the Soviet Union: the isolated and professionally unattractive nature of rural practice. In Japan these problems were, and still are, exacerbated by the private ownership of most hospitals and clinics. The majority of these facilities were owned and managed by doctors and run as profit-making institutions. In light of the deteriorating economic situation in the rural areas and the high degree of indebtedness, many physicians found it economically impossible to remain in these areas.

Despite the obvious need for a rural health care policy to stimulate the supply of medical facilities and personnel and to alleviate the personal financial burden of health costs, a proposal in 1934 for a national system of health insurance met strong opposition from the medical profession and mutual aid associations. More critically, the Ministry of Finance, concerned about the costs of the proposed scheme, vetoed the plan before it reached the Diet.

The plan for a national health insurance program thus lay dormant until 1937–8, when it was revitalized and eventually enacted as the National Health Insurance Law on March 2, 1938.[10] The reason for the plan's newfound support was simple and reminiscent of the British experience. In the 1930s Japan embarked upon an era of military expansionism. Physical examinations of recruits for the military draft revealed a high rejection rate because of poor physical condition. The War Ministry became concerned about its ability to meet the military's manpower needs. In 1937 the War Ministry put its support behind the national health insurance plan. It should be noted that the law applied not only to rural residents but to many categories of people not covered by the Health Insurance Law of 1922. Nevertheless, the intention and effect of the law were primarily rural in nature, organization, and scope. For this reason, much of the following discussion focuses on the rural sector.

The National Health Insurance (NHI) Law differed in several significant ways from the Employee's Health Insurance (EHI) Law of 1922. It was based upon two traditional Japanese social institutions: the family and the village. Because over 95 percent of the rural population was self-employed, the workplace as the unit for organizing the population under NHI was obviously inappropriate. Instead, the government chose the family as represented by individual households as the insurable unit. The choice of the village as the basic administrative unit was dictated by the fact that in rural Japan of the 1930s the village was the most significant suprafamilial socioeconomic unit. Perhaps most importantly, life in the village was characterized by extensive religious, social, and economic cooperative efforts. Families cooperated in planting and harvesting rice, building and repairing public works projects and private homes, extending aid during emergencies, and so on.[11] The village thus provided a logical and convenient administrative unit for implementing a program that appeared to be an extension of village cooperative behavior.

The original scheme worked in the following manner. Householders interested in joining the program voluntarily organized a nonprofit insurance association. Insurance benefits were automatically extended to all members of the family once the head of the household joined an association. There were three types of insurance associations: ordinary, substitute, and special. The most numerous were ordinary associations, called "national health insurance associations." These were established specifically and exclusively for the purpose of organizing and administering NHI in a geographical area (e.g., a village or town). The substitute associations, too, were geographically based, but were preexisting organizations, such as agricultural or fishing cooperatives, which took on the added function of providing health insurance. The special associations were craft- or trade-based, rather than geographically based, and included persons from the same trade or profession, but not necessarily the same locality. Approval by the prefectural (i.e., provincial) governor was required for the establishment and operation of a health insurance association. Local governmental supervision over these associations was generally accomplished by requiring the town mayor or village headman to act as chairman of an association's board of directors. The administrative and supervisory role of the national government was minimal, in keeping with the local emphasis on the scheme.

The original law left each association considerable discretion in terms of the scope and duration of benefits to be provided. Its primary responsibility was to provide medical and dental care in the event of sickness or injury and maternity care. If finances permitted, it could also provide funeral benefits. Medical care was available on either an out-patient or in-patient basis. Some of the substitute (i.e., cooperative) associations owned and operated their own clinics and hospitals, but more typically in-patient care was provided by an authorized (i.e., contracted) private hospital or clinic. Doctors, too, were contracted by the insurance associations to provide medical care to members. Doctors and hospitals were reimbursed in part by patient fees and in part on the basis of a system by which every medical procedure was assigned a point value (e.g., 600 points for an appendectomy or 45 points for an ordinary medical examination). The number of points was then multiplied by a set yen value per point (e.g., 0.30 yen x 600 = 180 yen). The point value of each procedure was determined by the Japan Medical Association; the set yen value per point was negotiated by the physicians, dentists, and the insurance associations. The patient paid the doctor 30 to 50 percent of the bill, depending on the financial circumstances of his insurance association, and the doctor collected the remainder from the association.

The program was financed from two sources: (1) health insurance premiums and (2) national and local government subsidies. The insurance premium was based on a family's ability to pay as measured by property and the size of the family. The government subsidy was not fixed by law – until after World War II – but was extended "within the limits of the budget." The ratio of contributions between the two components varied over time, but in general 60 to 75 percent of the financing came from the household premiums.

Membership in the program grew gradually in the first years of operation: about 500,000 in 1938; over 3 million in 1940. In 1942, with the Pacific war in full swing, the law was amended to allow prefectural governors to require participation in those areas not yet covered by NHI. The result was a quantum leap in membership: 23 million in 1942; 41 million in 1944. Another important feature of the 1942 amendment was that doctors and dentists were compelled to serve in the program, whereas previously such participation was voluntary. Thus, virtually all doctors and dentists became insurance practitioners, although many did so reluctantly.

One final noteworthy feature of the NHI Law was that insurance carriers were encouraged through various financial inducements to provide preventive and educational facilities and services. Specific encouragement was given to tuberculosis testing, maternal and infant health care services, and vaccinations. Among the more important additional services supplied by many health insurance associations was the provision of public health nurses in the rural areas. This contribution to rural health was particularly significant, given the shortage of rural doctors.

The National Health Insurance Law of 1938 continues as one of the major pillars of Japanese health care policy. Like the EHI Law of 1922, it has been amended often and undergone considerable alteration. These changes are discussed in a subsequent section of the chapter. The NHI Law once again illustrates the important impact of situational factors (e.g., an economic depression and war), cultural values (e.g., use of the family and village structures), and economic structure (e.g., private medical practice) on the substance, coverage, and operation of health care policy.

Before we examine the impact of the American occupation on Japanese health care policy, two additional features of the prewar policy should be noted. The first is the establishment in 1938 of the Ministry of Welfare. Much like the NHI Law, the creation of a separate Welfare Ministry was seen by the military as a vital step in improving the nation's overall physical vitality and preparing it for the conflict ahead. In the announcement justifying the creation of the ministry, the Privy Council noted that "the level of physical health of the people has been declining every year. Moreover, this has contributed to a decline in national strength and economic productivity. The future seems grim. Therefore, by all means we must strive to promote the level of public health immediately."[12]

The second development is passage of the Seamen's Insurance Law and the Personnel Health Insurance Law, both in 1939. The former affected over 200,000 seamen serving on large fishing and merchant vessels. The law provided medical and income insurance similar to that provided under EHI. Because of the peculiar working conditions of this group, the law was and continues to be administered and operated separately from either the NHI or EHI system. The Personnel Health Insurance Law covered salaried workers in certain commercial, financial, and advertising enterprises.

In summation, by the beginning of World War II, Japan had established a widespread but diverse national health care policy. Approximately 60 million of Japan's 71 million people were covered by some form of government-sponsored and/or -operated insurance scheme. The effort to bring medical care to the entire population was making headway: By 1945, the number of doctorless communities had declined to 1,534 from the 1938 level of 3,232. Finally, an effort had been made, with the establishment of the Ministry of Welfare, to rationalize the administration of the health care system.

Health care policy and the American occupation

Although the impact of the American occupation on the Japanese health care system may not have been as profound and certainly was not as celebrated as its effects in the area of political and constitutional changes, it was nevertheless far-reaching. Only the most important aspects are noted here.

Aside from the important substantive changes introduced, two points concerning the policy-making process are noteworthy. The first is that the occupation is an obvious, albeit extraordinary, illustration of the impact of external influence on domestic policy making. Although the occupation authorities were sensitive to Japanese culture and tradition, in this policy area, as in many others, the policy changes reflected American values and the effort to transplant American institutions to Japanese soil. The second point is that the changes or "reforms" were initiated either directly by the occupation command or indirectly through a Japanese agency such as the Welfare Ministry. There was thus a reinforcement of the important role government had played in shaping the nature of health care in Japan.

It is not difficult to understand why the occupation government – the Supreme Commander of the Allied Powers (SCAP) – played such a prominent role in the health policy area. Japan had suffered great destruction from conventional and atomic bombings. Epidemics caused by inadequate housing, food, water, sewage, disposal, medicine, and medical facilities were both a real and a potential danger. Under such circumstances, large-scale radical action was obviously necessary. The point must be stressed that the United States authorities intended to go beyond simply providing emergency health services and preparing the Japanese for a return to normalcy. SCAP authorities intended to institute a major reform of the preexisting health care system. The leader of the effort was General Crawford Sams, chief of the Public Health and Welfare Section of SCAP. In order to help him formulate policy, Sams invited several "missions" to Japan representing American educational, medical, and social security groups.

One of the first areas with which the occupation authorities dealt was medical education and licensing. American authorities believed that the quality of Japanese medical education and the resulting quality of the physicians were inadequate and inferior. General Sams directed the formation of the Japanese Council on Medical Education and asked it to suggest reforms. Among the recommendations submitted and adopted were the lengthening of the medical school program; greater emphasis on practical training, including a 1-year medical internship; and a national medical examination as a requirement for licensing.

The introduction of the internship requirement provides a nice illustration of the clash between American values and practice and Japanese institutions and practice. Most hospitals in Japan permitted only full-time staff doctors to practice in them. Thus, there was considerable reluctance by hospital staff doctors to accept and help train interns. In 1949 General Sams noted in this regard: "Under the Japanese closed hospital system with complete paid staffs, interns were not only without a function to perform but were actually resented by many members of the staff who were not interested in training these young men . . . Only time will determine whether the intern system has a place in Japanese medical education."[13] The internship did survive, but in a form quite different from its American model. Most interns in Japan have little opportunity actually to treat or care for patients and generally use the year to prepare for the licensing examination. The internship system has been described by one observer as "the weakest link in medical education in Japan."[14]

The SCAP government also sponsored a reorganization of hospital administration. The Medical Service Law of July 1948 provided for, among other things, the inspection, classification, and licensing of hospitals by the Health and Welfare Ministry. The law also "opened" *public* hospitals, permitting qualified physicians to admit and treat patients in them.

Among the more extensive reforms during the period were those that dealt with the health insurance system. These reforms were prompted by a partial breakdown of the NHI scheme and a developing sentiment among the Japanese for constructing a welfare-oriented society. This latter sentiment found expression in the 1946 Constitution, which stated in Article 25: "All people shall have the right to maintain standards of wholesome and cultural living. And the State shall use its endeavors for the promotion and extension of social welfare and security and of public health." Under these twin mandates – restoring the NHI system and extending social insurance principles – SCAP and Japanese authorities in the Ministry of Health and Welfare prepared plans to implement the program. Although the occupation government and its various advisory missions considered reforms of existing health insurance programs and offered recommendations, the ultimate revisions to the program were largely the work of Japanese officials in the Insurance Bureau of the Ministry of Health and Welfare.[15]

The primary concern of both the Japanese and Allied authorities was to revitalize the NHI system. The problems of the system were many; some were a direct result of the war, others were more fundamental. A major problem derived from overextension, when in 1942 membership became compulsory. As a result, the number of insurance carriers increased from 937 in 1940 to 6,596 in 1942 to 10,474 in 1944. The accelerated extension of insurance carriers and insured persons was followed by an equally precipitous decline following the war. In 1948 the number of insurance carriers was down to 5,446 and the number of insured persons was about 26 million compared with 41 million in 1944. This decline represents the precarious financial condition of many of the insurance carriers, the unpopularity of compulsory membership by some rural inhabitants, and the overall economic instability that plagued Japan in the immediate postwar years.

In 1948, SCAP authorities encouraged amendments to the National Health Insurance Law that would make the program fiscally sound, popularly attractive, and democratically operated. The underlying principle of the amendments was to incorporate the concept of municipal management. With this in mind, primary responsibility for operation of the NHI was transferred from the ordinary and substitute national health insurance associations to city, town, and village governments. National health insurance associations could also be insurance carriers as long as local assemblies did not choose to adopt local control. Membership in the scheme by a community was to be an all or nothing affair: If a majority agreed to participate, all had to participate; if a majority was lacking, there would be no program. The purpose of this provision was to get a large enough insurance pool to ensure a sufficient distribution of risk. Along these lines, two or more communities were allowed to operate a scheme jointly in order to ensure adequate membership for risk sharing. The principle of local control was also manifested in provisions allowing fiscal supervision by prefectural governors.

The democratization of the insurance scheme found expression in the form of meaningful administrative oversight by local citizens' advisory councils. These councils, appointed by local authorities, consisted of insurance carriers, doctors, and members of the community. Their purpose was to make recommendations about the operation of the insurance program, hear complaints, and generally publicize the program. In addition, NHI appeals boards were set up at the prefectural level to hear any complaints that might arise. These boards were representative of all concerned parties.

Lastly, it should be noted that under a SCAP directive in May 1946 the Welfare Ministry was reorganized. Included in the reorganization program was the introduction of four new bureaus: for health, medical treatment, preventive medicine, and social affairs. This reorganization provided the basis for the current structure of the Welfare Ministry.[16]

To sum up, the major impact of the Allied occupation (1945–52) on the Japanese health care system, aside from the initial public health concern, occurred in the areas of (1) regulating the medical profession and medical institutions, (2) operation of the National Health Insurance program and to a lesser extent other health insurance schemes, and (3) administrative organization of the health care system. The overriding themes in the Allied effort were improvement in the quality of medical care in Japan, ensuring fiscal stability in the health insurance program, and democratization of the system. Although many compromises and concessions were made, for better or worse, the American occupation of Japan, unlike the Allied occupation of Germany, had a lasting and profound impact on Japan's health care system.

Current politics and policies in Japanese medical care

Since the end of the American occupation in 1952, the major issues and trends in Japanese health care policy have involved the extension in scope and membership of state-sponsored or state-operated health insurance programs and the role of the medical profession in the overall health care system.

Health insurance for the whole nation

From 1948 on, but especially since the end of the occupation, the trend in Japanese health care policy has been in the direction of creating a universal, compulsory, and comprehensive medical care system. Beginning in 1948, medical insurance coverage was extended by specific legislation to various categories of workers not covered by existing EHI or NHI laws. Included among the newly covered persons were national government employees (1948); day laborers, including seasonal and temporary employees (1953); private school teachers (1953); public corporation employees such as railway, telephone, and telegraph workers (1956); and local government employees (1962).

In 1961 the government of Prime Minister Nobusuke Kishi formally announced the policy of Health Insurance for the Whole Nation. The Ministry of Health and Welfare was assigned the task of developing a 4-year plan to implement this commitment. Because membership in most employee-based insurance programs was compulsory, the main thrust of the effort was in extending the voluntary NHI system. With this in mind, the government radically amended the National Health Insurance Law in December 1958. The amendment specified that "a city, town, or village which has not at the time of enforcement of this Law administered National Health Insurance shall be required to establish a National Health Insurance program by April 1, 1961."[17] The effect of this amendment was to make NHI a compulsory program. Despite some problems, by April 1, 1961, virtually the entire nation was covered by some form of state-sponsored and / or state-managed health insurance program.

An outline of the insurance system, the relative distribution of members (as of 1975), and some indication of its complexity are presented in Table 8–1. As the table indicates, medical insurance programs in Japan can be divided into two general categories: (1) health insurance for workers or employees and their dependents and (2) national health insurance for all persons in cities, towns, and villages not covered by some form of employees' insurance. Of the major programs, EHI and NHI together cover almost 87 percent of the population. Given the preponderant role played by these two schemes, the following discussion of the coverage, financing, benefits, and administration of Japanese health insurance is limited to EHI and NHI.

There are, however, two points worth emphasizing about the other programs because of their relevance to an overall evaluation of health care in Japan. First, despite the fact that they cover only 12 percent of the population, these programs affect almost 15 million persons and, therefore, are an important part of the health care system. Second, these programs incorporate considerable variety in rates and methods of contri-

Table 8–1. *Health insurance programs in Japan, 1975*

Program	Date established	Number of persons covered	Percent of persons covered
Programs for employees			
Health Insurance	1922	53,294,000	47.5
Seamen's Insurance	1939	753,000	0.7
Day-Laborers' Health			
Insurance	1953	752,000	0.7
Mutual Aid Association[a]		13,475,400	12.0
Program for self-employed			
National Health			
Insurance	1938	43,853,000	39.1
Total		112,127,400	100.0

[a]Includes National Public Service (1948), Private School Teachers and Employees (1953), Public Enterprise Staffs (1956), and Local Public Services (1962) mutual aid associations.
Source: Outline of Social Insurance in Japan (Tokyo: Social Insurance Agency, 1976).

bution and in scope and content of benefits. As we will note shortly, this almost chaotic variation is one of the most serious shortcomings in the Japanese system.

Employee's and national health insurance

The following discussion compares the provisions of the two major forms of health insurance.[18] Although specific comparison is not always made with the original content of these two laws, the reader may wish to refer back to the appropriate discussions to make such comparisons.

Coverage

As noted above, approximately 87 percent of the population in Japan is covered by one of these two schemes. EHI is a compulsory program available to any person employed in a place of work (e.g., firm, factory, hospital, mine) where five or more persons are usually employed. In essence, EHI covers virtually every kind of worker and his or her dependents. In 1975, 47.5 percent of all Japanese were covered by EHI (Table 8–1). NHI is a residual program intended to cover all persons not eligible for EHI or one of the more specialized insurance programs. Because NHI is residentially rather than occupationally based, there is no distinction between worker and dependent. In 1975, 39.1 percent of the population was covered by NHI.

Benefits

One observer of the Japanese health care system notes that "the sick person as a rule fares best under a [insurance] society-managed EHI plan, slightly less well under the Government managed EHI program, and not as well under NHI."[19] This comment suggests that although the range of benefits under these and most other programs is essentially the same, significant differences do exist between and (even within EHI) programs. For example, a cash sickness benefit is available under EHI but not under NHI. In addition, some plans, provided by the wealthier health insurance societies, offer extra health promotion and prevention services. Aside from these differences and certain cost-sharing differences mentioned below, basic medical benefits are the same for all health insurance plans. Generally, medical care benefits include medical consultations and examinations; medicines and other therapeutic materials (excluding eyeglasses); medical treatment, surgery, and therapy; hospitalization and in-patient clinic care; nursing; medically related transportation costs; and dental care. There are no durational limits on any of these benefits.

Differences between the major schemes exist in the area of insurance premiums. Under EHI, insured persons and their dependents must pay a first consultation fee of 200 yen ($1.00 at 1979 exchange rate) and, in the event of hospitalization, 60 yen (33 cents) per day for the first month. Beyond these nominal fees, the worker pays nothing for benefits and his dependents pay 30 percent of the total medical bill. The cost-sharing fee for dependents represents a decrease instituted under a revision of the Health Insurance Law in 1973. Prior to the revision, dependent liability was 50 percent of medical care costs. Another component of the 1973 insurance revision provides that EHI covers all expenses in excess of 30,000 yen (about $150) in 1 month. Those covered by NHI pay 30 percent of all medical costs.

Financing

Financing of health insurance in Japan varies according to program. The medical care costs for NHI are paid from three sources: direct cost-sharing fees paid to the doctor, dentist, or pharmacist at time of service; a subsidy from the national treasury; and money collected from a national health insurance tax. As noted above, persons covered by NHI pay 30 percent of all medical expenses. Of the remaining 70 percent, the national government pays 40 to 45 percent of the costs of the program to the local insurance carrier, usually the local government. The standard subsidy is 40 percent, which the national government can increase by 5 percent for less affluent communities. The remaining 25 to 30 percent of the insurance costs is paid through the national health insurance tax. The tax, which is assessed on each household, is based upon (1) household income, (2) property value, (3) number of persons in the household, and (4) a flat rate for each household. The maximum amount of NHI tax any one household may pay is 120,000 yen per year ($600). The average annual tax paid in 1974 was 25,858 yen ($129). Finally, all administrative costs of the program are borne by the national government.

In the case of EHI, aside from cost sharing, there are two sources of financing: employee-employer contributions and a national government subsidy. In terms of the employee-employer component, the rate of contribution of each party is different in the government-managed and insurance-society-managed programs. Under the government-managed EHI program, worker and employer each contributes an equal amount per month based upon a percentage of the employee's income. The combined contribution rate is set by the Health and Welfare Ministry within a statutory range of 6.8 to 8.0 percent. Since November 1974, the rate has been 7.6 percent, or 3.8 percent of a worker's salary contributed by the worker and by the employer. The government subsidy, too, is set by law and since October 1973 has been 10 percent of the medical care costs of the government-managed EHI program.

In the case of society-managed EHI programs, the rate of employee-employer contributions is determined by each society's by-laws, within a range of 3 to 9 percent. The rate must be approved by the Ministry of Health and Welfare. Each society may increase the employer's share, but the contribution rate of a worker may not exceed 4 percent of his salary. In 1975 the average employer contribution was 4.03 percent and the average employee contribution was 2.96 percent (i.e., lower than the 3.8 percent for government-managed schemes) for a combined total of 6.99 percent. The implications of the differing contributory rates among the NHI and EHI programs are examined when we evaluate the Japanese health care system at the conclusion of this chapter.

Administration of health insurance programs

Management of the NHI program is done locally by approximately 3,200 city-, town-, and village-run NHI offices throughout the country. Immediate control over these local offices is vested in the prefectural government. The local offices administer NHI for approximately 41 million of the 43.8 million persons covered by the scheme. In addition, there is a small number (188 in 1975) of private NHI associations, which represent local residents with occupational or trade affiliations. Each of these associations must have at least 300 members and be approved by the prefectural governor. In 1975, approximately 2.5 million persons were insured through NHI associations.

The EHI program is administered either directly by the national government through the Ministry of Health and Welfare or by legally authorized health insurance societies. The government-managed programs cover about 52 percent of the workers and dependents insured by EHI. The remaining 48 percent are covered by one of approximately 1,600 health insurance societies. Approval to establish a health insurance society is limited to establishments employing 300 or more persons – although the tendency in recent years has been to grant approval only to firms with 1,000 or more employees.[20] At least one-half of the employees and the Health and Welfare Ministry must approve the establishment of a society. The societies are governed and policy determined by a "conference" and an executive board of directors representing the employer and employees.

Ultimate policy authority for the entire health insurance system rests with the national government. The prime minister receives advice and recommendations on overall social security and health legislation from the 40-member Social Security Advisory Council, which is made up of 10 members from the Diet, 10 from private (insurance) organizations, 10 from "scholars and persons of experience," and 10 vice-ministers. In addition, the Ministry of Health consults with the Social Insurance Council on matters concerning the administration and operation of health insurance programs. At the local level, citizens' advisory councils, appointed by the local mayor or headman with approval of the local assembly, are responsible for monitoring the operation of the local health insurance program. Lastly, there are social insurance referees in every prefecture and the national Appeals Committee, which can investigate benefit complaints.

The provision of medical care

Medical services under Japanese health insurance are provided by doctors, dentists, and pharmacists at "designated health insurance medical care facilities" (i.e., hospitals, clinics, and pharmacies). Both medical personnel and facilities must register with, and be approved for participation in the health insurance system by, prefectural governors. Over 95 percent of the hospitals (i.e., institutions with 20 beds or more), clinics (i.e., fewer than 20 beds), as well as doctors, dentists, and pharmacists are registered for participation in the health insurance system. Generally, patients have complete freedom in choosing medical personnel and facilities. In some instances where health insurance societies own and operate their own hospitals or clinics, patients are expected to use these facilities.

As noted earlier, most Japanese hospitals work on a closed-system basis: only salaried staff physicians may treat patients in a hospital. Approximately two-thirds of the hospitals are privately owned and, therefore, are closed to nonstaff physicians. As a result, most physicians have set up their own private clinics, which by law may include up to 19 beds for in-patient care. Virtually all clinics are privately owned and are well equipped with x-ray and laboratory facilities and ancillary medical personnel. Most physicians are reluctant to refer a patient to a hospital because they can no longer treat or derive income from him. Therefore, even minor surgery is commonly performed in these clinics.

Reimbursement for medical services is based in part upon direct, cost-sharing contributions to the physicians or medical facility as specified under each health insurance plan: for example, 30 percent of the medical bill under NHI. The remainder of the charges is covered by health insurance. Reimbursement for the health insurance portion is based on a fee-for-service system by which every medical procedure is assigned a certain point value. The fee is computed by multiplying the total number of points by a set unit cost (e.g., 10 yen or 5 cents). A doctor who has examined a patient (45 points), performed a urinalysis (25 points), taken and read an x-ray (100 points), and ultimately performed an appendectomy (600 points) sends a bill to the appropriate fee-paying agency for 770 points times 10 yen or 7,770 yen ($38.85). The bill is examined by a medical consultant at either the Medical Care Fee Payment Fund for EHI patients or the Federation of National Health Insurance Organization for NHI patients to check for unnecessary charges or procedures. Generally, the doctor is reimbursed within 45 days after submitting the bill.

Summary

The Japanese health care system represents a compromise between the essentially free market system of the United States and the completely socialized national health services of the Soviet Union and Great Britain. Coverage is universal and compulsory, and the state plays a major administrative and financial role. On the other hand, medical practice is predominantly private, and two-thirds of the hospitals and over 95 percent of the clinics are privately owned. Freedom of choice is enjoyed by most patients. Management of part of the administrative system, about one-half of EHI and a small part of NHI, is undertaken by insurance carriers run by employee-employer groups. Furthermore, doctors are free to practice and patients to receive health care outside the insurance system, although in fact a very small percentage (about 3 percent) of most physicians' incomes are from noninsurance practice.

Health care policy and the Japan Medical Association

No discussion of the Japanese health care system is complete without some attention to the role of the Japan Medical Association (JMA). Physicians in Japan began organizing as early as 1879, when *kampo* doctors formed an association to protect their interests in light of the Westernization campaign. The first association of Western style doctors, the Tokyo Medical Society, was organized in 1887. The current Japan Medical Association was officially formed in 1923, although its origins can be traced back to the

Greater Japan Medical Association, which was organized in 1916. The formation of the JMA in 1923 was in response to an amendment to the Medical Practitioners Law (1906). The amendment provided for the formation of a "Japan Medical Association." The amendment was followed by a set of implementing rules from the Home Ministry detailing the conditions of formation and organization of the association. Among the rules was the provision that if the JMA made any decision or took any action that violated existing laws or were "deemed detrimental to the public welfare" the Home Ministry could take control of or dissolve the association.[21] Thus, the Japan Medical Association initially came into existence with the encouragement of the national government and subject to its scrutiny. This is quite contrary to the totally private nature of the British and American medical associations.

Although the JMA enjoyed some degree of professional autonomy by the 1930s, as the nation began mobilizing for war greater government control was exercised over the association. The association was reorganized in 1942 under the wartime National Medical Care Law. The law provided for the compulsory formation of regional medical associations to be controlled by the JMA, and required membership by all practitioners. In addition, the JMA was given the mandate "to work for the achievement of improved medical care and guidance of health, and to cooperate with national policy for the improvement of the people's physical strength."[22] Officers of the association were appointed by the cabinet upon recommendation of the Health and Welfare Ministry. Thus, the JMA became a governmental body for controlling the medical profession.

In keeping with the policy of democratizing Japanese institutions, SCAP officials consulted with members of the Japanese medical profession and the Health and Welfare Ministry with a view to reorganizing the JMA. Following several months of discussions, the "old" JMA was dissolved on October 31, 1947, and the "new" JMA was officially established the following day. The constitution of the association was patterned after that of the American Medical Association. Membership in the association is voluntary, officers are popularly elected, and the organization is conducted along democratic lines.[23]

Since its rebirth in 1947, the Japanese Medical Association has become, in the words of one Japanese commentator, "one of the nation's most active and aggressive pressure groups."[24] Much of the activity of the JMA has been related to two main issues: the operation of the health insurance system and the right of doctors to prescribe *and* sell medicine.[25]

The issue of selling medicine is interesting and, as far as we can determine, unique to Japan. Since the introduction of Western-style medicine in Japan, doctors and dentists have not only prescribed but have prepared and sold medicine to their patients. Doctors and dentists have jealously guarded the right to sell medicine for the simple reason that the sales have always provided a significant part of their incomes. In fact, by 1969 almost 50 percent of the total average point score in clinics was based on the preparation and sale of medicine; the figure in hospitals was about 30 percent. "It is a standing joke that when visiting a doctor, one must carry with him a big bag in which to put all the medicine he will receive."[26]

The right of physicians and dentists to prepare and sell medicine became an issue during the occupation and produced the first postwar political activity by the Japan Medical Association. General Sams, with the support of a report from a mission of American pharmacists, concluded that Japan should follow the American practice of separating the prescription from the preparation and sale of medicine. SCAP directed the Japanese Health and Welfare Ministry to draft a bill to this effect. Despite the objections of both the JMA and the Japan Dental Association (JDA), the bill to separate the prescription and sale of medicine was introduced in March and passed by the Diet in June 1951.[27] It was scheduled to take effect on January 1, 1955.

As the date of implementation approached, the JMA asserted its opposition more vigorously. Its effectiveness was improved by removal of the American influence following the end of the occupation in 1952. In 1954 and 1955, the JMA engaged in a variety of pressure group tactics ranging from meetings with public officials to a sitdown strike in the Diet. Ultimately, the association was successful. The bill was first postponed until April 1, 1956, and later effectively modified.[28] Although the law permitted and encouraged Japanese pharmacists to prepare and sell prescriptions, it also allowed physicians and dentists to continue to do so. Today, most prescriptions filled in Japan are sold by doctors. The JMA defends this practice as necessary to supplement the "meager" incomes earned by physicians under the health insurance system.

Although the sale of medicine has been an important issue for the JMA, the most persistent concern of the association has involved the health insurance system. The subissues involved include the rate of remuneration for medical services, questions of clinical freedom, the burden of paperwork associated with health insurance, and the role of the profession and the association in health insurance administration and policy making. The major protagonists have been the JMA (usually allied with the JDA) on one side and the Health and Welfare Ministry and the insurance societies on the other. On two occasions the conflict between the government and the JMA resulted in nationwide action by the association in the form of a 1-day "medical holiday" on February 19, 1961, and mass resignation from insurance practice from July 1 to July 30, 1971. In both cases, the single most prominent personality was Dr. Taro Takemi, who has been president of the JMA since 1957. It was during this period that the JMA became one of the nation's strongest and most successful interest groups.

In the first case, the conflict began on August 18, 1960, when a delegation from the JMA visited the Health and Welfare Ministry to deliver a list of four demands relating to the health insurance system. The doctors demanded (1) elimination of various restrictions on medical practice imposed by the health insurance laws, (2) a 30 percent increase in medical fees, (3) reduction and simplification of insurance paperwork, and (4) elimination of a dual system of fees – one for large hospitals and one for small clinics. From August 1960 until July 31, 1961, when a compromise on the demands was reached, the JMA and JDA engaged in negotiations, demonstrations, and compromise with the ruling Liberal Democratic Party (LDP) leadership and the Welfare Ministry. The most celebrated episode of the campaign occurred on February 19, 1961 – a Sunday, when medical and dental clinics are normally closed – when the JMA and JDA declared a 1-day "medical holiday." During that day, it was estimated that approximately 80 to 90 percent of the associations' members participated in various meetings and demonstrations throughout Japan, the purpose of which was to educate the public on the issues involved.

The events of February 19 were followed by threats of more "holidays" and, if necessary, a mass resignation from the health insurance system. Discussions, demonstrations, and threats continued. On July 19, 1961, the three professional associations (the JMA, JDA, and, interestingly enough, the Japan Pharmacists Association) announced their intention of submitting previously collected letters of resignation from the health insurance system by the nation's doctors, dentists, and pharmacists. The unified position of the three associations and the obviously serious implications of the threat caused the LDP leadership and the Welfare Ministry to renew negotiations. Finally, on July 31, 1961, a compromise agreement was signed. The agreement provided for (1) an increase in medical fees, which eventually amounted not to 30 percent but to 2.3 percent; (2) a considerable reduction in the volume of health insurance forms; (3) elimination of important restrictions on medical treatment under health insurance; and (4) a promise to integrate the two fee schedules (this was never achieved).

Clearly, the medical profession did not get all it wanted. Nevertheless, it did prove that it could act in a forceful, unified fashion and that it was a political force not to be ignored. The unresolved issues, particularly increased medical fees, would await another day.

That day came one decade later in July 1971. The dispute, according to Dr. Takemi, had its roots in the failure of the government and the LDP to live up to their pledge of 1961 to reform the insurance system and increase medical fees.[29] At the heart of the dispute was an increase in medical fees. When an agreement over the fee issue could not be reached by July 1, 1971, 65,000 of the JMA's 87,000 members, who had submitted their resignations from the system on May 31, withdrew from the health insurance system. These doctors continued to provide medical service, but on a private patient basis. Citizens could still receive medical care under health insurance in the nation's public hospitals.

JMA president Takemi met with welfare minister Saito on several occasions during July, including one meeting open to the press. Finally, on July 29 in a meeting between Prime Minister Eisaku Sato, Welfare Minister Saito, and Dr. Takemi, an agreement was reached ending the month-long boycott. The agreement included a promise to raise medical fees in accordance with cost-of-living increases, greater government aid to medical schools, and a complete reexamination of the health insurance system. The agreement was described by the *Japan Times* of July 30, 1971, as "a complete victory for the JMA." Medical fees were raised about 14 percent and a major revision of the health insurance law was passed by the Diet in September 1973.

These two episodes confirm an earlier characterization of the JMA as one of Japan's most aggressive and successful interest groups. One should not conclude from these episodes that the JMA engages only in dramatic and extraordinary behavior. In fact, the JMA maintains close contact with appropriate government agencies in order to influence health insurance administration and policy. In addition, the JMA, through its political arm, the Japan Doctors League, endorses and finances political candidates sympathetic to its interests. Although the league is not formally a part of the JMA, it is financed by the association, and the separate organizational structure is a thinly veiled subterfuge to get around the legal requirement prohibiting "public interest" organizations from engaging in overt political activity. However, it is universally recognized that the JMA and Japan Doctors League are "one and the same."[30]

Thus, in a variety of ways the Japan Medical Association, under the strong leadership of Taro Takemi, has exercised considerable influence over the operation and substance of Japanese health care policy.

The performance of the Japanese health care system

In evaluating the performance of the Japanese health care system, we focus on two issues. The first is the record of accomplishment of Japanese health and health care as measured by standard, quantitative health indicators. The second is an assessment of the Japanese health insurance system.

The state of health and health care

There are two general ways in which one can judge the relative accomplishments of the Japanese or any other health care system. One is to make within-nation comparisons over time to determine the rate and nature of improvement in the health and health care of a people. The other is to compare the status of health and health care in Japan with their status in other nations. We can make both comparisons, beginning with the intranational longitudinal data.

Unlike Germany, Great Britain, and the Soviet Union, each of which displays one or two convenient and easily discernible political and health policy benchmarks (e.g., 1883 in Germany, 1912 and 1948 in Great Britain, 1917 in the USSR), Japan has, not one or two, but several such historical points. There were, for example, the Meiji restoration (1868), introduction of Employee's Health Insurance (1927) and National Health Insurance (1938), the American occupation (1945–52), and Health Insurance for the Whole Nation (1961). In addition, whereas in Great Britain and the Soviet Union there has been political regime continuity during the twentieth century, in Japan, as in Germany, there have been fundamental regime changes. Thus, it is necessary to examine several points in time in order to detect the influence of events on Japan's health care situation.

Because data are scant for the period prior to 1900 and virtually nonexistent prior to 1868, the analysis begins with the health situation in 1900. As Table 8–2 indicates, progress in selected health areas during the first four decades of the twentieth century was generally slow and erratic. For example, average life expectancy at birth for males increased by only 3 years (from 43.9 to 46.9) between 1900 and 1936. This compares with an increase in the Soviet Union of 16 years over roughly the same period (from 32 years average life expectancy to 48.4 years). Infant mortality from 1900 to 1940 declined 42 percent compared with a decline in Great Britain of 63 percent during the same period. Thus, in those areas where there was improvement, it was occurring at a slower pace than in the Soviet Union or Great Britain.

There were, however, areas in which no progress was made at all. Death rates from both dysentery and tuberculosis were actually one-third higher in 1940 than in 1900. In fact, during the first four decades of the twentieth century the mortality and morbidity profile of Japan more closely resembled that of a developing nation than that of an industrial one. For example, Japan had higher mortality rates than France, Germany, Great Britain, the Netherlands, and the United States for communicable diseases such as typhoid, measles, whooping cough, and tuberculosis. On the other hand, it had lower mortality rates than these other countries for such "modern" and "industrial" disorders as cancer and heart disease.

The postwar era marks a period of really impressive improvements in the health status of the Japanese. Life expectancy, which had increased by only 6.8 percent between 1900 and 1936, increased by 26.8 percent from 1936 to 1950. General mortality, which had declined by 21 percent in the first *four* decades of the century, declined 64 percent in the *two* decades

Table 8-2. *Health status in Japan, 1900-74*

Indicator	1900	1920	1930	1940	1950	1960	1974
Life expectancy (yr)[a]	43.9	42.0	44.8	46.9[b]	59.5	65.3	71.2
General mortality rate (per 1,000 population)	20.8	25.4	18.2	16.5	10.9	7.6	6.5[c]
Infant mortality rate (per 1,000 live births)	155.0	165.7	124.2	90.0	60.1	30.7	10.8
Tuberculosis mortality rate (per 100,000 population)	159.7	223.7	185.6	212.9	146.4	34.2	9.9
Dysentery mortality rate (per 100,000 population)	23.2	5.2	19.2	30.8	14.4	2.2	0.0
Physicians per 100,000 population	25.0	N.A.	69.4[d]	76.5[e]	91.9	110.4	116.7
Population (in millions)	43.8	55.9	64.4	71.9	83.1	93.4	112.1

N.A. = data not available.

[a]Males only. Female life expectancy was about 2 years longer from 1900 to 1940; about 5 years longer since 1960.

[b]1936; [c]1973; [d]1932; [e]1937.

Sources: F. Ohtani, *One Hundred Years of Health Progress in Japan* (Tokyo: International Medical Foundation of Japan, 1971); *Demographic Yearbook* (New York: United Nations, 1975).

between 1940 and 1960. The tuberculosis death rate, which had increased by one-third between 1900 and 1940, declined by 77 percent from 1950 to 1960 and another 71 percent from 1960 to 1964. Similarly, the mortality rate from dysentery declined 53 percent from 1940 to 1950 and 85 percent from 1950 to 1960.

The obvious question is: To what can we attribute the remarkable post–World War II health achievements compared with the more modest successes and failures prior to 1940? In Japan, as in other countries, part of the explanation lies in the progress of medical science. Take, for example, poliomyelitis. In 1960 there were 5,606 cases of polio in Japan. In 1961 the use of attenuated live polio vaccine was introduced. In 1962 there were 289 polio cases; in 1969, just 16 cases. Clearly, the Japanese government has been willing and able to apply the achievements of modern science. One should add here, however, that the availability of medical technology does not ensure its use. The ability (financial and administrative) and willingness of the public and/or private sectors to take advantage of such technology are an important part of a successful health program.

A second explanation for the improved health status of the nation lies in national health policy dealing with the control of infectious and communicable diseases. In 1948 the Ministry of Health and Welfare sponsored passage of the Preventive Vaccination Law, which required all persons under 30 years old to be inoculated against smallpox, typhoid, para-typhoid, diphtheria, whooping cough, and tuberculosis. Dramatic declines in the number of cases and the mortality rates from all but tuberculosis began almost immediately. Tuberculosis continued to provide Japanese health officials with one of their most intractable health problems. As a result of the obvious lack of progress in this area – the death rate in 1947 was virtually identical to that in 1933 – the government decided to take extraordinary action. In 1951 it sponsored the Tuberculosis Control Law, which provided for greater preventive measures, closer scrutiny of tuber-cular patients, and most significantly, assumption of medical expenses for tuberculosis patients by the national government. The results were dramatic: mortality rates for tuberculosis declined from 146.4 per 100,000 persons in 1950 to 34.2 in 1960. Clearly, specific governmental policy in the area of public health has contributed to the improved health status of the Japanese. Since the end of World War II there has been an apparent change in Japanese political attitudes in the direction of expecting the state to assume greater responsibility for protecting the health of the people.

Finally, it should be noted that the improved health status of the Japanese people is also related to the improved standard of living they enjoy. Japan has moved from the position of an industrializing nation in the early part of the century to the status of a fully modern, industrialized nation. In 1973 it ranked 15th among 132 nations in terms of per capita gross national product. Improvements in nutrition, including increased protein consumption, better sanitary facilities, higher personal income, and an associated increase in leisure time have contributed to the overall improvement in the health status of the nation.

Turning now to a comparison of health and health care in Japan and in other industrialized nations, we find that, in general, Japan compares quite favorably. Table 8–3, which repeats some of the data listed in Chapter 7 (Table 7–2), conveys the truly impressive comparative health status of the Japanese people. Japan has lower general and infant mortality rates, a longer life expectancy, and lower death rates from cancer and heart disease than any other nation for which we have data. The two exceptions to the impressive record are the higher mortality rates from tuberculosis (which if current trends continue should disappear) and stroke.

One of the most extraordinary and interesting findings in Table 8–3 is Japan's very low mortality rate from heart disease, compared with the United States, Great Britain, and Germany. This phenomenon has been studied by Y. Scott Matsumoto, who hypothesizes that it can be explained in large part by certain ''stress''-reducing mechanisms in Japanese life that ''tend to diminish the negative consequences of stress and presumably lead to lower coronary disease incidence.''[31] Among the social mechanisms

Table 8–3. *Health status in Japan, Germany, Great Britain, USSR, and the United States, ca. 1975*

Indicator	Japan	Germany	Great Britain	USSR	United States
Life expectancy (yr)	73.0	71.0	72.0	70.0	71.0
General mortality rate (per 1,000 population)	6.5	11.8	11.9	8.7	9.4
Infant mortality rate (per 1,000 live births)	11.0	21.0	16.0	28.0	17.0
Tuberculosis mortality rate (per 100,000 population)	9.6	5.7	2.6	N.A.	1.6
Cancer mortality rate (per 100,000 population)	123.6	239.8	247.5	N.A.	171.7
Heart disease mortality rate (per 100,000 population)	87.2	202.7	311.5	N.A.	301.7
Stroke mortality rate (per 100,000 population)	158.1	168.4	160.2	N.A.	91.1
Population per physician	862.0	517.0	728.0	361.0	604.0
Population per hospital bed	96.0	88.0	106.0	89.0	138.0

N.A. = data not available.
Sources: Demographic Yearbook (New York: United Nations, 1977); Ruth L. Sivard, *World Military and Social Expenditures: 1977* (Leesburg, Va.: WMSE, 1977).

mentioned are greater group dependency, orientation, and solidarity in contrast to the individual competitiveness of Americans; paternalism in the workplace; and the popularity of after-work socializing. Matsumoto does acknowledge that there is also a lower fat intake in the Japanese than in the American diet, but tends to minimize its importance. He does not, however, examine the high rate of stroke, which is also related to stress and tension. In any case, it appears that at least part of the health care accomplishments of the Japanese relative to other nations relates to cultural rather than health policy factors. This should not minimize, however, the fact that compared with the nations listed here, and indeed, with most other modern nations, the Japanese enjoy impressively good health.

Lastly, in terms of health care personnel and facilities, we find that while Japan compares favorably in the provision of hospital beds per population – it ranks ahead of the United States and Great Britain but behind the USSR and Germany – it does not compare as well in terms of physicians per population. Of the five nations listed in Table 8–3, Japan ranks last. Critics within Japan, and especially within its medical profession, claim that the conditions of medical practice imposed by the health insurance system tend to discourage young people from entering the medical profession. There is no evidence either to support or to refute this position. It is true, however, that in 1973 Japan ranked 27th among 28 industrialized nations in terms of physicians per population.

The health insurance system

Virtually everyone in Japan today receives medical care through a state-sponsored or state-operated insurance scheme. How well does the system work? If one begins with the assumption that the primary purpose of any health care delivery system – public, private or mixed – is to contribute to the well-being of a people, we have to conclude that the Japanese system is apparently working quite well. With much of the financial burden removed, the majority of the people have access, without fear of serious financial consequences, to competent and comprehensive medical care. We do not have the data to prove conclusively that the development of a universal health insurance system has contributed to the improved health status of the Japanese. It is, however, a reasonable assumption. We do know that since 1961, when the entire population became eligible for some form of health insurance, two things have happened: (1) within 5 years of introducing health insurance for the whole nation, there was a one-third increase in the number of patients attending hospitals and clinics, mainly because of the enactment of the compulsory medical insurance policy for the nation,[32] and (2) the health status of the people as measured by standard health indexes continued to improve, in some cases at an accelerated rate.

Despite the apparent success of the system, serious problems and criticisms persist. Foremost among these are the inequalities in benefits and contributions among insurance schemes and rapidly rising medical costs.

Inequities among programs

The health insurance system in Japan has changed considerably since 1927. New programs were established to meet the needs or demands of particular groups or circumstances in Japanese society. Depending upon the calculation, there are between five and nine programs with different provisions, benefits, contributions, and so on. In terms of the major plans, it is worth repeating an earlier observation that in Japan, ''the sick person as a rule fares best under a [insurance] society managed EHI plan, slightly less well under the Government managed EHI program, and not as well under NHI.'' The explanation for the difference between programs is that each scheme bases its benefits on, and derives its funding from, different sectors of the population. For example, the NHI program primarily serves the lower-income population and older people, particularly in agricultural areas. As a result, NHI has a poorer base on which to finance its benefits and, therefore, must impose greater qualifying conditions. Thus, under NHI, all persons must pay 30 percent of their medical expenses. Under EHI only dependents, not workers, must pay 30 percent of each medical bill.

There are also important contribution and benefit rate differences between persons covered by the government-managed EHI program and the various insurance-society-managed EHI programs operated by industrial enterprises. In 1975, employees in the government-managed plan paid an average monthly premium of 3.8 percent of their incomes for health insurance; the average contribution in the society-managed programs was 2.9 percent. Despite the lower premiums, workers and dependents under society-managed schemes generally receive more generous benefits than those under the government-run program. Many society-managed schemes offer medical benefits beyond the minimum required by law and provide health and recreational facilities unavailable to those in the government-managed scheme. The reason is that company-based insurance societies tend to represent large industrial enterprises of 300 or more persons in which incomes are higher and the average worker's age is lower than those in enterprises covered by the government-run program. The government-managed scheme tends to cover smaller enterprises with workers in lower income groups who have less generous retirement programs and, therefore, stay on the job longer. In short, the government-run program covers a high-illness-risk population, which provides a small financial base because of lower incomes. As a result of these factors, the costs, number of persons seeking medical care, and duration of treatment have consistently been higher in the government-managed EHI program than in the more affluent, younger, and less illness-prone society-managed groups.

As the Japanese health insurance system is now constituted, the poorer segments of the population consisting of farmers and lower-income urban workers and their dependents pay proportionately more in premiums and receive comparatively less in benefits than the younger, more affluent, and healthier urban workers. This paradoxical situation has by no means escaped the attention of the government. However, periodic proposals either to integrate the two major programs of EHI and NHI or, even more radically, to create a single, unified national health system have been met with strong and effective opposition. The strongest objections have come from the company-based insurance societies and the labor unions that maintain loyalty to the company. These groups fear loss of control over the current system as well as a leveling down of benefits and a leveling up of costs if a single or integrated system is created. Despite periodic changes in the laws upgrading less favored segments of the system, political opposition has prevented a fundamental change in the Japanese health care delivery system.

Health care costs

Health care costs in Japan, as in Germany and Great Britain, have increased astronomically over the last few years. In 1965, for example, the average daily medical fee for a person covered by NHI was 558 yen ($2.79). In 1974 the fee was 2,131 yen ($10.65). In 1 year alone, 1973–4, daily medical fees increased 37 percent under NHI and between 30 and 40 percent under the various EHI plans. Overall costs for the government-managed health insurance system increased from 828.2 billion yen ($4.14 billion) in 1971 to 1.6 trillion yen ($8 billion) in 1974 or an increase of 49 percent. (In these figures, billion and trillion are used in the American sense.)

Clearly, some of the increase is the result of the inflation that has affected medical care costs worldwide. However, critics of the Japanese health insurance system contend that much of this increase resulted from the fee-for-service remuneration system, whereby doctors are reimbursed for each separate medical procedure. The point system, the critics argue, leads to abuses such as prolonging medical treatment, requiring unnecessary tests and procedures (as the physician is paid for the actual cost of the test *and* its administration and preparation), and unnecessary or excessive medication of patients. With regard to the last point, according to one source: "Many cases of over-medication are found within the social health insurance program where all fees are covered by insurance."[33] These charges are denied by the JMA, and in all fairness, we were unable to find empirical evidence to document the claims of abuse. It is certainly a claim, however, that has as wide a currency in the literature on the Japanese health insurance system as it does in the literature on the German health insurance system.

Conclusion

The Japanese health care system is by far the most complex of the four systems examined in this book. It is complex in the dual sense that there is no single unified system, as in Great Britain or the Soviet Union, and in that it is a mixed system of public and private administration, operation, financing, and delivery. This complexity is a result of the almost spasmodic developments in health care in which new programs and institutions were introduced when circumstances demanded them. Each new component has been tacked on to the existing structures, creating a complex and in some respects inequitable system.

What then can one conclude about the Japanese health care system? In the final analysis the question to be answered is: Does the system provide for all who want it, adequate, accessible, and competent medical care?

Based upon this measure, the Japanese system, for all its complexity and shortcomings, performs amazingly well. The Japanese people enjoy one of the highest standards of health in the world today, and that is quite an accomplishment.

Accounting for Japanese health care policy

The history of Japanese health care policy is replete with almost textbook illustrations of the impact of situational, environmental, cultural, and structural factors on public policy.

Situational factors

Watershed events in Japanese political history have had direct and immediate impact on health care policy. The two most outstanding illustrations are the decision to Westernize medicine following the Meiji restoration of 1868 and the reforms in medical education, public health, and the organization of the Japan Medical Association following World War II and the American occupation. In addition, there was the impact of the preparation for war and the worldwide depression, which resulted in the National Health Insurance Act of 1937.

Environmental factors

The Japanese case also illustrates, more than the others, the enormous impact that policy diffusion and conscious imitation can have on the internal policy process of a nation. The Meiji ruler adopted, in almost wholesale fashion, the German model of medical practice, organization, and education. That impact is still apparent over one century after the original importation. The current dilution of the German influence is the result of still another policy-imitating experience: the American occupation. In this situation, of course, policy was as much imposed as imitated. Nevertheless, the point that it emanated from without remains valid.

Cultural factors

Although there is no denying the extraordinarily imitative nature of the Japanese health policy, the health care system is still very much a product of Japanese culture and tradition. Traditional forms of medicine were not abolished by the modernizing Meiji elite and are still practiced today. The imposition of a medical internship has been modified and its purpose negated by the traditional organization of private clinics. Finally, and perhaps most importantly, the health insurance systems have been built upon traditional Japanese social and economic institutions: the family, the village, and paternalism in industrial employee-employer relations.

Structural factors

Japanese health care policy also illustrates the importance of socio-economic and political structures in the policy process. Among the more significant of these has been the impact of the free market economy on the role of the medical profession. Despite a tradition of state regulation of medical practices, the relationship between doctor and patient in Japan has remained essentially a private one. Clinics and hospitals are mainly privately owned, doctors are paid on a fee-for-service basis, and all parties have freedom of choice. Political structure, too, has influenced the nature of the health care system. Since the democratization of the Japanese political system, public policy has been forged in an atmosphere of aggressive interest group behavior, legislative and partisan debate, and informed public opinion. The openness of the policy-making process since 1952 is in direct contrast to the situation of the 1930s, when Japanese authoritarianism prevailed and popular input into the policy process was limited. Lastly, the Japanese case illustrates that a fundamental and enduring influence on the policy process is the legacy of previous policy decisions. The importance of policy inheritance is particularly obvious in the development of health insurance in Japan. In virtually every instance of new insurance programs or reforms, existing policy has provided the point of departure. The apparent reluctance of the Japanese to abandon old policy mechanisms is a major problem of the system.

In summary, Japanese health care policy in the last 100 years has been a product of major political events and external influences. However, these situational and environmental factors have been interpreted within a cultural and structural context that has produced a health care system that is uniquely Japanese.

9

Summary and implications
for health care policy
in the United States

We intend to do two things in this chapter: (1) summarize the major findings of the study, and (2) suggest the implications of some of these findings for an understanding of health care policy in the United States.

Summary

This summary does not review or repeat all that has been discussed in the preceding pages. It merely notes certain points that bear recapitulation and reemphasis.

The areas of policy examined in this book show clearly that no single factor is likely to provide the key to an understanding of why governments do what they do. The policy-making process is an extraordinarily complicated one involving, in terms of our analytical framework, the interaction of situational, environmental, cultural, and structural factors. Nevertheless, certain general tendencies appear in the course of the analysis that can be summarized below and perhaps tested by others for different policy areas.

One such general finding is that the type of political regime (a structural variable) appears to be relatively unimportant in certain policy areas in explaining differences and similarities in public policy among nations. For example, there are far fewer significant differences than one might expect between military and civilian, and socialist and nonsocialist, regimes in terms of levels of expenditure for defense, health, and education. In addition, regime type does not appear to have influenced the introduction of national health care policies – at least not in our small sample of four countries. National health insurance was first introduced in Germany under a conservative, authoritarian regime. Later on, and at roughly the same time, it was adopted in communist Russia, democratic Great Britain, and fascist Japan. The differences in political regime *did* play an important role in shaping the content, operation, and evolution of these health care systems, but the basic principle of a state-sponsored national health insurance system was adopted by significantly different regimes. If we had examined policy areas such as civil rights and civil liberties, the results would have been much different. The political abuse of medicine in the Soviet Union and Nazi Germany provides us with some indication of that. In addition, we are certainly *not* suggesting that politics is unimportant. In the final analysis politics always prevails in the sense that authoritative actors must ultimately make decisions. What we are saying is that formal political structure may not be as important as the emphasis placed on it in comparative politics courses suggests.

If type of political structure is not as important as one might expect, what *is* important in accounting for the actions of governments? One of the conclusions of the study is that dramatic situational factors such as wars, international crises, epidemics, and economic depressions, as well as more commonplace events such as change in political party, have profound impact on public policy. In the case of expenditures for national defense, the big spenders are those nations actively engaged in "hot" wars, those plagued with difficulties in maintaining internal order, and the participants in the cold war. Although this conclusion seems obvious, we remind the reader of the rhetoric from both the Left and the Right about the militaristic tendencies of various types of political systems. In the case of the development of health care policy, the study demonstrates how, in Germany, Great Britain, the Soviet Union, and Japan, events such as inflation, economic depression, epidemic, or an election played a key role in the policy process. Public policy making appears to be an extraordinarily reactive process.

Public policy making also appears to be an extraordinarily imitative process. We suggest that part of the explanation for the levels of educational spending among nations may be the result of imitating or trying to "keep up with the Joneses" – in this case the advanced nations. It is conclusively demonstrated that policy imitation and diffusion are important in accounting for health care policy in Great Britain, Russia, and Japan, although there is a difference between the cloistered nature of policy making in the Soviet Union and the compulsively imitative nature of Japanese health policy making, with Great Britain falling between the two extremes. In each country, except Germany, environmental factors played an important role in the initiation and content of health care policy. One question that begs an answer is: Under what circumstances does true policy innovation rather than imitation occur? Why was health care policy innovative in Germany but imitative in Tsarist Russia, Japan, and Great Britain? We cannot answer this question. We can outline the socioeconomic and political factors that led Bismarck to his pathbreaking social reforms, but additional case studies of policy innovation are needed before we can generalize about the circumstances under which such innovation occurs.

A nation's political culture or ideology and its general cultural values are also important in the determination of public policy. Once again this conclusion is based on the four case studies. The most outstanding illustrations are the impact of communist ideology on the content and organization of the Soviet health care system and the influence of nazism on health care during the Third Reich. Similarly, in Great Britain the move to the Left, in the form of general acceptance of the ideology of the modern welfare state, was instrumental in the change from National Health Insurance to National Health Service. Finally, in the case of Japan, the traditional values and institutions of the family, industrial paternalism, and the role of the village became integrated into, and helped form the nature of, the Japanese health care system.

Among the structural variables found to be of considerable importance in accounting for public policy is the economic wealth or level of economic development of a nation. This factor is particularly important in the areas of education and health spending. Simply stated, wealthier nations are more likely to allocate larger proportions of their incomes to education and health policy than are poorer nations. This conclusion coincides with the findings of several other cross-national, aggregate policy studies. A political structural variable of importance in the policy process is the impact of interest groups. In Germany, Great Britain, and Japan, interest groups such as the medical profession, insurance carriers, and benevolent associations exercised considerable influence over the content and administration of health care policy. It is important to note, however, that interest groups became important only *after* the issue of state health care had become part of the policy agenda.

The final point we wish to emphasize concerns the impact of inherited policy, procedures, and experience on present and future policies. The major conclusion is that both present and future policies are frequently anchored in the past. In this vein, we remind the reader of budgetary incrementalism (a structural policy process variable) both as a description of the rate or magnitude of expenditure change and as the decision-making procedure by which budget makers actually process expenditure policy. Chapter 4 does not demonstrate incrementalism because the expenditure data are for 1 year only. Nevertheless, the incremental nature of expenditure change is illustrated for a small number of nations, and we are convinced, based upon other research, that changes in levels of public spending, in most nations, are of an incremental nature and that policy is made in an incremental fashion: Policy makers accept existing policy as given and make marginal adjustments, either of a monetary or a substantive nature, in existing policy. This point is demonstrated in the changes in health care policy in each of the four nations discussed. Even in the Soviet Union there was, and to some degree continues to be, reliance on past tsarist institutions and health care procedures as well as on past Soviet policy. The German and Japanese cases illustrate the tenacious unwillingness of policy makers to abandon existing policy and their preference for tacking on new components to existing policy. Finally, in the British case, the National Health Service, in appearance a radical concept, was really a logical extension of existing health care policy.

These, then, are the major findings of the study. The reader should not interpret this brief summary as an attempt to minimize the importance of some of the other factors (e.g., demographic structure, public opinion) that are discussed as significant in accounting for the similarities and differences in the public policies of nations. The summary simply underscores the most salient findings of the study.

A comparative approach to understanding United States health care policy

Comparative policy analysis holds considerable promise for the study of both comparative politics and public policy. A comparative policy perspective enlarges the base for comparing and evaluating political systems; it allows us to test the relationship between public policy and various independent variables more conclusively than do intranational policy studies; and it provides students and policy makers an opportunity to examine the experiences of different nations in trying to find policy solutions to common public problems.

The last point is particularly important. In this book we try to demonstrate that in the "real world" policy makers engage in comparative analysis all the time. They compare either their own current problems with those of other nations or their present conditions and options with those in their own past. The resulting decisions usually bear a remarkable resemblance to those made earlier by others. If comparison is part of the policy-making process, students of comparative public policy can do no less than use the same frame of reference as the decision makers themselves in trying to account for public policy.

In the remainder of this chapter we practice what we preach and apply some of the findings concerning health care policy making in the four countries studied here to an understanding of the future course of health care policy, and its implications, in the United States. We hasten to add that this is not an exercise in prediction. At this moment we are reluctant even to predict *if*, much less *when* and *how*, the United States will adopt a comprehensive national health care program. Pundits, politicians, and political scientists have been heralding the imminent arrival of such a program for about 30 years. Like countless observers before us, we believe the United States eventually will adopt some form of comprehensive health care program. The long history of the issue should make even the most fearless or prescient observer reluctant to predict the date of arrival or the specific content of a national health care program. Nevertheless, the experiences of Germany, Great Britain, the Soviet Union, and Japan provide the basis for making informed comments about the future course of American health care policy.

The context of American health care policy making

Federally sponsored national health insurance was first proposed in 1912 – a year after the British National Health Insurance Act – by former President Theodore Roosevelt, who was seeking reelection under the banner of the Progressive Party. Three decades later, President Franklin D. Roosevelt seriously considered including health insurance in his Social Security Bill – a policy reaction to the Great Depression – but abandoned the idea for fear it would endanger passage of his entire program. In the post–World War II era, presidents ranging in ideology from Truman to Nixon proclaimed their commitment to some form of health insurance program. As a candidate in 1976 and as president in 1977, Jimmy Carter became the most recent enthusiastic proponent of national health insurance. Carter directed secretary of health, education and welfare, Joseph Califano, to draw up a proposal for a comprehensive national health insurance (NHI) program. The year 1978 ended without consideratoin of the administration's proposal or of several other bills sponsored by members of Congress. We should add here that public opinion polls consistently have shown that a majority of Americans – today about two-thirds – favor such a program.

In recent years the debate over NHI has taken on a new dimension and sense of urgency. This has been occasioned by a proclaimed – although not undisputed – "crisis" in American medicine and health care. The crisis – and the term must be qualified out of deference to those who deny its existence[1] – has several features, most of which are familiar to the reader.

There is, to begin, the problem of access to and distribution of health services. As in every country studied here, there are regional inequalities: In 1974 Mississippi and Alabama had 96 and 100 physicians per 100,000 people, respectively; Maryland and New York had 253 and 245 doctors per 100,000 population. Similarly, there are significant inequalities between urban and rural areas. In 1977 there were approximately 150, mostly rural, counties in the United States without a resident physician and 250 counties with only one physician.[2] In addition, persons in rural areas were much less likely than their urban counterparts to have specialist care available to them: In 1973 there were 79 specialists per 100,000 people in nonmetropolitan areas compared with 172 per 100,000 in metropolitan areas.³ American doctors, like their German, British, Soviet, and Japanese colleagues, prefer the financial, cultural, and professional advantages associated with urban medical practice.

Inequalities in access manifest themselves in their most intolerable form as differences in life chances among social classes and racial groups. There are fewer doctors per person, and higher mortality and morbidity rates, in the predominantly black urban ghettos than in any other part of the country. In 1974, the infant mortality rates were 14.8 per 1,000 live births among whites and 24.9 per 1,000 live births among nonwhites. In the same year, the rates of maternal death (during delivery or from complications associated with pregnancy) per 100,000 were 10.0 for white women and 35.1 for nonwhites. By now the reader should be aware that differential mortality and morbidity rates among social classes and racial groups are determined more by differences in education, degree of health awareness, nutrition, housing, income, and so on than by access to health care. Nevertheless, popular misconception and political pressure and expediency have combined to attribute these differences to the health care crisis rather than to the broader and more relevant issue area of racial and social discrimination and inequality.

A second dimension of the health care crisis involves the quality of medical care. Frequently mentioned in this regard is the allegation that American doctors prescribe more medicine and perform more surgery than is either necessary or healthy for the public. One highly publicized report by a congressional subcommittee claimed that in 1974 there were 2.4 million unnecessary surgical procedures resulting in 11,900 deaths.⁴

However, the issue of quality of American medical care has become most closely associated with the mushrooming of malpractice suits against American physicians. Since 1970, malpractice suits have increased at an annual rate of 12 percent.⁵ In 1960, American surgeons paid a total of $19.7 million in malpractice insurance premiums; in 1970, they paid $206.7 million. In 1960, the average premium for a surgeon was $229 per year; in 1972 it was $2,307 per year. Several factors, other than increasing incompetence among the medical profession, explain these extraordinary increases – although incompetence and carelessness cannot be ruled out. Among the more prominent factors are (1) a general increase in consumer awareness and willingness to hold "sellers" accountable for actual or perceived poor service; (2) "the growth in skepticism toward social institutions in furthering the public interest";⁶ (3) greater use of medical services, which allows greater error; (4) a changing legal environment that has facilitated, and perhaps encouraged, recourse to litigation; and (5) a bandwagon effect produced by the publicity and knowledge about malpractice suits and particularly about highly celebrated big settlements. Whatever the reasons, malpractice suits both reflect and contribute to the disillusionment and increasing hostility toward the medical community and constitute part of the health care crisis.

But when most Americans talk of a crisis in American health care, they are thinking not of the accessibility or distribution of health services, or of malpractice suits, but rather of the explosion in health care costs. And the evidence indeed suggests that if there is no crisis, there is certainly a big problem. In 1950, Americans spent $12 billion (American billion) on health care; in 1976 they spent just under $140 billion. These figures represent an increase from 4.6 percent of the gross national product to 8.4 percent. For the average American family, health care costs have risen from $830 per year in 1965 to $2,200 in 1975.[7] If health care costs continue to rise at their current rate of about 12 percent per year, the cost will double every 6 years.[8]

Although a large proportion of the American people have some form of private or public (i.e., Medicaid or Medicare) health insurance, coverage is not universal, does not apply to all types of medical procedures, and generally does not pay the entire medical bill. For example, in 1975 about one-fourth of all Americans had no hospital insurance, 41 percent had no insurance for nonhospital physician care, one-third had no insurance to cover the cost of prescribed drugs, and 85 percent had no insurance for dental care.[9]

This, then, is the crisis in American health care: rapidly rising costs and inadequate insurance to pay for them. The solution most frequently offered to solve these, and other, health care problems is a national health insurance system.

National health insurance in the United States

If the experiences of the other nations studied here are relevant – and we think they are – NHI is not likely to solve the crisis in American health care. First, NHI, even if it includes appropriate and attractive incentives, is not likely to lure physicians out of the metropolitan areas and into the rural areas, or out of comfortable upper- and middle-class neighborhoods and into urban ghettos. We need only remind the reader of the inability of the Soviet regime to accomplish a geographical redistribution of health personnel, despite its substantial coercive capability, to suggest the magnitude of the task and the futility of such a hope. It is possible to be slightly more sanguine about the impact of national health insurance on improving access to health care among disadvantaged segments of the population. Theodore Marmor reports that following the adoption of national health insurance in Canada there was a "moderate" redistribution of access from the rich to the poor.[10] The evidence, however, is neither overwhelming nor complete. Our findings concerning the continued problem of access by the British lower class lead us to be cautious about expressing optimism over the prospects that NHI will substantially reduce inequalities.

Second, there seems no reason to expect national health insurance to improve the quality of health care. The experiences of Germany and Japan suggest that, if anything, a fee-for-service-based national health insurance system – which is probably what the United States will adopt – leads to more, not less, unnecessary surgery, office visits, and overprescribing of drugs. Recent revelations concerning physician abuses within the federal-state Medicaid program seem to corroborate our evidence and offer an unpromising picture of the future. Although malpractice is not mentioned as a serious problem in any of the countries studied here, Marmor's research on the Canadian experience suggests that NHI will not be the solution to increasing litigation over real or alleged medical abuses.

Lastly, in terms of health care costs, the evidence seems most clear – and damning. The experiences of Germany and Japan, which are most relevant here, clearly demonstrate that national health insurance will not hold down health care costs. Indeed, there is ample evidence to suggest that in the absence of some cost-control mechanism just the opposite will occur. This will probably result from increased use of medical facilities and personnel, particularly by poorer persons and, again with Medicaid in mind, increased abuses. Such increases are by no means ordained or inevitable. A cost-control mechanism, such as the establishment of a ceiling on health care expenditures financed by NHI as proposed in the Health Security Act sponsored by Senator Kennedy and Congressman Corman, could control costs. Similarly, various quality-control mechanisms – perhaps along the lines used in the German system – might minimize the abuses of overtreatment. Nevertheless, even its staunchest supporters hold little hope for the prospects of either cost control or abuse control under NHI.

One final issue should be raised concerning the probable impact of national health insurance on health care in the United States. Most people tend to equate *health care* with *health*. This equation is not valid. Chapter 4 demonstrates at the aggregate level the absence of a positive relationship between health personnel and infant mortality rates. In describing the experiences of Germany, Great Britain, the Soviet Union, and Japan, we repeatedly remind the reader that improvements in the health status of the people in these nations are linked with a host of social, cultural, economic, and personal behavior factors. We believe that, when first introduced in the latter part of the nineteenth and early twentieth centuries, national health insurance did contribute significantly to improving the health status of people. There were millions of people in all four nations who rarely, if ever, had seen a doctor prior to the introduction of NHI. For these people, access to health care did mean healthier and longer lives.

Conditions in the United States today are not analogous to those of the late nineteenth and early twentieth centuries. Few people in the United States today have never been to a physician or cannot have access to one. Furthermore, the contribution modern medicine makes to the health prospects of an individual (i.e., morbidity, mortality, and life expectancy) is relatively small. Aaron Wildavsky estimates that only about 10 percent of the improvement in personal health (i.e., longer life and fewer illnesses and deaths) can be attributed to the medical system. The remaining 90 percent depends upon the socioeconomic and behavioral factors discussed before.[11] In short, a national health insurance system will not make most people healthier.

One appropriately may ask at this point: Then why bother? If NHI will not significantly reduce costs or abuses, or improve access and distribution, how can one justify its adoption? There are several possible reasons. First, although it is true that access to medical care will not substantially, if at all, improve peoples' health, it can alleviate the physical pain and the mental anguish that often accompany illness. There are many people in this country who postpone or avoid seeing a physician because of financial considerations. Many illnesses resolve themselves without significant long-term implications for the health of the individual. But in many instances, the individual has needlessly suffered pain and anxiety that could have been minimized by medical care. In addition, there are certainly cases when delay in getting medical attention does have serious, and sometimes fatal, consequences.

A second reason for adopting NHI relates to the financial consequences of illness. For many Americans, illness, particularly a chronic illness or one requiring hospitalization, can spell financial disaster. And because 25 million Americans, in 1977, had no medical insurance at all, and 56 million had no hospital insurance, such disasters are not at all unusual. Most Americans without hospital insurance tend to be poor, and for them $134 per day for a hospital stay (in 1975) is simply beyond their means. Beyond the dollar costs of medical care there are, of course, the incalculable costs associated with the fear of a mammoth and ruinous medical bill. In the chapter on Great Britain, we quote one source that cites as a major achievement of the National Health Service that it "removed a burden of anxiety about ability to meet doctors' bills or hospital charges, which in the past preyed heavily on many people of low or modest means."[12] We reiterate the point made then: It is impossible to put a price tag on the peace of mind associated with the freedom from fear of medical bills.

A third reason that has been offered for establishing a NHI system is both the most fundamental and the most controversial. Senator Edward Kennedy, a consistent and vocal supporter of national health insurance, put it this way: "All Americans have come to expect health care as one of the basic rights of citizenship."[13] The proposition is clearly overstated. Not *all* Americans believe that health care is a basic right of citizenship in the sense that freedom of speech, assembly, and religion, and the right to vote, are. But it is probably accurate to say that a majority of Americans believe this. The notion that every person should have access to competent and adequate health care *regardless of ability to pay* is certainly part of the positive or general-welfare state ideology that has developed in the course of the twentieth century in most industrial and many developing nations of the world. The issue is still, however, a matter of considerable debate in the Congress of the United States. And one has to consider to what extent the right of all Americans to have adequate and competent health care conflicts with the right of physicians to practice medicine as they choose without interference from the state. The reconciliation of these conflicting rights should be no more intractable – and no less difficult – than it was in Germany, Great Britain, and Japan. But they can be reconciled.

It seems to us that the ultimate question is this: Is the availability of adequate health care, regardless of ability to pay, a fundamental right of citizenship? If it is judged to be so by a majority of the American people, then a national health insurance system should be adopted. The remaining issues of quality and cost control, though important, are secondary.

The future of American health care policy

What will be the future course of American health care policy and policy making? It will probably not be too dissimilar from the experiences of the other nations studied here. The United States already has begun creating a national health insurance system in the form of Medicare (health care for those over 65 years old) and Medicaid (health care for the needy). Like their German, British, and Japanese predecessors, American policy makers have begun by introducing health insurance to relatively small but vulnerable segments of the population. And like these earlier programs, the case of Medicaid provides an illustration of the use of social policy to diffuse political discontent. Medicaid was adopted in 1965 in the wake of political assassinations and urban violence. In addition, it was championed by a newly elected (in his own right) president, Lyndon Johnson, who had just received an extraordinary popular mandate. Thus, in the United States, as in the other countries, situational factors of a rather extraordinary nature ushered in the era of publicly sponsored health insurance.

Based upon the experiences of other nations, we can expect that in the future health care policy will use existing institutions and policies as the basis for further development. Health care probably will be incrementally extended to larger segments of the population and expanded in terms of increasing benefits. Furthermore, as in Germany, Great Britain, and Japan, political expediency and the power of interest groups can be expected to dictate the use of established agencies and institutions in the administration of the system. It seems likely that private insurance carriers, like Blue Cross and Blue Shield, and existing administrative agencies, will play a prominent role in any future national health care program.

And it is certain that at every stage of the health policy-making process, the American Medical Association, like its German, British, and Japanese counterparts, will play a major role in determining the content and administration of policy. The experiences of these other nations suggest that activity and influence will be as great *after* policy has been set as during the deliberative stage. The experiences of these other nations also suggest that ultimately the medical profession will become reconciled to, and indeed prosper under, a national health insurance system.

Experience also has shown that whatever its problems and shortcomings, national health care typically enjoys widespread popular support and favor.

Appendixes: defense, education, and health policies in various nations, 1973

Appendix 1. *Defense policy: expenditure and output for 127 nations, 1973*

Country[a]	Military expenditure as percent of GNP		Population per soldier		Level of economic development[b]
	Rank	%	Rank	No.	
Israel	1	37.6	1	28	1
Egypt	2	18.8	34	120	3
Yemen People's Republic	3	17.1	44	156	3
North Vietnam	4	16.7	6	39	4
South Vietnam	5	16.4	5	35	3
Syria[c]	6	15.7	11	52	3
Jordan	7	15.6	4	35	3
Cambodia	8	14.9	7	40	4
Saudi Arabia	9	13.4	50	180	1
Iraq	10	13.2	25	102	2
North Korea	11	11.4	3	32	3
USSR	12	10.7	16	73	1
Albania	13	9.6	15	62	2
Iran	14	9.5	43	148	2
Laos	15	9.0	9	43	4
China	16	8.3	69	281	3
Taiwan	17	8.0	2	31	2
Mongolia	18	6.9	10	47	2
Pakistan	19	6.7	46	171	4
Burma[c]	20	6.3	55	198	4
Somalia[c]	21	6.2	48	176	4
United States	22	6.1	23	93	1
Portugal	23	5.6	8	42	1
Chad	24	5.5	104	968	4
Cuba	25	5.4	18	82	2
East Germany	26	5.3	39	129	1
Singapore	27	5.3	27	104	1
Nigeria[c]	28	5.1	85	454	3

Country[a]	Military expenditure as percent of GNP		Population per soldier		Level of economic development[b]
	Rank	%	Rank	No.	
Equatorial Guinea	29	5.0	74	300	3
United Kingdom	30	5.0[d]	45	159	1
Sudan[c]	31	4.8	84	433	3
Turkey	32	4.3	19	82	2
Yemen Arab Republic	33	4.2	73	296	4
Greece	34	4.2	13	56	1
Congo[c]	35	4.1	62	250	3
Malaysia	36	4.1	56	210	2
Yugoslavia	37	4.0	21	87	1
Zaire	38	3.8	87	471	3
Czechoslovakia	39	3.8	17	77	1
Peru[c]	40	3.7	67	276	2
Guinea	41	3.7	98	702	3
France	42	3.7	26	103	1
South Korea	43	3.7	12	52	3
Zambia	44	3.6	71	290	3
Sweden	45	3.5	29	109	1
West Germany	46	3.4	40	130	1
Indonesia	47	3.3	82	391	4
Netherlands	48	3.3	34	120	1
Australia	49	3.2	50	180	1
Lebanon	50	3.2	54	191	2
Poland	51	3.1	32	119	1
Norway	52	3.1	30	110	1
Spain	53	3.1	33	119	1
India	54	3.1	95	606	3
Morocco	55	3.0	72	291	3
Uganda	56	3.0	101	832	3
Italy	57	3.0	38	128	1
Thailand	58	3.0	58	219	3
Belgium	59	2.7	28	108	1
Rwanda[c]	60	2.6	114	1,337	4
Uruguay[c]	61	2.5	41	142	2
Mali[c]	62	2.5	115	1,345	4
Bulgaria	63	2.5	14	57	1
Chile	64	2.5	46	171	2
Ethiopia	65	2.5	92	590	4
Brazil[c]	66	2.4	88	488	2
South Africa	67	2.4	91	551	1
Tanzania	68	2.3	107	1,027	3
Central African Republic[c]	69	2.3	102	855	3
Mauritania	70	2.3	95	630	3
Hungary	71	2.3	24	101	1
Denmark	72	2.1	37	126	1

Country[a]	Military expenditure as percent of GNP		Population per soldier		Level of economic development[b]
	Rank	%	Rank	No.	
Canada	73	2.0	65	276	1
Bolivia[c]	74	2.0	61	242	3
Burundi[c]	75	2.0	118	1,790	4
Ecuador[c]	76	2.0	75	306	3
Argentina	77	2.0	50	180	1
Switzerland	78	1.9	53	186	1
Rhodesia	79	1.9	112	1,180	3
Paraguay	80	1.9	49	178	3
Cameroon	81	1.9	108	1,035	3
Honduras	82	1.8	86	463	3
Venezuela	83	1.8	76	314	1
Kuwait	84	1.8	22	88	1
New Zealand	85	1.8	59	228	1
Ghana[c]	86	1.7	89	490	3
Romania	87	1.7	36	123	1
Afghanistan	88	1.7	57	218	4
Algeria	89	1.7	62	250	2
Libya[c]	90	1.7	20	86	1
Gabon	91	1.6	64	260	1
Philippines	92	1.6	103	935	3
Dominican Republic	93	1.6	68	277	2
Ireland	94	1.5	66	275	1
Togo[c]	95	1.5	110	1,060	3
Finland	96	1.5	31	117	1
Tunisia	97	1.5	60	228	3
Dahomey[c]	98	1.4	116	1,455	3
Malagasy[c]	99	1.4	119	1,815	3
Kenya	100	1.4	117	1,783	3
Nicaragua	101	1.4	70	287	2
Guyana	102	1.4	81	385	3
Haiti	103	1.3	97	644	3
Upper Volta[c]	104	1.3	121	1,913	4
Senegal	105	1.3	99	705	3
Bangladesh	106	1.3	123	4,261	4
Niger	107	1.2	122	2,150	3
El Salvador	108	1.2	96	643	3
Malta	109	1.1	e	e	1
Ivory Coast	110	1.1	111	1,160	2
Cyprus	111	1.1	77	315	1
Colombia	112	1.0	80	368	3
Liberia	113	1.0	78	332	3
Sri Lanka	114	0.9	106	1,019	3
Austria	115	0.9	42	145	1
Japan	116	0.9	83	407	1

Country[a]	Military expenditure as percent of GNP		Population per soldier		Level of economic development[b]
	Rank	%	Rank	No.	
Luxembourg	117	0.9	79	350	1
Sierra Leone	118	0.8	113	1,335	3
Guatemala	119	0.8	90	504	3
Mexico	120	0.7	100	765	2
Malawi	121	0.6	124	4,790	3
Nepal	122	0.6	93	601	4
Costa Rica	123	0.6	120	1,870	2
Jamaica	124	0.5	105	990	2
Trinidad and Tobago	125	0.3	109	1,060	1
Mauritius	126	0.3	e	e	3
Panama	127	0.1	e	e	2

[a]Italic indicates nations with communist or militant socialist regimes.

[b]Level of economic development (per capita GNP in U.S. dollars): 1 (First World) = $1,000 + ; 2 (Second World) = $500–$999; 3 (Third World) = $100–$499; 4 (Fourth World) = less than $100.

[c]Under direct military rule in 1973.

[d]The figure for the United Kingdom is 4.99 and for Equatorial Guinea 5.0. Owing to rounding, each is assigned the same score. In these and other cases where ties occur, the proper rank order is listed.

[e]None or too few to calculate.

Source: Based on data in Ruth L. Sivard, World Military and Social Expenditures, 1976 (Leesburg, Va.: WMSE Publications, 1976), pp. 20–9.

Appendix 2. *Education policy: expenditure, output, and performance for 132 nations,*
1973

Country[a]	Expenditure: education expenditure as percent of GNP		Output: school-age population in school		Output: school-age population per teacher		Performance: literacy rate		Level of economic development[b]
	Rank	%	Rank	%	Rank	No.	Rank	%	
Canada	1	8.5	2	85	3	21	26	94	1
Algeria	2	8.3	85	45	83	79	88	26	2
Sweden	3	8.0	7	80	7	22	1	99	1
Denmark	4	7.6	17	67	3	21	1	99	1
Netherlands	5	7.4	38	62	36	37	1	99	1
Ivory Coast	6	7.0	95	39	105	110	100	20	2
USSR	7	6.9	24	66	22	29	1	99	1
Malagasy[c]	8	6.8	88	42	102	109	89	39	3
Zambia	9	6.8	67	53	83	79	77	40	3
Libya[c]	10	6.8	42	60	29	32	96	22	1
Belgium	11	6.7	10	71	7	22	13	98	1
Congo[c]	12	6.5	52	58	44	43	100	20	3
Finland	13	6.3	17	67	20	28	1	99	1
Yemen People's Republic	14	6.3	100	35	71	66	111	10	3
Tunisia	15	6.0	42	60	72	67	84	32	3
United Kingdom	16	5.9	3	83	11	24	13	98	1
Guyana	17	5.8	15	68	39	40	44	83	3
Swaziland	18	5.8	58	56	88	85	81	36	3
France	19	5.8	11	70	11	24	1	99	1
Malta	20	5.7	24	66	10	23	65	60	1
Morocco	21	5.7	110	26	101	103	99	21	3
United States	22	5.7	1	90	13	25	1	99	1
Saudi Arabia	23	5.4	108	27	98	97	108	15	1
Norway	24	5.4	17	67	3	21	1	99	1
Costa Rica	25	5.4	30	65	36	37	34	89	2
Kenya	26	5.4	95	39	75	73	91	25	3
Malaysia	27	5.3	67	53	60	53	76	43	2
Jamaica	28	5.3	40	61	68	60	37	86	2
Australia	29	5.2	3	83	18	26	13	98	1
Guinea	30	5.1	116	20	106	111	111	10	3
Cuba	31	5.0	14	69	32	34	39	85	2
Yugoslavia	32	5.0	55	57	41	41	25	93	1
Austria	33	4.9	24	66	28	31	1	99	1
Italy	34	4.8	35	64	13	25	27	93	1
Iceland	35	4.7	6	82	1	20	13	98	1
New Zealand	36	4.6	3	83	20	28	13	98	1
Sudan[c]	37	4.5	116	20	117	165	109	12	3

Country[a]	Expenditure: education expenditure as percent of GNP		Output: school-age population in school		Output: school-age population per teacher		Performance: literacy rate		Level of economic development[b]
	Rank	%	Rank	%	Rank	No.	Rank	%	
East Germany	38	4.5	24	66	13	25	13	98	1
West Germany	39	4.5	15	68	23	30	1	99	1
Poland	40	4.5	42	60	32	34	13	98	1
Iraq	41	4.4	88	42	58	52	88	26	2
Panama	42	4.4	17	67	36	37	47	79	2
Japan	43	4.3	11	70	23	30	1	99	1
Dahomey[c]	44	4.3	121	18	124	214	100	20	3
Venezuela	45	4.3	64	54	51	48	46	82	1
Switzerland	46	4.3	9	75	7	22	1	99	1
Trinidad and Tobago	47	4.3	42	60	46	46	34	89	1
Ireland	48	4.3	30	65	23	30	13	98	1
Egypt	49	4.3	88	42	89	88	88	26	3
Luxembourg	50	4.2	11	70	19	27	13	98	1
Zaire	51	4.2	81	46	94	91	109	12	3
Lesotho	52	4.2	71	51	81	78	65	60	4
Cameroon	53	4.1	91	41	91	90	111	10	3
Gabon	54	4.1	17	67	53	50	87	30	1
Botswana	55	4.1	95	39	78	76	100	20	4
Mongolia	56	4.0	42	60	52	49	24	95	2
Bolivia[c]	57	4.0	77	48	53	50	74	45	3
South Vietnam	58	3.9	72	50	91	90	63	65	3
Peru[c]	59	3.9	58	56	56	51	55	72	2
North Vietnam	60	3.9	72	50	90	89	57	70	4
China	61	3.9	36	63	47	47	24	95	3
Syria[c]	62	3.8	55	57	80	77	86	31	3
Cambodia	63	3.8	92	40	110	145	69	59	4
Taiwan	64	3.8	24	66	60	53	39	85	2
Mauritania	65	3.8	127	11	112	146	129	5	3
Sierra Leone	66	3.8	116	20	102	109	111	10	3
Equatorial Guinea	67	3.8	86	44	91	90	100	20	3
Chad	68	3.7	124	14	127	358	128	6	4
Iran	69	3.7	81	46	74	71	80	37	2
Ecuador[c]	70	3.7	77	48	67	59	60	68	3
Israel	71	3.6	42	60	3	21	42	84	1
Uruguay[c]	72	3.6	60	55	23	30	30	91	2
Bulgaria	73	3.6	52	58	34	35	31	90	1
Czechoslovakia	74	3.6	55	57	31	33	13	98	1
Sri Lanka	75	3.6	30	65	39	40	49	76	3
Albania	76	3.5	24	66	35	36	52	75	2
Tanzania	77	3.5	113	21	121	204	106	18	3
Burma[c]	78	3.4	67	53	96	93	65	60	4
Hungary	79	3.4	70	52	29	32	13	98	1
Ghana[c]	80	3.4	86	44	65	58	91	25	3

Country[a]	Expenditure: education expenditure as percent of GNP		Output: school-age population in school		Output: school-age population per teacher		Performance: literacy rate		Level of economic development[b]
	Rank	%	Rank	%	Rank	No.	Rank	%	
Rhodesia	81	3.3	92	40	83	79	91	25	3
Central African Republic[c]	82	3.3	102	33	110	145	125	8	3
El Salvador	83	3.3	80	47	99	99	71	57	3
Chile	84	3.2	8	79	64	57	31	90	2
Brazil[c]	85	3.2	72	50	56	51	62	66	2
Gambia	86	3.2	120	19	116	160	111	10	3
Uganda	87	3.1	113	21	114	154	91	25	3
Senegal	88	3.0	108	27	118	169	111	10	3
Honduras	89	3.0	81	46	69	63	74	45	3
Thailand	90	3.0	81	46	70	64	57	70	3
Rwanda[c]	91	2.9	102	33	120	192	111	10	4
Turkey	92	2.9	76	49	73	69	73	51	2
Kuwait	93	2.9	42	60	13	25	72	55	1
North Korea	94	2.8	42	60	96	93	39	85	3
Indonesia	95	2.8	101	34	87	84	65	60	4
South Korea	96	2.8	30	65	78	76	36	88	3
Philippines	97	2.8	17	67	47	47	55	72	3
Mali[c]	98	2.8	124	14	122	211	111	10	4
Romania	99	2.6	30	65	23	30	31	90	1
Singapore	100	2.6	38	62	43	42	52	75	1
Liberia	101	2.6	110	26	95	92	111	10	3
Mauritius	102	2.6	40	61	47	47	64	62	3
Ethiopia	103	2.6	128	10	129	420	127	7	4
Mexico	104	2.6	64	54	63	56	49	76	2
Lebanon	105	2.6	77	48	1	20	37	86	2
Cyprus	106	2.6	60	55	53	50	49	76	1
Jordan	107	2.5	42	60	60	53	84	32	3
Malawi	108	2.5	112	24	114	154	96	22	3
Togo[c]	109	2.5	99	37	102	109	111	10	3
Guatemala	110	2.4	104	32	107	123	79	38	3
Burundi[c]	111	2.4	123	15	125	220	111	10	4
Colombia	112	2.4	92	40	75	73	54	74	3
Nicaragua	113	2.2	72	50	77	75	70	58	2
Upper Volta[c]	114	2.2	132	5	131	515	129	5	4
Argentina	115	2.2	42	60	13	25	27	93	1
Spain	116	2.0	36	63	41	41	26	94	1
Niger	117	2.0	131	6	132	543	129	5	3
Somalia[c]	118	1.9	130	7	128	380	129	5	4
Nigeria[c]	119	1.9	116	20	123	212	91	25	3
Greece	120	1.9	17	67	47	47	42	84	1
Paraguay	121	1.8	60	55	58	52	47	79	3
Dominican Republic	122	1.8	64	54	83	79	60	68	2

Country[a]	Expenditure: education expenditure as percent of GNP		Output: school-age population in school		Output: school-age population per teacher		Performance: literacy rate		Level of economic development[b]
	Rank	%	Rank	%	Rank	No.	Rank	%	
India	123	1.8	95	39	65	58	83	34	3
Bangladesh	124	1.8	106	29	113	149	96	22	4
Portugal	125	1.7	52	58	44	43	57	70	1
Pakistan	126	1.6	106	29	109	134	107	16	4
Laos	127	1.6	105	30	108	133	100	20	4
South Africa	128	1.6	60	55	81	78	82	35	1
Yemen Arab Republic	129	1.2	129	9	130	470	111	10	4
Afghanistan	130	0.9	126	13	126	261	125	8	4
Nepal	131	0.7	122	16	99	99	124	9	4
Haiti	132	0.7	113	21	119	188	111	10	3

[a]Italic indicates nations with communist or militant socialist regimes.

[b]Level of economic development (per capita GNP in U.S. dollars): 1 (First World) = $1,000 + ; 2 (Second World) = $500–$999; 3 (Third World) = $100–$499; 4 (Fourth World) = less than $100.

[c]Under direct military rule in 1973.

Source: Based on data in Ruth L. Sivard, *World Military and Social Expenditures, 1976* (Leesburg, Va.: WMSE Publications, 1976), pp. 20–9.

Appendix 3. *Health policy: expenditure, output, and performance for 132 nations,*
1973

Country[a]	Expenditure: health expenditure as percent of GNP		Output: population per physician		Performance: infant mortality rate (per 1,000 live births)		Performance: life expectancy		Level of economic development[b]
	Rank	%	Rank	No.	Rank	Rate	Rank	Yr	
Sweden	1	6.5	22	690	1	10	5	73	1
Canada	2	6.0	18	615	13	17	10	72	1
New Zealand	3	4.9	25	740	11	16	10	72	1
West Germany	4	4.6	10	532	21	20	20	71	1
Netherlands	5	4.6	23	696	4	12	1	74	1
Zaire	6	4.4	121	28,802	111	160	98	44	3
Denmark	7	4.4	13	591	7	13	1	74	1
United Kingdom	8	4.3	26	756	13	17	10	72	1
France	9	4.2	21	677	9	15	5	73	1
Finland	10	4.0	29	832	1	10	27	70	1
Belgium	11	4.0	15	599	13	17	5	73	1
Luxembourg	12	3.6	35	933	11	16	20	71	1
Panama	13	3.5	44	1,340	44	47	47	66	2
Malta	14	3.4	36	941	25	24	20	71	1
Japan	15	3.4	31	864	4	12	5	73	1
Poland	16	3.3	16	607	33	28	27	70	1
USSR	17	3.3	2	369	29	26	27	70	1
Austria	18	3.3	7	509	25	24	20	71	1
Czechoslovakia	19	3.2	3	432	23	21	36	69	1
East Germany	20	2.9	12	580	17	18	5	73	1
Taiwan	21	2.8	68	2,967	17	18	36	69	2
United States	22	2.8	17	612	17	18	20	71	1
Costa Rica	23	2.8	47	1,413	46	54	39	68	2
Zambia	24	2.7	98	12,211	108	157	98	44	3
Hungary	25	2.7	8	518	35	34	27	70	1
Venezuela	26	2.6	34	925	45	50	49	65	1
Ireland	27	2.6	30	842	17	18	10	72	1
Swaziland	28	2.5	85	7,188	98	149	98	44	3
Chile	29	2.5	53	1,836	55	71	50	63	2
Switzerland	30	2.5	14	597	7	13	10	72	1
Cuba	31	2.5	39	1,115	28	25	27	70	2
Guyana	32	2.4	74	3,820	37	40	39	68	3
Dominican Republic	33	2.4	55	1,926	67	98	62	58	2
Jamaica	34	2.2	64	2,750	29	26	27	70	2
Egypt	35	2.2	50	1,516	70	103	78	52	3
Libya[c]	36	2.2	42	1,244	87	130	71	53	1
Tunisia	37	2.1	81	5,460	85	128	68	54	3
Lesotho	38	2.0	112	21,522	125	181	92	46	4

Country[a]	Expenditure: health expenditure as percent of GNP		Output: population per physician		Performance: infant mortality rate (per 1,000 live births)		Performance: life expectancy		Level of economic development[b]
	Rank	%	Rank	No.	Rank	Rate	Rank	Yr	
Trinidad and Tobago	39	2.0	59	2,120	36	35	27	70	1
Botswana	40	2.0	105	14,545	66	97	98	44	4
Yemen Arab Republic	41	2.0	119	25,347	104	152	94	45	4
Portugal	42	1.9	37	973	42	45	39	68	1
Nicaragua	43	1.9	48	1,436	80	123	71	53	2
Romania	44	1.9	27	817	37	40	45	67	1
Australia	45	1.8	28	821	13	17	10	72	1
Sri Lanka	46	1.8	73	3,681	42	45	39	68	3
Malaysia	47	1.8	80	5,341	56	75	61	59	2
Guinea	48	1.8	114	22,394	131	216	110	41	3
Bolivia[c]	49	1.7	62	2,487	71	108	91	47	3
Mauritius	50	1.7	70	3,192	53	64	47	66	3
Dahomey[c]	51	1.7	123	30,632	129	185	110	41	3
Yemen People's Republic	52	1.7	95	10,400	104	152	94	45	3
Bulgaria	53	1.7	5	490	29	26	10	72	1
Congo[c]	54	1.6	82	6,173	123	180	98	44	3
Gambia	55	1.6	117	24,500	117	165	120	40	3
Ivory Coast	56	1.6	103	13,257	116	164	98	44	2
Somalia[c]	57	1.5	108	15,544	121	177	110	41	4
Kenya	58	1.5	90	8,914	91	135	82	50	3
Rhodesia	59	1.5	83	6,556	99	122	78	52	3
Guatemala	60	1.5	76	3,957	61	79	71	53	3
Morocco	61	1.5	104	13,592	98	149	71	53	3
Liberia	62	1.4	101	12,576	109	159	92	46	3
Saudi Arabia	63	1.4	75	3,870	104	152	74	45	1
Paraguay	64	1.4	54	1,907	62	84	53	62	3
Gabon	65	1.4	78	5,200	132	229	110	41	1
El Salvador	66	1.4	72	3,676	48	58	62	58	3
Turkey	67	1.4	58	2,018	76	119	66	57	2
Algeria	68	1.4	88	8,200	85	128	71	53	2
Tanzania	69	1.4	116	23,967	114	162	98	44	3
Central African Republic[c]	70	1.3	122	28,983	115	163	110	41	3
Kuwait	71	1.3	38	1,035	41	44	45	67	1
Mali[c]	72	1.3	124	35,867	119	168	126	38	4
Equatorial Guinea	73	1.3	92	10,000	117	165	98	44	3
Iceland	74	1.2	20	656	1	10	1	74	1
Chad	75	1.2	127	43,483	111	160	126	38	4
Burma[c]	76	1.2	84	6,906	83	126	82	50	4
Italy	77	1.2	9	527	29	26	10	72	1

Country[a]	Expenditure: health expenditure as percent of GNP		Output: population per physician		Performance: infant mortality rate (per 1,000 live births)		Performance: life expectancy		Level of economic development[b]
	Rank	%	Rank	No.	Rank	Rate	Rank	Yr	
Uganda	78	1.2	91	9,008	111	160	82	50	3
Senegal	79	1.2	106	14,739	109	159	120	40	3
Ghana[c]	80	1.1	94	10,344	107	156	98	44	3
Mauritania	81	1.1	111	17,746	93	137	126	38	3
Jordan	82	1.1	65	2,822	68	99	71	53	3
Cambodia	83	1.1	110	16,978	84	127	94	45	4
Uruguay[c]	84	1.1	33	879	37	40	27	70	2
Peru[c]	85	1.1	52	1,818	72	110	67	56	2
Iran	86	1.1	67	2,953	95	139	81	51	2
Greece	87	1.1	11	568	25	24	10	72	1
Singapore	88	1.1	45	1,369	21	20	27	70	1
Norway	89	1.1	19	639	4	12	1	74	1
Sierra Leone	90	1.0	109	15,706	92	136	98	44	3
Sudan[c]	91	1.0	100	12,528	97	141	88	49	3
Honduras	92	1.0	71	3,523	74	115	68	54	3
Cameroon	93	1.0	120	27,000	93	137	110	41	3
Niger	94	1.0	126	43,000	130	200	126	38	3
Yugoslavia	95	1.0	32	873	40	43	39	68	1
Albania	96	1.0	40	1,175	63	87	36	69	2
Mongolia	97	1.0	6	504	56	75	55	61	2
China	98	1.0	87	8,142	47	55	53	62	3
Spain	99	1.0	24	726	9	15	10	72	1
Togo[c]	100	1.0	113	22,316	122	179	110	41	3
Rwanda[c]	101	1.0	129	52,763	90	133	110	41	4
Cyprus	102	1.0	41	1,195	34	33	20	71	1
Malawi	103	1.0	131	68,429	76	119	110	41	3
Iraq	104	0.9	63	2,525	68	99	71	53	2
Colombia	105	0.9	60	2,184	58	76	55	61	3
Argentina	106	0.9	4	467	50	60	39	68	1
Upper Volta[c]	107	0.9	130	59,792	127	182	126	38	4
Malagasy[c]	108	0.9	97	10,568	78	120	98	44	3
India	109	0.8	77	4,399	95	139	81	50	3
Ethiopia	110	0.8	132	73,750	125	181	126	38	4
Burundi[c]	111	0.7	128	44,750	100	150	125	39	4
Haiti	112	0.7	89	8,640	100	150	82	50	3
South Vietnam	113	0.6	96	10,500	100	150	120	40	3
North Vietnam	114	0.6	99	12,500	100	150	89	48	4
Lebanon	115	0.6	43	1,330	49	59	50	63	2
Ecuador[c]	116	0.6	69	3,059	59	78	60	60	3
Nepal	117	0.6	125	42,929	120	169	98	44	4
Israel	118	0.5	1	361	23	21	20	71	1

Country[a]	Expenditure: health expenditure as percent of GNP		Output: population per physician		Performance: infant mortality rate (per 1,000 live births)		Performance: life expectancy		Level of economic development[b]
	Rank	%	Rank	No.	Rank	Rate	Rank	Yr	
Mexico	119	0.5	46	1,392	52	61	50	63	2
Syria[c]	120	0.5	66	2,906	64	93	68	54	3
Thailand	121	0.5	86	8,041	54	65	62	58	3
Philippines	122	0.4	49	1,490	59	78	62	58	3
Nigeria[c]	123	0.4	115	23,753	123	180	110	41	3
Laos	124	0.4	102	12,720	80	123	120	40	4
South Africa	125	0.4	57	2,012	75	117	78	52	1
Bangladesh	126	0.3	93	10,009	88	132	132	36	4
Brazil[c]	127	0.3	51	1,811	65	94	55	61	2
Afghanistan	128	0.2	107	15,242	127	182	120	40	4
South Korea	129	0.2	56	1,983	50	60	55	61	3
North Korea	130	0.2	61	2,286	72	110	55	61	3
Indonesia	131	0.1	118	24,553	82	125	89	48	4
Pakistan	132	0.1	79	5,284	88	132	82	50	4

[a]Italic indicates nations with communist or militant socialist regimes.

[b]Level of economic development (per capita GNP in U.S. dollars): 1 (First World) = $1,000 + ; 2 (Second World) = $500–$999; 3 (Third World) = $100–$499; 4 (Fourth World) = less than $100.

[c]Under direct military rule in 1973.

Source: Based on data in Ruth L. Sivard, *World Military and Social Expenditures, 1976* (Leesburg, Va.: WMSE Publications, 1976), pp. 20–9.

Notes

Chapter 1. Introduction

1 Henry C. Burdett, *Hospitals and Asylums of the World* (1893), pp. 3, 55–6, 613, quoted in Brian Abel-Smith, "The History of Medical Care," *Comparative Development in Social Welfare*, ed. E. W. Martin (London: Allen & Unwin, 1972), p. 220.

2 Quoted in Karl de Schweinitz, *England's Road to Social Security* (New York: Barnes, 1961), p. 142.

3 Quoted in Samuel Mencher, *Poor Law to Poverty Program: Economic Security Policy in Britain and the United States* (Pittsburgh: University of Pittsburgh Press, 1967), p. 247.

4 Charles W. Anderson, "System and Strategy in Comparative Policy Analysis: A Plea for Contextual and Experiential Knowledge," *Perspectives on Public Policy-Making*, ed. William B. Gwyn and George C. Edwards, III (New Orleans: Tulane Studies in Political Science, 1975), p. 219.

5 The periodic and monographic literature is already too voluminous to allow a definitive listing. Among the recent monographs are: Cynthia Enloe, *The Politics of Pollution in a Comparative Perspective* (New York: McKay, 1975); T. Alexander, *The Comparative Policy Process* (Santa Barbara: Clio Press, 1975); Arnold J. Heidenheimer, Hugh Heclo, and Carolyn Adams. *Comparative Public Policy: The Politics of Social Choice in Europe and America* (New York: St. Martin's Press, 1975); Craig Liske, William Loehr, and John McCamant, *Comparative Public Policy: Issues, Theories, and Methods* (New York: Halsted Press, 1975); Richard L. Siegel and Leonard Weinberg, *Comparing Public Policies* (Homewood, Ill.: Dorsey Press, 1977). Prominent among the periodical literature are: Charles Anderson, "System and Strategy in Comparative Policy Analysis"; Richard Rose, "Concepts for Comparison," *Policy Studies Journal*, 1 (spring 1973), 14–17; Arthur Cyr and Peter de Leon, "Comparative Policy Analysis," *Policy Sciences*, 6 (December 1975), 375–84; Hugh Heclo, "Review Article: Policy Analysis," *British Journal of Political Science*, 2 (1972), 83–108.

6 Even here, however, significant progress has been made. For example, Almond and Powell, in the second edition of their highly influential book on comparative politics, have added *policy* to the subtitle and devoted nearly one-third of the book to public policy. See Gabriel Almond and G. Bingham Powell, *Comparative Politics: System, Process and Policy*, 2nd ed. (Boston: Little, Brown, 1978).

7 See, for example, Thomas R. Dye, *Politics, Economics and the Public* (Chicago: Rand McNally, 1966); Richard E. Dawson and James A. Robinson, "Inter-Party Competition, Economic Variables and Welfare Policies in the American

States," *State Politics*, ed. Robert E. Crew, Jr. (Belmont, Calif.: Wadsworth, 1968), pp. 459–78; Richard I. Hofferbert, *The Study of Public Policy* (Indianapolis: Bobbs-Merrill, 1974).

8 James E. Alt, "Some Social and Political Correlates of County Borough Expenditures," *British Journal of Political Science*, 1 (January 1971), 49–62; Robert C. Fried, "Communism, Urban Budgets, and the Two Italies: A Case Study in Comparative Urban Government," *Journal of Politics*, 33 (November 1971), 1008–51; James B. Hogan, "Social Structure and Public Policy: A Longitudinal Study of Mexico and Canada," *Comparative Politics*, 4 (July 1972), 477–509; B. Guy Peters, "Public Policy, Socioeconomic Conditions and the Political System: A Note on Their Developmental Relationship," *Polity*, 5 (winter 1972), 277–84.

9 Howard M. Leichter, "Comparative Public Policy: Problems and Prospects," *Policy Studies Journal*, 5 (summer 1977), 83–96.

10 Hofferbert, *Study of Public Policy*, p. 10.

11 Elliot J. Feldman, "Comparative Public Policy: Field or Method?" *Comparative Politics*, 10 (January 1978), 288.

12 See, for example, Robert Alford, *Bureaucracy and Participation* (Chicago: Rand McNally, 1969), pp. 1–2; Heclo, "Review Article."

13 Heclo, "Review Article," p. 85. Emphasis added.

14 James E. Anderson, *Public Policy-Making* (New York: Praeger, 1975), p. 3.

15 Samuel P. Huntington, *Political Order in Changing Societies* (New Haven: Yale University Press, 1968), p. 47.

16 *Houston Chronicle*, August 16, 1976.

17 Anthony King, "Ideas, Institutions and the Policies of Governments: A Comparative Analysis," Parts I–III, *British Journal of Political Science* (October 1973), 291–313, 409–23.

18 Naomi Caiden and Aaron Wildavsky, *Planning and Budgeting in Poor Countries* (New York: Wiley, 1974), p. xvi.

19 Frederic L. Pryor, *Public Expenditures in Communist and Capitalist Nations* (Homewood, Ill.: Richard Irwin, 1968). Pryor found a statistically significant difference in public spending between economic systems in the area of education, but not for defense, welfare, or health.

20 B. Guy Peters, "The Development of Social Policy in France, Sweden and the United Kingdom: 1850–1965," *Politics in Europe*, ed. Martin Hiesler (New York: McKay, 1972), pp. 257–92.

21 See Enloe, *Politics of Pollution;* Hugh Heclo, *Modern Social Politics in Britain and Sweden* (New Haven: Yale University Press, 1974).

22 Almost one-third of these references appear in the following illuminating sentence: "The 1960 scores on the Schutz coefficient and the Social Welfare Index for the United States, Canada and the United Kingdom are no higher than those for a large number of other countries such as Argentina and Israel." Robert W. Jackman, *Politics and Social Equality: A Comparative Analysis* (New York: Wiley, 1975), p. 57.

23 Philips Cutright, "Political Structure, Economic Development and Social Security Programs," *American Journal of Sociology*, 70 (March 1965), 547.

24 Howard M. Leichter, *Political Regime and Public Policy in the Philippines* (DeKalb, Ill.: Center for Southeast Asian Studies, 1975).

25 James A. Bill and Robert L. Hardgrave, Jr., *Comparative Politics: The Quest for Theory* (Columbus, Ohio: Merrill, 1973), pp. 33–7.

26 Arthur L. Kalleberg, "The Logic of Comparison: A Methodological Note on

the Comparative Study of Political Systems," *World Politics,* 19 (October 1966), 73.

Chapter 2. The origins and evolution of the positive state

1 The term *general welfare* state is used by Sidney Fine and connotes a positive exertion of state authority for promoting the welfare of all citizens. Sidney Fine, *Laissez-Faire and the General Welfare State: A Study of Conflict in American Thought, 1865-1901* (Ann Arbor: University of Michigan Press, 1956), p. 167.

2 Reinhold A. Dorwart, *The Prussian Welfare State Before 1740* (Cambridge, Mass.: Harvard University Press, 1971), p. vii.

3 Quincy Wright, *A Study of War,* 2nd ed. (Chicago: University of Chicago Press, 1965), p. 651.

4 Charles Tilly, "Reflections on the History of European State Making," *The Formation of National States in Western Europe,* ed. Charles Tilly (Princeton: Princeton University Press, 1975), p. 74.

5 See Pitirim A. Sorokin, *Social and Cultural Dynamics,* Vol. III (New York: American Book, 1937), pp. 409–72.

6 Daniel Bell, "The Public Household–On 'Fiscal Sociology' and the Liberal Society," *Public Interest,* 37 (fall 1974), 35.

7 Gabriel Ardant, "Financial Policy and the Economic Infrastructure of Modern States and Nations," *Formation of National States,* ed. Tilly, p. 181.

8 Rudolf Braun, "Taxation, Sociopolitical Structure, and State-Building: Great Britain and Brandenburg-Prussia." *Formation of National States,* ed. Tilly, pp. 243–327.

9 Barrington Moore, Jr., *Social Origins of Dictatorship and Democracy* (Boston: Beacon Press, 1967), p. 317.

10 Charles Tilly, "Food Supply and Public Order in Modern Europe," *Formation of National States,* ed. Tilly, pp. 412, 453.

11 Moore, *Social Origins,* p. 205.

12 R. T. Holt and J. E. Turner, *The Political Basis of Economic Development* (Princeton: Van Nostrand, 1966), pp. 72, 120–1.

13 See Dorwart, *Prussian Welfare State,* pp. 35–48.

14 A classic and indispensable treatment of mercantilism is Eli F. Heckscher, *Mercantilism,* rev. ed. (New York: Macmillan, 1955), 2 vols.

15 Holt and Turner, *Political Basis,* p. 184.

16 Dorwart, *Prussian Welfare State,* pp. 49, 295.

17 Holt and Turner, *Political Basis,* p. 122.

18 Derek Fraser, *The Evolution of the British Welfare State: A History of Social Policy Since the Industrial Revolution* (London: Macmillan, 1973), p. 28.

19 For a discussion of the concept of "medical police," see George Rosen, *From Medical Police to Social Medicine* (New York: Science History Publication, 1974). Especially relevant is "Cameralism and the Concept of Medical Police," pp. 120–41.

20 Bernice Q. Madison, *Social Welfare in the Soviet Union* (Stanford: Stanford University Press, 1968), pp. 5–9; Fraser, *Evolution of the British Welfare State,* p. 30.

21 Dorwart, *Prussian Welfare State,* p. 102.

22 Adam Smith, *Inquiry into the Wealth of Nations,* quoted in Fine, *Laissez-Faire and the General Welfare State,* p. 7.

23 Karl Polanyi, *The Great Transformation* (Boston: Beacon Press, 1957), p. 140.
24 Thomas Malthus, quoted in Fine, *Laissez-Faire and the General Welfare State*, p. 7.
25 Gaston V. Rimlinger, *Welfare Policy and Industrialization in Europe, America and Russia* (New York: Wiley, 1971), p. 39.
26 Ibid., p. 48.
27 For a discussion of these and other changes, see Eugene N. Anderson and Pauline R. Anderson, *Political Institutions and Social Change in Continental Europe in the Nineteenth Century* (Berkeley: University of California Press, 1967).
28 Frank J. Coppa, "Industrialization and Urbanization: European Style," *Cities in Transitions: From the Ancient World to Urban America*, ed. Frank J. Coppa and Philip C. Dolce (Chicago: Nelson-Hall, 1974), p. 70.
29 Ibid., p. 71.
30 Excerpts from "Minutes of Samuel Coulson," in Fraser, *Evolution of the British Welfare State*, pp. 234–5.
31 Quoted in Heinrich Braun, *Industrialisation and Social Policy in Germany* (Cologne: Heymanns, 1956), p. 16.
32 Fraser, *Evolution of the British Welfare State*, p. 84.
33 Quoted in Rosen, *From Medical Police*, p. 64.
34 For a thorough discussion of the public health reform movement, see Rosen, *From Medical Police*, pp. 60–119.
35 Walter A. Friedlander, *Individualism and Social Welfare: An Analysis of the System of Social Security and Social Welfare in France* (New York: Free Press, 1962), p. 23.
36 Brian Abel-Smith, "The History of Medical Care," *Comparative Development in Social Welfare*, ed. E. W. Martin (London: Allen & Unwin, 1972), pp. 222–3.
37 Friedlander, *Individualism and Social Welfare*, p. 21.
38 Fraser, *Evolution of the British Welfare State*, p. 31.
39 See E. Dubois, "Child Labor in Belgium," *Annals*, 20 (July–December 1902), 203–20.
40 Fraser, *Evolution of the British Welfare State*, pp. 72–3.
41 G. A. Rennison, *We Live Among Strangers: A Sociology of the Welfare State* (Melbourne: Melbourne University Press, 1970), p. 87.
42 Gaston V. Rimlinger, "Social Security and Society: An East-West Comparison," *Social Science Quarterly*, 50 (December 1969), 494.
43 Sidney B. Fay, "Bismarck's Welfare State," *Current History*, 18 (January 1950), 1–7.
44 Rimlinger, "Social Security and Society," p. 494.
45 T. H. Marshall, "Citizenship and Social Class," *Class, Citizenship and Social Development*, ed. T. H. Marshall (Garden City, N.Y.: Doubleday [Anchor Books], 1965), p. 91.

Chapter 3. Accounting for public policy

1 Quotations in this section all come from Robert Alford, *Bureaucracy and Participation: Political Culture in Four Wisconsin Cities* (Chicago: Rand McNally, 1969), p. 2.
2 See B. Guy Peters, "The Development of Social Policy in France, Sweden, and the United Kingdom, 1850–1965," *Politics in Europe*, ed. Martin Heisler (New York: McKay, 1972), pp. 257–92.

3 Alan T. Peacock and Jack Wiseman, *The Growth of Public Expenditures in the United Kingdom* (Princeton: Princeton University Press, 1961), p. 93.

4 James W. Wilkie, "Bolivian Public Expenditure Since 1952," *Statistics and National Policy,* ed. James W. Wilkie (Los Angeles: UCLA Latin American Center, 1974), p. 89.

5 Rolland G. Paulston, "Education," *Revolutionary Change in Cuba,* ed. Carmelo Mesa-Logo (Pittsburgh: University of Pittsburgh Press, 1971), pp. 375–97.

6 Peter Sederberg, "National Expenditures as an Indicator of Political Change in Ghana," *Journal of Developing Areas,* 7 (December 1972), 37–56.

7 Irma Adelman and Cynthia Taft Morris, *Economic Growth and Social Equity in Developing Countries* (Stanford: Stanford University Press, 1973), p. 41.

8 B. U. Ratchford, *Public Expenditures in Australia* (Durham, N.C.: Duke University Press, 1959), p. 12.

9 Charles E. Lindblom, *The Policy-Making Process* (New York: Prentice-Hall, 1968), p. 4.

10 Adelman and Morris, *Economic Growth,* p. 64.

11 Richard A. Musgrave, *Fiscal Systems* (New Haven: Yale University Press, 1969), p. 79.

12 Gunnar Myrdal, *Asian Drama: An Inquiry into the Poverty of Nations,* Vol. III (New York: Pantheon Books, 1968), p. 478.

13 Beverly Pooley, "The Modernization of Law in Ghana," *Ghana and the Ivory Coast: Perspectives on Modernization,* ed. Philip Foster and Aristede R. Zolberg (Chicago: University of Chicago Press, 1971), p. 179.

14 Joyce M. Mitchell and William C. Mitchell, *Political Analysis and Public Policy* (Chicago: Rand McNally, 1969), pp. 56–8.

15 "An Agenda for Comparative European Policy Research," *European Workshop on Policy Studies* (University of Strathclyde, June 18–23, 1972).

16 Harrell Rodgers, "The Supreme Court and School Desegregation: Twenty Years Later," *Political Science Quarterly,* 89 (winter 1974–5), 753.

17 See Roland J. Pennock, "Agricultural Subsidies in Britain and America," *Policy-making in Britain,* ed. Richard Rose (New York: Free Press, 1969), pp. 199–200.

18 David Easton and Jack Dennis, *Children in the Political System* (New York: McGraw-Hill, 1969), p. 59.

19 Eric A. Nordlinger, "Soldiers in Mufti: The Impact of Military Rule upon Economic and Social Change in the Non-Western World," *American Political Science Review,* 64 (December 1970), 1135.

20 R. D. McKinlay and A. S. Cohan, "A Comparative Analysis of the Political and Economic Performance of Military and Civilian Regimes: A Cross-National Aggregate Study," *Comparative Politics,* 8, No. 1 (October 1975), 17.

21 Ibid., p. 25. Emphasis added.

22 Alexander J. Groth, *Comparative Politics: A Distributive Approach* (New York: Macmillan, 1971), p. 11.

23 Ibid., Chapter 6.

24 Aaron Wildavsky, *Budgeting: A Comparative Theory of Budgetary Processes* (Boston: Little, Brown, 1975), p. 6.

25 Charles E. Lindblom, "The Science of Muddling Through," *Public Administration Review,* 19 (spring 1959), 84.

26 Wildavsky, *Budgeting,* p. 225.

27 Cynthia Enloe, *The Politics of Pollution in a Comparative Perspective* (New York: McKay, 1975), pp. 82–3.

28 Lawrence C. Mayer, *Comparative Political Inquiry* (Homewood, Ill.: Dorsey Press, 1972), p. 166.
29 Gabriel A. Almond and Sidney Verba, *The Civic Culture* (Boston: Little, Brown, 1963), pp. 308–9.
30 David Easton, *A Systems Analysis of Political Life* (New York: Wiley, 1965), p. 103.
31 Anthony King, "Ideas, Institutions and the Policies of Governments: A Comparative Analysis," Part III, *British Journal of Political Science* (October 1973), 418.
32 Ibid., p. 418.
33 Myrdal, *Asian Drama*, Vol. II, p. 1516.
34 Enloe, *Politics of Pollution*, pp. 54–5.
35 Jesse Burkhead and Jerry Miner, *Public Expenditures* (Chicago: Aldine, 1971), p. 2.
36 Bruce Russett, "Who Pays for Defense?" *American Political Science Review*, 63 (June 1969), 417.
37 Margaret Daly Hayes, "Policy Consequences of Military Participation in Politics: An Analysis of Trade Offs in Brazilian Federal Expenditures," *Comparative Public Policy: Issues, Theories and Methods*, ed. Craig Liske, William Loehr, and John McCamant (New York: Halsted Press, 1975), pp. 48–9.
38 David A. Caputo, "New Perspectives on the Public Policy Implications of Defense and Welfare Expenditures in Four Modern Democracies: 1950–1970," *Policy Sciences*, 6 (December 1975), 439. Emphasis added.
39 Charles W. Anderson, *The Political Economy of Modern Spain* (Madison: University of Wisconsin Press, 1970), p. 9.
40 Anthony King, "On Studying the Impacts of Public Policies: The Role of the Political Scientist," *What Government Does*, ed. Matthew Holden, Jr., and Dennis L. Dresang (Beverly Hills: Sage Publications, 1975), pp. 298–316.
41 Anderson, *Political Economy of Modern Spain*, p. 247.
42 Ernest Barker, *The Development of Public Services in Western Europe: 1660–1930* (Hamden, Conn.: Archon Books, 1966), p. 93.
43 T. Van Waasdijk, *Public Expenditure in South Africa* (Johannesburg: Witwatersrand University Press, 1964), p. 154.
44 Enloe, *Politics of Pollution*, p. 136.
45 Ronald T. Libby, "External Co-Optation of a Less Developed Country's Policy Making: The Case of Ghana, 1969–1972," *World Politics*, 29, No. 1 (October 1976), 67–89.

Chapter 4. Comparing policy priorities

1 Joyce M. Mitchell and William C. Mitchell, *Political Analysis and Public Policy* (Chicago: Rand McNally, 1969), pp. 595–6.
2 Alexander J. Groth, *Comparative Politics: A Distributive Approach* (New York: Macmillan, 1971), p. 68.
3 Frederic L. Pryor, *Public Expenditures in Communist and Capitalist Nations* (Homewood, Ill.: Irwin, 1968), p. 88.
4 U.S. Department of the Army, *Japan: Analytical Bibliography* (Washington, D.C.: GPO, 1972), p. 198.
5 Jerome Stromberg, "Community Involvement in Solving Local Health Problems in Ghana," *Inquiry*, 12 (suppl.) (June 1975), 148–55.
6 See Kim Q. Hill, "Distributional and Impact Analysis of Public Policy: A Two

Nation Study for Education and Health Policy" (Ph.D. dissertation, Department of Political Science, Rice University, 1974).

7 See Pryor, *Public Expenditures in Communist and Capitalist Nations;* Richard M. Bird, *the Growth of Government Spending in Canada* (Toronto: Canadian Tax Foundation, 1970).

8 Charles W. Anderson, Fred R. Von der Mehden, and Crawford Young, *Issues of Political Development,* 2nd edition (Englewood Cliffs, N.J.: Prentice-Hall, 1974). Chapter 11.

9 Bird, *Growth of Government Spending,* p. 151.

10 Cyril E. Black, et al., *Neutralization and World Politics* (Princeton: Princeton University Press, 1968), p. xiii.

11 *SIPRI Yearbook of World Armaments and Disarmament: 1968/69* (Stockholm: Almqvist & Wiksell, 1969), pp. 359–73.

12 Ruth L. Sivard, *World Military and Social Expenditures: 1976* (Leesburg, Va.: WMSE Publications, 1976), p. 16.

13 André Garcia, "The Financing of Education Under a Centralized System: France," *Financing of Education for Economic Growth,* ed. Lucille Reifman (Paris: OECD, 1966), pp. 154–5.

14 See Friedrich Edding and Dieter Berstecher, *International Developments of Educational Expenditure: 1950–1965* (Paris: UNESCO, 1969), pp. 51–61.

15 R. D. McKinlay and A. S. Cohan, "A Comparative Analysis of the Political and Economic Performance of Military and Civilian Regimes: A Cross-National Aggregate Study," *Comparative Politics,* 8, No. 1 (October 1975), 1–30.

16 Edding and Berstecher, *International Developments,* p. 52.

17 Frederick Harbison and Charles Myers, *Education, Manpower and Economic Growth: Strategies of Human Resource Development* (New York: McGraw-Hill, 1964), p. 203. Emphasis added.

Introduction to Part II

1 For a discussion of the role of case studies in comparative research and their various types, see Arend Lijphart, "Comparative Politics and the Comparative Method," *American Political Science Review,* 65 (September 1971), 682–93.

2 See Adam Przeworski and Henry Teune, *The Logic of Comparative Social Inquiry* (New York: Wiley, 1970).

Chapter 5. Germany: the pioneer in national health care

1 Although modern usage favors the term *health* insurance, the German word *Krankenversicherung* is literally translated "sickness insurance." This is the term generally used by scholars, although the most recent English translation of the *Survey of Social Security in the Federal Republic of Germany* (Bonn: Federal Minister for Labour and Social Affairs, 1972) uses the term *health insurance.* In this chapter we will follow the more traditional and widely used translation.

2 See, for example, "The Position of the Medical Practitioner Under the National Insurance Scheme of Germany," *Lancet* (October 28, 1911), 1216–20. For a rare note of praise, see George P. Forrester, "State Insurance in Germany," *Lancet* (April 27, 1912), 1152–3.

3 Gustav Hartz, "Don't Copy Germany's Mistakes!" *Ohio State Medical Journal*, 32 (January 1936), 67–71. For an earlier attack on the German system in a popular magazine, see Madge C. Jenison, "The State Insurance of Germany," *Harper's Magazine*, 119 (1909), 727–34.

4 Walter Sulzbach, *German Experience with Social Insurance* (New York: National Industrial Conference Board, 1947), p. 39.

5 See Heinrich Braun, *Industrialisation and Social Policy in Germany* (Cologne: Heymenns, 1956), pp. 13–14. For one of the most authoritative and detailed studies of economic development in Germany, see J. H. Clapham, *The Economic Development of France and Germany, 1815–1914*, 4th ed. (Cambridge: Cambridge University Press, 1963).

6 Gustav Stolper, *German Economy 1870–1940: Issues and Trends* (London: Allen & Unwin, 1940), p. 42.

7 Karl Born, "Structural Changes in German Social and Economic Development at the End of the Nineteenth Century," *Imperial Germany*, ed. James J. Sheehan (New York: New Viewpoints, 1976), p. 28.

8 Clapham, *Economic Development of France and Germany*, p. 279.

9 Braun, *Industrialisation and Social Policy*, p. 16.

10 Gaston V. Rimlinger, *Welfare Policy and Industrialization in Europe, America and Russia* (New York: Wiley, 1971), p. 103.

11 English-born German free trade leader, John Prince-Smith, quoted in ibid.

12 Braun, *Industrialisation and Social Policy*, p. 71.

13 For an account of the early history of the movement, see Gunther Roth, *The Social Democrats in Imperial Germany* (Totowa, N.J.: Bedminster Press, 1963).

14 Lassalle had died in 1864.

15 William D. P. Bliss and Rudolph M. Binder (eds.), *The New Encyclopedia of Social Reform* (New York: Arno Press, 1970), p. 538.

16 William Harbutt Dawson, *Social Insurance in Germany 1883–1911* (London: Unwin, 1912), p. 11.

17 William Harbutt Dawson, *Bismarck and State Socialism* (New York: Fertig, 1973), p. 111. Emphasis added.

18 Translated and quoted in Braun, *Industrialisation and Social Policy*, p. 76.

19 The following discussion draws heavily upon the works of Dawson, *Bismarck and State Socialism* and *Social Insurance in Germany*.

20 See Rimlinger, *Welfare Policy and Industrialization*, p. 117.

21 Ibid., p. 120.

22 Henry E. Sigerist, "From Bismarck to Beveridge," *Bulletin of the History of Medicine*, 13 (1943), quoted in Sulzbach, *German Experience with Social Insurance*, p. 33.

23 "The Medical Profession in Germany," *British Medical Journal* (June 3, 1905), 1203.

24 Karl Jaffe, *Stellung und Aufgaben des Arztes auf dem Gebiete der Krankenversicherung* (Jena: Gustav Fischer, 1903), p. 5.

25 Although there was no direct subsidy, in practice there was local financial assistance. As noted below, some sickness funds were run by local authorities, who paid the administrative costs. In addition, much of the institutional health care was done in public hospitals, usually at a reduced rate for insurance patients. I. G. Gibbon, *Medical Benefit: A Study of the Experience of Germany and Denmark* (London: King, 1912), p. 511.

26 Friedrich von Muller "Memorandum on Medical Education," *Lancet* (November 11, 1911), 1353.

27 Dawson, *Social Insurance in Germany*, p. 35.
28 Ludwig Preller, *Sozialpolitik in der Weimarer Republik* (Stuttgart: Mittelbach, 1949), p. 285.
29 Sulzbach, *German Experience with Social Insurance*, p. 107.
30 Jaffe, *Stellung und Aufgaben des Arztes*, p. 164, notes 14 doctors' strikes between 1887 and 1903.
31 Wilhelm Thiele, "Zum Verständnis von Arzteschaft und Krankenkasse 1883 bis 1913," *Das Argument* (July 1974), 27.
32 Quoted in Julius Hadrich, *Die Arztfrage in der deutschen Sozialversicherung* (Berlin: Duncker & Humblot, 1955), p. 108.
33 Dawson, *Social Insurance in Germany*, p. 85.
34 Gibbon, *Medical Benefit*, p. 65.
35 *British Medical Journal* (November 8, 1913), 1234.
36 For an English translation of the agreement, see *British Medical Journal* (January 10, 1914), 96.
37 See Sulzbach, *German Experience with Social Insurance*, p. 35; Franz Goldman and Alfred Grotjahn, *Benefits of the German Sickness Insurance System from the Point of View of Social Hygiene* (Geneva: International Labor Office, 1928), pp. 19–20.
38 Goldman and Grotjahn, *Benefits of the German Sickness Insurance System*, p. 20.
39 W. J. Potts, "Socialized Medicine in Germany," *American Medical Association Bulletin*, 26 (October 1931), 158.
40 Foreign Office and Ministry of Economic Warfare, "The Nazi System of Medicine and Public Health Organisation," (London, 1944), p. 229.
41 "New Law for Regulation of the Medical Profession," *Journal of the American Medical Association*, 111 (January 1938), 222.
42 Foreign Office and Ministry of Economic Warfare, "The Nazi System of Medicine," p. 250.
43 Richard Grunberger, *The 12-Year Reich: A Social History of Nazi Germany* (New York: Holt, Rinehart & Winston, 1971), p. 221.
44 See Albert Holler, "Die Entwicklung der sozialen Krankenversicherung in den Jahren 1945 bis 1975," *Sozialpolitik nach 1945: Geschichte und Analysen*, ed. Reinhart Bartholomai and Wolfgang Bodenbender (Bonn-Bad Godesberg: Verlag Neue Gesellschaft, 1977), pp. 305–6.
45 Ibid., p. 306.
46 Rimlinger, *Welfare Policy and Industrialization*, p. 143.
47 Holler, "Die Entwicklung der sozialen Krankenversicherung," pp. 308–10.
48 William Safran, *Veto Group Politics: The Case of Health Insurance Reform in West Germany* (San Francisco: Chandler, 1967), pp. 49–50.
49 Ibid., p. 50.
50 Oscar Umrath, "Sickness Insurance Schemes in the Federal Republic of Germany," *Bulletin of the International Social Security Association*, 12 (March 1959), 118–21.
51 For a discussion of recent changes in the sickness insurance system, see Holler, "Die Entwicklung der sozialen Krankenversicherung," pp. 310–14; Dieter Schewe, Klaus Schenke, Anne Meurer, and Karl-Wermer Hermsen, *Uebersicht über die Soziale Sicherung* (Bonn: Bundesminister für Arbeit und Sozialordnung, 1977), pp. 179–210.
52 Alan Maynard, *Health Care in the European Community* (Pittsburgh: University of Pittsburgh Press, 1975), pp. 19–20.

53 The exception to this is the miners' fund, in which the miners have two-thirds representation and the employees one-third.
54 See William A. Glaser, *Paying the Doctor: Systems of Remuneration and Their Effects* (Baltimore: Johns Hopkins Press, 1970), p. 124.
55 Derick Fulcher, *Medical Care Systems: Public and Private Health Coverage in Selected Industrial Countries* (Geneva: International Labor Office, 1974), p. 75.
56 Ibid.
57 There are obvious exceptions to this generalization. Mortality and morbidity rates for cancer, stroke, and heart disease are frequently higher in modern, industrialized nations than in many poorer nations. In general, however, in terms of gross indicators such as general and infant mortality rates, as well as mortality rates for most diseases, the principle does apply.
58 Fulcher, *Medical Care Systems*, p. 78.
59 Christa Altenstetter, *Health Policy Making and Administration in West Germany and the United States* (Beverly Hills: Sage Publications, 1974), p. 69.
60 Maynard, *Health Care*, p. 35.
61 See Gordon K. MacLeod, "National Health Insurance in the Federal Republic of Germany and Its Implications for U.S. Consumers," *Public Health Report*, 90 (July–August 1976), 345; F. Kastner, *Monograph on the Organisation of Medical Care within the Framework of Social Security: Federal Republic of Germany* (Geneva: International Labor Office, 1968), pp. 65–6.
62 Maynard, *Health Care*, p. 35.
63 MacLeod, "National Health Insurance in the Federal Republic of Germany," p. 344. For specific survey data, see Kastner, *Monograph on the Organisation of Medical Care*, p. 63.
64 Glaser, *Paying the Doctor*, p. 143.
65 See Gibbon, *Medical Benefit*, Chapter 10; Potts, "Socialized Medicine in Germany," pp. 160–1; Hartz, "Don't Copy Germany's Mistakes!," p. 70; F. G. Dickinson, "German Experience with Social Insurance," *Journal of the American Medical Association*, 138, No. 1 (September 1948), 149–50; H. J. Hamburg, "Health Insurance in West Germany," *Medical World*, 91 (September 1959), 249–50.
66 See, for example, L. L. Bigelow (trans.), "Socialized Medicine as Part of a Program of Social Insurance: Data and Comparisons in France and Germany," *Ohio State Medical Journal*, 25 (September 1929); Potts, "Socialized Medicine in Germany."
67 M. Pflanz, "German Health Insurance: The Evolution and Current Problems of the Pioneer System," *International Journal of Health Services*, 1, No. 4 (November 1971), 318–19.
68 Fulcher, *Medical Care Systems*, pp. 76–77.
69 Holler, "Die Entwicklung der sozialen Krankenversicherung," p. 113.

Chapter 6. Great Britain: health care in a modern welfare state

1 Reported in the *International Herald Tribune*, July 7, 1978.
2 Wyndham Davies, *Health or Health Service?* (London: Charles Knight, 1972), p. 111.
3 Throughout this chapter we will deal only with development of health care policy in England and Wales. Separate, although virtually identical, programs developed in Scotland and Northern Ireland.

4 One of the best accounts of this period and the development of the National Health Insurance Act is Bentley B. Gilbert, *The Evolution of National Insurance in Great Britain* (London: Michael Joseph, 1966). This section relies heavily upon Gilbert's work.

5 Ibid., p. 87.

6 Ibid., p. 60.

7 Quoted in J. R. Hay, *The Origins of the Liberal Welfare Reforms: 1906–1914* (London: Macmillan, 1975), pp. 54–5.

8 Asa Briggs, "The Welfare State in Historical Perspective," *Social Welfare Institutions: A Sociological Reader*, ed. Mayer N. Zald (New York: Wiley, 1965), p. 60.

9 Ibid., pp. 62–3.

10 Hay, *Origins of the Liberal Welfare Reforms*, p. 62.

11 Gaston V. Rimlinger, *Welfare Policy and Industrialization in Europe, America, and Russia* (New York: Wiley, 1971), pp. 9–10.

12 Dr. Thomas Jones, quoted in Odin Anderson, *Health Care: Can There Be Equity? – The United States, Sweden, and England* (New York: Wiley, 1972), p. 58.

13 Harry Eckstein, *The English Health Service* (Cambridge, Mass.: Harvard University Press, 1964), p. 21.

14 Gilbert, *Evolution of National Insurance*, p. 320.

15 See Eckstein, *English Health Service*, p. 24.

16 See Jeane L. Brand, *Doctors and the State* (Baltimore: Johns Hopkins Press, 1965), pp. 216–21.

17 Gilbert, *Evolution of National Insurance*, pp. 408–9.

18 For complete details of the National Health Insurance Act provisions, see Douglas W. Orr and Jean Walker Orr, *Health Insurance and Medical Care: The British Experience* (New York: Macmillan, 1938).

19 Aneurin Bevan, House of Commons, July 30, 1958. Quoted in Pauline Gregg, *The Welfare State* (London: Harrap, 1967), p. 63.

20 Eckstein, *English Health Service*, p. 9.

21 Richard M. Titmuss, *Problems of Social Policy* (London: HMSO and Longmans, Green, 1950), p. 73.

22 For a complete account of the problems facing the E.M.S. see Ibid., pp. 54–86.

23 Quoted in ibid., pp. 64–5.

24 Quoted in ibid., p. 508.

25 Sir William Beveridge, *Social Insurance and Allied Services* (New York: Macmillan, 1942), pp. 158, 159.

26 Quoted in Gregg, *Welfare State*, p. 22.

27 Almont Lindsey, *Socialized Medicine in England and Wales: The National Health Service, 1948–1961* (Chapel Hill: University of North Carolina Press, 1962), pp. 27–8.

28 Eckstein, *English Health Service*, p. 118.

29 Ibid., p. 144.

30 Ibid., p. 132.

31 Lindsey, *Socialized Medicine in England and Wales*, p. 45.

32 In 1977 the Labour government announced its intention of abolishing reserved beds in NHS hospitals.

33 U.S. Congress, Senate, Government Committee on Labor and Public Welfare, *Medical Care Systems in Industrialized Countries*, 93rd Cong., 1974, p. 84.

34 Alan Maynard, *Health Care in the European Community* (Pittsburgh: University of Pittsburgh Press, 1975), p. 203.

35 R. G. S. Brown, *The Changing National Health Service* (London: Routledge & Kegan Paul, 1973), p. 3.

36 Anderson, *Health Care*, p. 158.

37 William Stewart and Philip Enterline, "Effects of the NHS on Physician Utilization and Health in England and Wales," *New England Journal of Medicine*, 265 (December 1961), 1194.

38 Anderson, *Health Care*, p. 143.

39 J. F. Sleeman, *The Welfare State: Its Aims, Benefits, and Costs* (London: Allen & Unwin, 1973), p. 92.

40 *Social Trends 1977* (London: Central Statistical Office, 1977), p. 143.

41 Ibid., p. 136.

42 Peter Townsend, "Inequality and the Health Service," *Lancet*, 1 (June 1974), 1179–90; see 1183.

43 Rudolf Klein, "The Political Economy of National Health," *Public Interest*, 26 (winter 1972), 120.

44 Roger M. Battistella and Theodore E. Chester, "The 1974 Reorganization of the British National Health Service – Aims and Issues," *New England Journal of Medicine*, 289 (1973), 610–15.

45 U.S. Congress, House Committee on Ways and Means, *National Health Resource Book*, 93rd Congress, p. 388.

46 Brown, *Changing National Health Service*, p. 6.

47 *Public Expenditure to 1979–80* (London: HMSO, 1976), pp. 94–5.

Chapter 7. The Soviet Union: health care in a communist state

1 Alex Inkeles, *Public Opinion in Soviet Russia* (Cambridge, Mass.: Harvard University Press, 1950), p. xii.

2 See, for example, Henry Sigerist, *Medicine and Health in the Soviet Union* (Bombay, India: Jaico Publishing House, 1947); Michael L. Ravitch, *The Romance of Russian Medicine* (New York: Liveright, 1937); W. Horsley Gantt, *Russian Medicine* (New York: Hoeber, 1937); Sir Arthur Newsholme and John A. Kingsbury, *Red Medicine: Socialized Health in Soviet Russia* (Garden City, N.Y.: Doubleday, 1933).

3 Gordon Hyde, *The Soviet Health Service: A Historical and Comparative Study* (London: Lawrence & Wishart, 1974), p. 18.

4 Y. Lisitsin, *Health Protection in the U.S.S.R.* (Moscow: Progress Publishers, 1972), p. 50.

5 Mark G. Field, *Soviet Socialized Medicine* (New York: Free Press, 1967), p. 27.

6 Nancy M. Frieden, "Physicians in Pre-Revolutionary Russia: Professionals or Servants of the State?" *Bulletin of the History of Medicine*, 49, No. 1 (spring 1975), 21.

7 Lisitsin, *Health Protection*, p. 19.

8 N. A. Semashko, *Health Protection in the U.S.S.R.* (New York: Putnam, 1935), p. 12.

9 Ibid., p. 13.

10 Hyde, *Soviet Health Service*, p. 17.

11 Frieden, "Physicians in Pre-Revolutionary Russia," pp. 23–4.

12 Ibid., pp. 24–5.

13 Mark G. Field, *Doctor and Patient in Soviet Russia* (Cambridge, Mass.: Harvard University Press, 1957), p. 1.

14 Frieden, "Physicians in Pre-Revolutionary Russia," p. 20.

15 Field, *Doctor and Patient*, p. 3.
16 Sigerist, *Medicine and Health*, p. 16.
17 K. V. Maystrakh, *The Organization of Public Health in the U.S.S.R.*, U.S. Department of Health, Education, and Welfare, 4th ed., (Moscow: State Publishing House for Medical Literature, 1956), p. 14.
18 Frieden, "Physicians in Pre-Revolutionary Russia," p. 28.
19 Quoted in Field, *Doctor and Patient*, p. 15.
20 Ibid., p. 16.
21 Hyde, *Soviet Health Service*, p. 31.
22 Lisitsin, *Health Protection*, p. 24.
23 Sigerist, *Medicine and Health*, p. 28.
24 Ravitch, *Romance of Russian Medicine*, p. 179.
25 Quoted in Semashko, *Health Protection in the U.S.S.R.*, pp. 39–40.
26 Sigerist, *Medicine and Health*, p. 28.
27 Hyde, *Soviet Health Service*, pp. 38–9.
28 A. P. Zhuk, *Public Health Planning in the U.S.S.R.*, trans. U.S. Department of Health, Education and Welfare, Publication No. (NIH) 79-999 (Washington: U.S. Government Public Health Service, National Institutes of Health, 1976), p. 28.
29 Mark G. Field, "Health as a 'Public Utility' or the 'Maintenance of Capacity' in Soviet Society," *Social Consequences of Modernization in Communist Societies*, ed. Mark G. Field (Baltimore: Johns Hopkins Press, 1976), p. 237.
30 Sigerist, *Medicine and Health*, p. 108.
31 Gaston V. Rimlinger, *Welfare Policy and Industrialization in Europe, America, and Russia* (New York: Wiley, 1971), pp. 265–6.
32 Hyde, *Soviet Health Service*, p. 23.
33 Milton Roemer, "Highlights of Soviet Health Services," *Milbank Memorial Fund Quarterly*, 40, No. 4 (October 1962), 396.
34 Newsholme and Kingsbury, *Red Medicine*, p. 211.
35 Ravitch, *Romance of Russian Medicine*, pp. 180–1.
36 Roemer, "Highlights of Soviet Health Services," pp. 396–7.
37 John Fry and L. Crome, "Medical Care in the U.S.S.R.," *International Medical Care: A Comparison and Evaluation of Medical Care Services Throughout the World*, ed. John Fry and W. A. J. Farndale (Wallingford, Pa.: Washington Square East, 1972), p. 183.
38 John Fry, *Medicine in Three Societies* (New York: Elsevier, 1970), p. 28.
39 Hyde, *Soviet Health Service*, 142–3.
40 Ibid., p. 148.
41 William M. Mandel, *Soviet Women* (Garden City, N.Y.: Doubleday [Anchor Books], 1975), 128–9.
42 *New York Times*, August 9, 1976.
43 Bernard de Fréminville, "Place des femmes medécins dans le monde," *Concours médical*, 88, No. 46 (November 1966), quoted in William A. Glaser, *Paying the Doctor: Systems of Remuneration and Their Effects* (Baltimore: Johns Hopkins Press, 1970), p. 249.
44 Hyde, *Soviet Health Service*, pp. 191–4.
45 Glaser, *Paying the Doctor*, p. 206; William Mandel, *Russia Re-Examined*, rev. ed. (New York: Hill & Wang, 1967), p. 130.
46 Roemer, "Highlights of Soviet Health Services," p. 381.
47 Ibid., p. 381.
48 Hedrick Smith, *The Russians* (New York: Quadrangle, 1976), pp. 74–5.

49 D. Venediktov, "Union of Soviet Socialist Republics," *Health Service Prospects: An International Survey*, ed. Douglas Wilson and Gordon McLaughlan (London: Lancet, 1973), p. 237.
50 Glaser, *Paying the Doctor*, p. 232.
51 Zhores A. Medvedev and Roy A. Medvedev, *A Question of Madness* (New York: Knopf, 1971), p. 202.
52 Ibid., p. 116.
53 Ibid., p. 194.
54 Lisitsin, *Health Protection*, p. 41.
55 Fry and Crome, "Medical Care in the U.S.S.R.," pp. 202–3.
56 Ari Kiev (ed.), *Psychiatry in the Communist World* (New York: Science House, 1968), p. 12.
57 Ibid., p. 12.
58 Roemer, "Highlights of Soviet Health Services," p. 393.
59 Kiev, *Psychiatry in the Communist World*, p. 17.
60 Mike Gorman, "Soviet Psychiatry and the Russian Citizen," *International Journal of Psychiatry*, 8 (November 1969), 847.

Chapter 8. Japan: health care in an Asian nation

1 Edwin O. Reischauer, *Japan: Past and Present* (New York: Knopf, 1964), pp. 116–17.
2 John Z. Bowers, *Medical Education in Japan* (New York: Hoeber, 1965), pp. 87–8.
3 F. Ohtani, *One Hundred Years of Health Progress in Japan* (Tokyo: International Medical Foundation of Japan, 1971), p. 20.
4 William E. Steslicke, "Doctors, Patients, and Government in Modern Japan," *Asian Survey*, 12, No. 11 (November 1972), 913–31.
5 Masataka Sugi, "Medical Manpower in Contemporary Japan," *Journal of Medical Education*, 46, No. 2 (February 1971), 150–5.
6 Frank Langdon, *Politics in Japan* (Boston: Little, Brown, 1967), pp. 42–4.
7 Ohtani, *One Hundred Years*, pp. 47–8.
8 Langdon, *Politics in Japan*, p. 48.
9 T. Higuchi, "Medical Care Through Social Insurance in the Japanese Rural Sector," *International Labor Review*, 109, No. 3 (March 1974), 251–74.
10 This section relies heavily on the discussions of national health insurance by George F. Rohrlich, "National Health Insurance in Japan," *International Labor Review*, 61, No. 4 (April 1950), 337–66; Higuchi, "Medical Care Through Social Insurance," pp. 251–74.
11 See John F. Embree, *Suye Mura: A Japanese Village* (Chicago: University of Chicago Press, 1939), especially Chapter 4.
12 Quoted in William E. Steslicke, "The Politics of Medical Care: A Study of the Japan Medical Association" (Ph.D. dissertation. Department of Political Science, University of Michigan, 1965), pp. 90–1.
13 Crawford F. Sams, "Medical Care Aspects of Public Health and Welfare in Japan," *Journal of the American Medical Association*, 141, No. 8 (October 22, 1949), 527–31.
14 Bowers, *Medical Education in Japan*, p. 101.
15 Rohrlich, "National Health Insurance," pp. 357–62.
16 Steslicke, "Politics of Medical Care," pp. 93–5.
17 Quoted in ibid., p. 141.

18 The data for this section are based largely on *Outline of Social Insurance in Japan* (Tokyo: Social Insurance Agency, 1976).

19 Paul Fisher, "Major Social Security Issues: Japan, 1972," *Social Security Bulletin*, 37 (March 1974), 34.

20 U.S. Congress, House Committee on Ways and Means, *National Health Insurance Resource Book*, 93rd Cong., 1974, p. 369.

21 Steslicke, "Politics of Medical Care," p. 230. This dissertation is the most informed study of the Japan Medical Association available in English.

22 Ibid., p. 231.

23 Ibid., pp. 232–6.

24 "Pressure Groups and Political Consciousness," *Journal of Social and Political Ideas in Japan*, 2, No. 3 (December 1964), 98.

25 Steslicke, "Politics of Medical Care," p. 236.

26 Mikio Yamamoto and Junshiro Ohmura, "The Health and Medical System in Japan," *Inquiry*, 12 (supplement), No. 2 (June 1975), 49.

27 Steslicke, "Politics of Medical Care," p. 64.

28 See Steslicke, "Politics of Medical Care," for a complete discussion of this issue.

29 *Japan Times*, August 4, 1971.

30 Steslicke, "Politics of Medical Care," p. 258.

31 Y. Scott Matsumoto, "Social Stress and Coronary Heart Disease in Japan: A Hypothesis," *Selected Readings on Modern Japanese Society*, ed. George Yamamoto and Tsuyoshi Ishida (Berkeley: McCutchan, 1971), p. 97.

32 Sugi, "Medical Manpower in Contemporary Japan," p. 154.

33 Yamamoto and Ohmura, "Health and Medical System in Japan," p. 49.

Chapter 9. Summary and implications for health care policy in the United States

1 See, for example, Keith Leffler, "National Health Insurance," *Current History*, 73, No. 428 (July–August 1977), 17–21, 36.

2 See Max W. Fine, "The Case for National Health Insurance," *Current History*, 73, No. 428 (July–August 1977), 14.

3 Mary W. Herman, "Health Care and the Patient's Needs," *Current History*, 73, No. 428 (July–August 1977), 3.

4 Ibid., p. 2.

5 Douglas Conrad, "Medical Malpractice Suits," *Current History*, 73, No. 428 (July–August 1977), 22–6, 36–7.

6 Ibid., p. 22.

7 Leffler, "National Health Insurance," p. 17.

8 See Herbert E. Klarman, "The Financing of Health Care," *Daedalus*, 106 (winter 1977), 216.

9 Fine, "Case for National Health Insurance," p. 16.

10 Theodore R. Marmor, "Rethinking National Health Insurance," *Public Interest*, No. 46 (winter 1977), 83.

11 Aaron Wildavsky, "Doing Better and Feeling Worse: The Political Pathology of Health Policy," *Daedalus*, 106 (winter 1977), 105.

12 J. F. Sleeman, *The Welfare State: Its Aims, Benefits, and Costs* (London: Allen & Unwin, 1973), p. 92.

13 Quoted in Merlin K. Duval, "The Provider, the Government, and the Consumer," *Daedalus*, 106 (winter 1977), 186.

Selected bibliography

This bibliography is intended to identify some of the most important works in the general field of comparative public policy as well as in the specific area of health care policy. Because comparative public policy is a relatively new area of study, much of the writing is in scholarly journals. For this reason we have included both book-length studies and journal articles. Unfortunately, a good deal of information on Soviet and Japanese health care policies is in relatively esoteric medical and public health journals and would be inaccessible to most students. The bibliographies for these two countries are, as a result, relatively short.

Comparative public policy

Adelman, Irma, and Morris, Cynthia Taft. *Economic Growth and Social Equity in Developing Countries.* Stanford: Stanford University Press, 1973.

Almond, Gabriel, and Powell, G. Bingham. *Comparative Politics: System, Process and Policy,* 2nd ed. Boston: Little, Brown, 1978.

Anderson, Charles W. *The Political Economy of Modern Spain.* Madison: University of Wisconsin Press, 1970.

Anderson, Charles W. "Comparative Policy Analysis: The Design of Measures." *Comparative Politics,* 4, No. 1 (October 1971), 117–31.

Anderson, Charles W. "System and Strategy in Comparative Policy Analysis: A Plea for Contextual and Experiential Knowledge." In *Perspectives on Public Policy-Making* (eds. William B. Gwyn and George C. Edwards, III). New Orleans: Tulane Studies in Political Science, 1975, pp. 219–41.

Barker, E. *The Development of Public Services in Western Europe: 1660–1930.* Hamden, Conn.: Archon Books, 1966.

Caputo, David A. "New Perspectives on the Public Policy Implications of Defense and Welfare Expenditures in Four Modern Democracies: 1950–1970." *Policy Sciences,* 6 (December 1975), 423–46.

Coulter, Philip B. "Comparative Community Politics and Public Policy: Problems in Theory and Research." *Polity,* 3 (fall 1970), 22–43.

Cutright, Philips. "Political Structure, Economic Development and National Social Security Programs." *American Journal of Sociology,* 70 (March 1965), 537–50.

Cyr, Arthur, and de Leon, Peter. "Comparative Policy Analysis." *Policy Sciences,* 6 (December 1975), 375–84.

Dolbeare, Kenneth M. "The Impacts of Public Policy." In *Political Science Annual,* Vol. 5 (ed. Cornelius P. Cotter). Indianapolis: Bobbs-Merrill, 1973, pp. 89–130.

Dorwart, Reinhold A. *The Prussian Welfare State Before 1740.* Cambridge, Mass.: Harvard University Press, 1971.

Dye, Thomas R. *Politics, Economics, and the Public.* Chicago: Rand McNally, 1966.

Enloe, Cynthia H. *The Politics of Pollution in a Comparative Perspective.* New York: McKay, 1975.

Fabricant, Solomon. *The Trend of Government Activity in the United States Since 1900.* New York: National Bureau of Economic Research, 1952.

Feldman, Elliot J. "Comparative Public Policy: Field or Method?" *Comparative Politics,* 10 (January 1978), 287–305.

Fenton, John H. and Chamberlayne, Donald. "The Literature Dealing with the Relationships Between Political Processes, Socioeconomic Conditions and Public Policies in the American States: A Bibliographical Essay." *Polity,* 1 (spring 1969), 388–404.

Fine, Sidney. *Laissez-Faire and the General Welfare State: A Study of Conflict in American Thought, 1865–1901.* Ann Arbor: University of Michigan Press, 1956.

Groth, Alexander J. *Comparative Politics: A Distributive Approach.* New York: Macmillan, 1971.

Heclo, Hugh. "Review Article: Policy Analysis." *British Journal of Political Science,* 2 (January 1972), 83–108.

Heclo, Hugh. *Modern Social Politics in Britain and Sweden.* New Haven: Yale University Press, 1974.

Heclo, Hugh. "Frontiers of Social Policy in Europe and America." *Policy Sciences,* 6 (December 1975), 403–21.

Heidenheimer, A. J. "The Politics of Public Education, Health and Welfare in the U.S.A. and Western Europe." *British Journal of Political Science,* 3 (July 1973), 315–40.

Heidenheimer, Arnold J.; Heclo, Hugh; and Adams, Carolyn. *Comparative Public Policy: The Politics of Social Choice in Europe and America.* New York: St. Martin's Press, 1975.

Hofferbert, Richard. *The Study of Public Policy.* Indianapolis: Bobbs-Merrill, 1974.

Holt, R. T., and Turner, J. E. *The Political Basis of Economic Development.* Princeton: Van Nostrand, 1966.

King, Anthony. "Ideas, Institutions and the Policies of Governments: A Comparative Analysis," Parts I and II. *British Journal of Political Science* (July 1973), 291–313.

King, Anthony. "Ideas, Institutions and the Policies of Governments: A Comparative Analysis," Part III. *British Journal of Political Science* (October 1973), 409–23.

King, Anthony. "On Studying the Impacts of Public Policies: The Role of the Political Scientist." In *What Government Does* (eds. Matthew Holden, Jr., and Dennis L. Dresang). Beverly Hills: Sage Publications, 1975, pp. 298–316.

Leichter, Howard M. "Comparative Public Policy: Problems and Prospects." *Policy Studies Journal,* 5 (summer 1977), 83–96.

Liske, Craig; Loehr, William; and McCamant, John. *Comparative Public Policy: Issues, Theories, and Methods.* New York: Halsted Press, 1975.

McKinlay, R. D., and Cohan, A. S. "A Comparative Analysis of the Political and Economic Performance of Military and Civilian Regimes: A Cross-National Aggregate Study." *Comparative Politics,* 8, No. 1 (October 1975), 1–30.

Mitchell, Joyce M., and Mitchell, William C. *Political Analysis and Public Policy.* Chicago: Rand McNally, 1969.

Moore, Barrington, Jr. *Social Origins of Dictatorship and Democracy.* Boston: Beacon Press, 1967.

Pennock, Roland J. "Political Development, Political Systems and Political Goods." *World Politics,* 18 (April 1966), 415–34.

Peters, B. Guy. "Economic and Political Effects on the Development of Social Expenditures in France, Sweden and the United Kingdom." *Midwest Journal of Political Science,* 16, No. 2 (May 1972), 225–38.

Pryor, Frederic. *Public Expenditures in Communist and Capitalist Nations.* Homewood, Ill.: Richard Irwin, 1968.

Rimlinger, Gaston V. *Welfare Policy and Industrialization in Europe, America and Russia.* New York: Wiley, 1971.

Rose, Richard. "Comparative Public Policy." In *Policy Studies in America and Elsewhere* (ed. Stuart S. Nagel). Lexington, Mass.: Heath, 1975, pp. 51–67.

Siegel, Richard, and Weinberg, Leonard. *Comparing Public Policies.* Homewood, Ill.: Dorsey Press, 1977.

Smith, T. Alexander. *The Comparative Policy Process.* Santa Barbara: Clio Press, 1975.

Tilly, Charles (ed.). *The Formation of National States in Western Europe.* Princeton: Princeton University Press, 1975.

Wildavsky, Aaron. *Budgeting: A Comparative Theory of Budgetary Processes.* Boston: Little, Brown, 1975.

Wilensky, Harold L. *The Welfare State and Equality.* Berkeley: University of California Press, 1975.

Wilensky, Harold L., and Lebaux, Charles N. *Industrial Society and Social Welfare.* New York: Free Press, 1965.

Health care policy: general

Abel-Smith, Brian. *Paying for Health Services: A Study of Costs and Sources of Finance in Six Countries.* Geneva: WHO, 1963.

Anderson, Odin W. *Health Care: Can There Be Equity? – The United States, Sweden, and England.* New York: Wiley, 1972.

Bowers, John Z., and Purcell, Elizabeth (eds.). *National Health Services.* New York: Macy Foundation, 1973.

Fry, John. *Medicine in Three Societies.* New York: Elsevier, 1970.

Fulcher, Derick. *Medical Care Systems: Public and Private Health Coverage in Selected Industrial Countries.* Geneva: International Labor Office, 1974.

Glaser, William. "Socialized Medicine in Practice." *Public Interest,* 3 (spring 1966), 90–106.

Glaser, William. *Paying the Doctor: Systems of Remuneration and Their Effects.* Baltimore: Johns Hopkins Press, 1970.

Klein, Rudolf. "The Political Economy of National Health." *Public Interest,* 26 (winter 1972), 112–25.

Maynard, Alan. *Health Care in the European Community.* Pittsburgh: University of Pittsburgh Press, 1975.

U.S. Department of Health, Education and Welfare, Social Security Administration. *National Health Systems in Eight Countries.* Washington, D.C.: GPO, 1975.

Wilson, Douglas, and McLaughlan, Gordon (eds.). *Health Service Prospects: An International Survey.* London: Lancet, 1973.

Health care policy: Germany

Altenstetter, Christa. *Health Policy Making and Administration in West Germany and the United States.* Beverly Hills: Sage Publications, 1974.

Bloch, Max. "Social Insurance in Post-War Germany." *International Labour Review*, 58 (August 1948), 306–44.

"Compulsory Sickness Insurance." *Studies and Reports*, No. 6. Geneva: International Labor Office, 1927.

Corwin, E. H. Lewinski. "State Medicine in Europe." *Bulletin of the American Hospital Association*, 6 (January 1932), 40–6.

Dawson, William Harbutt. *Social Insurance in Germany, 1883–1911*. London: Unwin, 1912.

Dawson, William Harbutt. *Bismarck and State Socialism*. New York: Fertig, 1973.

Fay, Sidney B. "Bismarck's Welfare State." *Current History*, 18, No. 101 (January 1950), 1–7.

Foreign Office and Ministry of Economic Warfare. *The Nazi System of Medicine and Public Health Organisation*. London: 1944, Chapters X and XI, pp. 227–75.

Gibbon, I. G. *Medical Benefit: A Study of the Experience of Germany and Denmark*. London: King, 1912.

Goldman, Franz, and Grotjahn, Alfred. *Benefits of the German Sickness Insurance System from the Point of View of Social Hygiene*. Geneva: International Labor Office, 1928.

Hadrich, Julius. *Die Aerztfrage in der deutschen Sozialversicherung*. Berlin: Duncker & Humblot, 1955.

Holler, Albert. "Die Entwicklung der sozialen Krankenversicherung in den Jahren 1945 bis 1975." In *Sozialpolitik nach 1945: Geschichte und Analysen* (eds. Reinhart Bartholomai and Wolfgang Bodenbender). Bonn-Bad Godesberg: Verlag Neue Gesellschaft, 1977, pp. 303–14.

Jaffe, Karl. *Stellung und Aufgaben des Arztes auf dem Gebiete der Krankenversicherung*. Jena: Gustav Fischer, 1903.

Kastner, F. *Monograph on the Organisation of Medical Care within the Framework of Social Security: Federal Republic of Germany*. Geneva: International Labor Office, 1968.

Pflanz, M. "German Health Insurance: The Evolution and Current Problems of the Pioneer System." *International Journal of Health Services*, 1, No. 4 (November 1971), 315–30.

Preller, Ludwig. *Sozialpolitik in der Weimarer Republik*. Stuttgart: Mittelbach, 1949.

Rimlinger, Gaston. *Welfare Policy and Industrialization in Europe, America and Russia*. New York: Wiley, 1971.

Safran, William. *Veto Group Politics: The Case of Health Insurance Reform in West Germany*. San Francisco: Chandler, 1967.

Schewe, Dieter; Nordhorn, Karlhugo; and Schenke, Klaus. *Survey of Social Security in the Federal Republic of Germany*. Bonn: Federal Minister for Labour and Social Affairs, 1972.

"Social Security Developments in the Federal Republic Since 1949." *International Labour Review*, 66 (November-December 1952), 485–501.

Sulzbach, Walter. *German Experience with Social Insurance*. New York: National Industrial Conference Board, 1947.

Thiele, Wilhelm. "Zum Verständnis von Aerzteschaft und Krankenkassen 1883 biz 1913." *Das Argument* (July 1974), 19–45.

Umrath, Oscar. "Sickness Insurance Schemes in the Federal Republic of Germany." *Bulletin of the International Social Security Association*, 12 (March 1959), 117–21.

Health care policy: Great Britain

Braithwaite, William J. *Lloyd George's Ambulance Wagons; Being the Memoirs of William J. Braithwaite, 1911–1912.* Ed. Henry N. Bunsbury. London: Methuen, 1957.

Brand, Jeane L. *Doctors and the State.* Baltimore: Johns Hopkins Press, 1965.

Brown, R. G. S. *The Changing National Health Service.* London: Routledge & Kegan Paul, 1973.

de Schweinitz, Karl. *England's Road to Social Security.* New York: Barnes, 1961.

Eckstein, Harry. *The English Health Service.* Cambridge, Mass.: Harvard University Press, 1964.

Eckstein, Harry. *The Evaluation of Political Performance: Problems and Dimensions.* Beverly Hills: Sage Professional Papers in Comparative Politics, 1971.

Fraser, Derek. *The Evolution of the British Welfare State: A History of Social Policy Since the Industrial Revolution.* London: Macmillan, 1973.

Gilbert, Bentley B. *The Evolution of National Insurance in Great Britain.* London: Michael Joseph, 1966.

Gregg, Pauline. *The Welfare State.* London: Harrap, 1967.

Harris, R. W. *National Health Insurance in Great Britain.* London: Allen & Unwin, 1946.

Hay, J. R. *The Origins of the Liberal Welfare Reforms: 1906–1914.* London: Macmillan, 1975.

Lindsey, Almont. *Socialized Medicine in England and Wales: The National Health Service, 1948–1961.* Chapel Hill: University of North Carolina Press, 1962.

Murray, D. Strak. *Blueprint for Health.* New York: Schocken Books, 1974.

Peacock, Alan T., and Wiseman, Jack. *The Growth of Public Expenditures in the United Kingdom.* Princeton: Princeton University Press, 1961.

Rennison, G. A. *We Live Among Strangers: A Sociology of the Welfare State.* Melbourne: Melbourne University Press, 1970.

Ross, James S. *The National Health Services in Great Britain.* London: Oxford University Press, 1952.

Sleeman, J. F. *The Welfare State: Its Aims, Benefits and Costs.* London: Allen & Unwin, 1973.

Titmuss, Richard M. *Essays on the Welfare State.* London: Allen & Unwin, 1958.

Titmuss, Richard M. *Commitment to Welfare.* New York: Pantheon Books, 1968.

Wade, Lord. *Europe and the British Health Service.* London: Bedford Square Press of the National Council of Social Service, 1974.

Willcocks, Arthur J. *The Creation of the National Health Service.* London: Routledge & Kegan Paul, 1967.

Health care policy: the Soviet Union

Field, Mark. G. *Doctor and Patient in Soviet Russia.* Cambridge, Mass.: Harvard University Press, 1957.

Field, Mark G. "Approaches to Mental Illness in Soviet Society: Some Comparisons and Conjectures." *Social Problems,* 7 (spring 1960), 277–97.

Field, Mark. G. *Soviet Socialized Medicine.* New York: Free Press, 1967.

Field, Mark G. "Health as a 'Public Utility' or the 'Maintenance of Capacity' in Soviet Society." In *Social Consequences of Modernization in Communist Societies* (ed. Mark G. Field). Baltimore: Johns Hopkins Press, 1976, pp. 234–64.

Gantt, W. Horsley. *Russian Medicine.* New York: Hoeber, 1937.

Fry, John, and Crome, L. "Medical Care in the U.S.S.R." In *International*

Medical Care: A Comparison and Evaluation of Medical Care Services Throughout the World (eds. John Fry and W. A. J. Farndale). Wallingford, Pa.: Washington Square East, 1972.

Hyde, Gordon. *The Soviet Health Service: A Historical and Comparative Study.* London: Lawrence and Wishart, 1974.

Kiev, Ari (ed.). *Psychiatry in the Communist World.* New York: Science House, 1968.

Lisitsin, Y. *Health Protection in the U.S.S.R.* Moscow: Progress Publishers, 1972.

Maystrakh, K. V. *The Organization of Public Health in the U.S.S.R.* (trans. U.S. Department of Health, Education and Welfare), 4th ed. Moscow: State Publishing House for Medical Literature, 1956.

Medvedev, Zhores A., and Medvedev, Roy A. *A Question of Madness.* New York: Knopf, 1971.

Newsholme, Sir Arthur, and Kingsbury, John A. *Red Medicine: Socialized Health in Soviet Russia.* Garden City, N.Y.: Doubleday, 1933.

Popov, G. A. *Principles of Health Planning in the U.S.S.R.* Public Health Paper No. 43. Geneva: WHO, 1971.

Roemer, Milton. "Highlights of Soviet Health Services." *Milbank Memorial Fund Quarterly,* 40, No. 4 (October 1962), 373–406.

Sigerist, Henry. *Medicine and Health in the Soviet Union.* Bombay, India: Jaico Publishing House, 1947.

Zhuk, A. P. *Public Health Planning in the U.S.S.R.* (trans. U.S. Department of Health, Education and Welfare). Washington, D.C.: U.S. Public Health Service, National Institutes of Health, 1976.

Health care policy: Japan

Akira, Ishihara. "Kampo: Japan's Traditional Medicine." *Japan Quarterly,* 9, No. 4 (October–December 1972), 429–37.

Bowers, John Z. *Medical Education in Japan.* New York: Hoeber, 1965.

Embree, John F. *Suye Mura: A Japanese Village.* Chicago: University of Chicago Press, 1939.

Emi, Koichi. *Government Fiscal Activity and Economic Growth in Japan: 1868–1960.* Tokyo: Kinokuniya Bookstore, 1963.

Fisher, Paul. "Major Social Security Issues: Japan, 1972." *Social Security Bulletin,* 37 (March 1974), 26–38.

Higuchi, T. "Medical Care Through Social Insurance in the Japanese Rural Sector," *International Labor Review,* 109, No. 3 (March 1974), 251–74.

Kiikuni, Kenzo. "Health Insurance Programs in Japan." *Inquiry,* 9 No. 1 (March 1972), 16–23.

Kuge, Katsuje. "Health Insurance in Japan." *Bulletin of the International Social Security Association,* 14, No. 4–5 (May 1961), 203–31.

Ohtani, F. *One Hundred Years of Health Progress in Japan.* Tokyo: International Medical Foundation of Japan, 1971.

Rohrlich, George F. "National Health Insurance in Japan." *International Labor Review,* 61, No. 4 (April 1950), 337–66.

Steslicke, William E. "Doctors, Patients, and Government in Modern Japan." *Asian Survey,* 12, No. 11 (November 1972), 913–31.

Steslicke, William E. *Doctors in Politics: The Political Life of the Japan Medical Association.* New York: Praeger, 1973.

Whitaker, Donald P., et al. *Area Handbook for Japan.* Washington, D.C.: GPO, 1974.

Index